Clinical Manual of Pediatric Psychosomatic Medicine

Mental Health Consultation With Physically Ill Children and Adolescents

Clinical Manual of Pediatric Psychosomatic Medicine

Mental Health Consultation With Physically Ill Children and Adolescents

Richard J. Shaw, M.B., B.S.

David R. DeMaso, M.D.

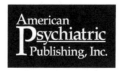

American Psychiatric Publishing, Inc.

Washington, DC
London, England

Copyright © 2006 American Psychiatric Publishing, Inc.
ALL RIGHTS RESERVED

Manufactured in the United States of America on acid-free paper
10   09   08   07   06   5   4   3   2   1
First Edition

Typeset in Adobe's Formata and AGaramond.

American Psychiatric Publishing, Inc., 1000 Wilson Boulevard, Arlington, VA 22209–3901; www.appi.org

Library of Congress Cataloging-in-Publication Data
Shaw, Richard J., 1958–
    Clinical manual of pediatric psychosomatic medicine : mental health consultation with physically ill children and adolescents / by Richard J. Shaw, David R. DeMaso.
—1st ed.
        p. ; cm.
    Includes bibliographical references and index.
    ISBN 1-58562-187-0 (pbk. : alk. paper)
    1. Medicine, Psychosomatic. 2. Pediatrics. I. DeMaso, David R. (David Ray), 1949– . II. Title.
    [DNLM: 1. Mental Disorders—complications. 2. Adolescent. 3. Child. 4. Mental Disorders—diagnosis. 5. Mental Disorders—therapy. 6. Psychophysiologic Disorders. 7. Referral and Consultation. WS 350 S535c 2006]
RC49.S53 2006
618.92—dc22   2006012000
British Library Cataloguing in Publication Data
A CIP record is available from the British Library.

Contents

Preface

$P_{ediatric\ psychosomatic\ medicine}$ refers to a specialized area of psychiatry whose practitioners have particular expertise in the diagnosis and management of emotional disorders and difficulties in physically ill children and adolescents (Gitlin et al. 2004). Patients commonly fall into one of the following three descriptive categories: 1) those with comorbid emotional and physical illnesses that complicate each other's management; 2) those with somatoform disorders; and 3) those with psychiatric symptoms that are a direct consequence of a primary physical illness or its treatment.

Over time, psychosomatic medicine has been designated by several names, including *medical-surgical psychiatry, pediatric psychiatry, psychological medicine, behavioral psychology, pediatric psychology,* and most commonly, *consultation-liaison psychiatry.* Johann Heinroth first introduced the term *psychosomatic* in 1818, whereas the term *psychosomatic medicine* was first used by Felix Deutsch in 1922 (Lipsitt 2001). In 1930, in a practice led by Leo Kanner, pediatric psychiatry fellowships were established for pediatricians who went on to develop child psychiatry units within pediatrics. An influential 1932 report on the relationship between pediatrics and psychiatry advocated for greater integration of mental health disciplines into the pediatric hospital. As a result of this report, consultation-liaison programs with psychiatrists were developed across the country to help increase awareness of the psychological issues affecting physically ill children (Fritz 1993; Work 1989). In 1935, the Rockefeller Foundation funded the development of several psychosomatic medicine inpatient units in teaching hospitals throughout the United States. Further growth occurred in the 1970s and 1980s as the National Institute of Mental Health funded new training and research grants in the specialty of psychosomatic medicine. In 2005, the American Board of Psychiatry and Neurology (ABPN) began certification in the subspecialty of psychosomatic medicine in order to establish this field as a definite area of subspecialization in psychiatry. Currently, training in pediatric psychosomatic medicine (or pediatric consultation-liaison psychiatry) is a mandatory requirement of training for all ABPN-accredited child and adolescent psychiatry residencies.

Parallel to psychiatry, psychology and pediatrics also have focused on psychosomatic medicine. In 1967, pediatric psychology emerged as a field defined by the concerns of psychologists and allied professionals who work in interdisciplinary settings such as children's hospitals, developmental clinics, pediatric or medical group practices, as well as traditional clinical child or academic arenas (Wright 1967). The Society of Pediatric Psychology (Also known as Division 54 of the American Psychological Association) was founded in 1968 to focus on the rapidly expanding role of behavioral medicine and health psychology in the care of children and adolescents. Currently, Division 54 has an annual forum for research and practice presentations in child health psychology. In 1982, the Society for Developmental and Behavioral Pediatrics was founded with a focus on the developmental and psychosocial aspects of pediatric health care. In 2002, pediatricians with special pediatric fellowship training in emotional, behavioral, and psychosomatic problems became eligible to receive American Board of Pediatrics certification in the specialty of developmental-behavioral pediatrics.

In addition to those already mentioned, there are a number of national and international organizations dedicated to the specialty of psychosomatic medicine, including the Academy of Psychosomatic Medicine, the American Psychosomatic Society, the European Association for Consultation-Liaison Psychiatry and Psychosomatics, and the International Organization for Consultation-Liaison Psychiatry. The American Academy of Child and Adolescent Psychiatry sponsors two committees, the Committee on the Physically Ill Child and the Committee on Liaison With Primary Care, that focus on clinical and research issues specifically related to pediatric psychosomatic medicine.

There are a number of journals that specialize in topics related to the field, including *Psychosomatic Medicine, Psychosomatics, Journal of Psychosomatic Research,* and *Journal of Pediatric Psychology,* as well as more specialized journals that focus on specific disorders (e.g., oncology and transplant psychiatry).

There are a number of outstanding textbooks of psychosomatic medicine, including *Psychiatric Care of the Medical Patient* (Stoudemire et al. 2000), *The American Psychiatric Publishing Textbook of Consultation-Liaison Psychiatry* (Wise and Rundell 2002), and *Handbook of Pediatric Psychology* (Roberts 2003). The most recent of these is the 2005 publication of *The American Psychiatric Publishing Textbook of Psychosomatic Medicine* (Levenson 2005), which has a chapter specifically focused on pediatric psychosomatic medicine.

This clinical manual aims to provide the practitioner with concise and pragmatic ways of organizing the key issues that arise in psychiatric consultation with physically ill children and a set of templates to help guide their clinical assessment and management. The book is organized into three sections. Chapters 1–4 provide an overview of pediatric psychiatry consultation, including legal and forensic issues, and a chapter on assessment principles. Chapters 5–12 are devoted to specific psychiatric symptoms and disorders in physically ill children and adolescents, with assessment templates that supplement the basic pediatric assessment described in Chapter 3. Chapters 13–16 address issues related to treatment and intervention.

Acknowledgements

There are innumerable people that we wish to thank for their encouragement, advice, and support in preparing this book. We cannot mention them all, but we hope they know of our gratitude. In particular, we acknowledge Robert Hales, Editor-in-Chief of American Psychiatric Publishing, Inc. (APPI); Drs. Hans Steiner and Alan Schatzberg in the Department of Psychiatry at Stanford University School of Medicine; and Dr. Oliver Sacks for their inspiration and support.

We have had many critical teachers and mentors who have supported our work on the interface of psychiatry and pediatrics. In psychiatry, there have been Drs. Myron Belfer, Keith Brodie, Leon Eisenberg, Carl Feinstein, Gregory Fritz, Frederick Melges, and Margaret Stuber. In pediatrics, there have been Drs. Harvey Cohen, Frederick Lovejoy, Alexander Nadas, and David Nathan. All of our colleagues and collaborators have been truly invaluable, although Drs. Pamela Beasley, William Beardslee, Michelle Brown, Leslie Campis, Julie Collier, Stuart Goldman, Joseph Gonzalez-Heydrich, Enrico Mezzacappa, Beth Steinberg, Allan Reiss, Barbara Sourkes, and Jane Newburger stand out. Drs. Paula Trzepacz and Susan Turkel provided expert assistance in the preparation of the chapter on delirium.

For their invaluable help in preparing the manuscript, we thank Richard Bourne, Josephine DeMaso, Christine DeMaso, Carolyn Kinnamon, Carrie Morris, and Kathryn Stockwell Skitt. We are especially grateful to our APPI editor, John McDuffie, for his support throughout the development and creation of this manual. We thank our families, who have helped in many practical as well as inspirational ways.

Finally, this book could not have been written without the many children and families with whom we have had the privilege of working. It is through the sharing of their lives with us in our work in pediatric psychosomatic medicine that we learned about the adversity and resiliency found in children and adolescents facing physical illnesses. It is our understanding of and responses to the stories of these families that form the bedrock of this manual.

References

Fritz GK: The hospital: an approach to consultation, in Child and Adolescent Mental Health Consultation in Hospitals, Schools, and Courts. Edited by Fritz GK, Mattison RE, Nurcombe B, et al. Washington, DC, American Psychiatric Press, 1993, pp 7–24

Gitlin DF, Levenson JL, Lyketsos CG: Psychosomatic medicine: a new psychiatric subspecialty. Acad Psychiatry 28:4–11, 2004

Levenson JL (ed): The American Psychiatric Publishing Textbook of Psychosomatic Medicine. Washington, DC, American Psychiatric Publishing, 2005

Lipsitt DR: Consultation-liaison psychiatry and psychosomatic medicine: the company they keep. Psychosom Med 63:896–909, 2001

Roberts MC (ed): Handbook of Pediatric Psychology, 3rd Edition. New York, Guilford, 2003

Stoudemire A, Fogel BS, Greenberg DB (eds): Psychiatric Care of the Medical Patient, 2nd Edition. Oxford, England, Oxford University Press, 2000

Wise MG, Rundell JR (eds): The American Psychiatric Publishing Textbook of Consultation-Liaison Psychiatry, 2nd Edition. Washington, DC, American Psychiatric Publishing, 2002

Work H: The "menace of psychiatry" revisited: the evolving relationship between pediatrics and child psychiatry. Psychosomatics 30:86–93, 1989

Wright L: The pediatric psychologist: a role model. Am Psychol 22:323–325, 1967

Pediatric Psychosomatic Medicine

Pediatric psychosomatic medicine, also referred to as *pediatric consultation-liaison psychiatry,* is the subspecialty of child and adolescent psychiatry that is dedicated to providing mental health services to physically ill pediatric patients. Lipowski (1967) has defined the specialty as those diagnostic, therapeutic, teaching, and research activities provided by psychiatrists in the nonpsychiatric part of the general hospital. Herzog and Stein (2001) outlined the following goals of a pediatric consultation-liaison psychiatry service: 1) to facilitate the early recognition and treatment of psychiatric disorders in physically ill children and adolescents; 2) to help differentiate psychological illnesses presenting with physical symptoms; 3) to help avoid unnecessary diagnostic tests and procedures; 4) to support pediatric patients and their families in coping with their disease and its treatment; and 5) to assist the medical team in understanding the reactions and behaviors of physically ill children, adolescents, and their families.

The term *consultation* generally refers to activities that involve patient-focused evaluations and recommendations that occur at the bedside. Table 1–1

Table 1–1.   Models of psychiatric consultation

Model	Consultation activity
Emergency response	Consultation request in response to acute situations, including safety issues such as the suicidal or delirious patient or child abuse.
Case finding	Practice of scrutinizing the pediatrician's caseload in joint rounds to identify patients requiring early psychiatric intervention.
Anticipatory	Identification and screening of high-risk patients for preventive psychiatric services (e.g., psychiatric consultation on bone marrow transplant patients for whom the stress of the treatment is expected to result in adjustment difficulties for the patient and family).
Continuing and collaborative care	Pediatrician and psychiatrist co-manage the patient's treatment (e.g., patient with eating disorders).
Education and training	Activities related to efforts to educate the pediatrician about the identification and management of psychiatric issues in the physically ill child.

Source.   Adapted from Lewis 1994.

summarizes some of the common models of psychiatric consultation. By contrast, *liaison* describes activities that focus on the medical team and its relationship with the patient. In its broadest interpretation, liaison may also include ongoing programmatic developments, policy and protocol issues, and research.

To have a significant impact in the pediatric setting, the consultant must assume an engaging, spontaneous, therapeutic stance and deviate from the more traditional anonymity, abstinence, and neutrality of therapy (DeMaso and Meyer 1996). The consultant should have expertise in the field of adjustment to acute and chronic illness as well as a firm grounding in developmental and family issues and psychiatric disorders specific to childhood. The consultant should have an in-depth understanding of medical illness and knowledge of procedures, medications, hospital routines, and medical outcomes for children and adolescents (Bronheim et al. 1998). The consultant must also appreciate the roles of the professional disciplines involved in the treatment of the physically ill child, some of which are listed in Table 1–2.

Roles of the Psychiatry Consultant

The psychiatry consultant has a complex position within the hospital. The position requires flexibility and adaptability to perform several roles: evaluation, advocacy, support, and education.

Evaluation

A primary role of the consultation psychiatrist is to make competent psychiatric evaluations to help identify comorbid psychiatric illness. The recognition of emotional illness is often more complicated in physically ill children and adolescents because the direct effects of their illnesses may mimic psychiatric symptoms (Kathol et al. 1990). Another important role of the consultant is to assist the pediatrician in the differential diagnosis of physical symptoms that may have a psychological basis and to avoid unnecessary diagnostic and therapeutic procedures. Lewis (1994) describes different levels at which the evaluation may occur. These include 1) the intrapsychic life of the child, 2) the relationship between the child and family, 3) the relationship between the family and the medical team, 4) interdisciplinary dynamics between members of the medical team, and 5) the relationship of the hospital with outside agencies.

Advocacy

A second important role is that of advocacy for the child, particularly with regard to the recognition of his or her developmental and emotional needs (Smith 1998). The consultant is often in the unique position of being able to provide insight into the child's view of his or her illness, which is influenced by the child's developmental stage. Adolescents with terminal illness, for example, may wish to be told about their prognosis or have strong opinions about whether to continue their treatment. The consultant can be a useful conduit for this information and can help promote consideration of the perspective of the child or adolescent. The consultant may also advocate on behalf of the family in their relationship with the medical team.

Support for the Pediatric Team

The consultant also supports the pediatrician during the difficult clinical situations that frequently arise in the pediatric setting. This might involve helping the pediatric team stay engaged with patients who are acting out or rejecting

Table 1–2.   Professional disciplines in the pediatric hospital

Professional discipline	Traditional role	Notes
Pediatrician	Leader of the medical team	Long established relationships with patient and family
	Development of diagnostic and treatment interventions	Oriented toward immediate concerns of patient
	Final medical responsibility for patient	Potential for ambivalent feelings toward the psychiatric consultant
House staff	Frontline clinician involved in assessment and management of the patient	Short-term clinical rotations with lack of continuity
	Trainee status as participant in residency training program	Frequently dealing with time constraints and excessive burden of clinical work
		Lack of familiarity with role of the psychiatric consultant
Nurses	Implementation of bedside treatment interventions	Most frequent, direct contact with patient
	Education of patient and family	Closest exposure to physical and emotional distress of the patient
	Psychosocial support for patient and family	Potential source of rich clinical information
	Liaison between family and the medical team	Lack of continuity due to shift changes and staffing issues
Social worker	Assistance with basic social services for the family	Long-established relationship with patient and family
	Liaison with outside agencies including child protective agencies in cases of abuse and neglect	Established relationship with the primary pediatric team
	Psychosocial support for patient and family	Potential for "turf" issues with psychiatric consultant due to overlap in clinical role
	Individual and family therapy	
	Referral and coordination of outpatient services	

Table 1–2. Professional disciplines in the pediatric hospital (*continued*)

Professional discipline	Traditional role	Notes
Occupational therapist	Support with activities of daily living	
	Rehabilitation of patients after surgery and medical illness	
	Treatment of feeding difficulties	
Physical therapist	Rehabilitation of patients after surgery and medical illness	
	Biofeedback	
Nutrition	Nutritional counseling and assistance with calculation of caloric needs	Important role in treatment of patients with eating disorders and pediatric feeding disorders
Child life/Recreation therapy	Preparation for hospitalization, surgery, and stressful or painful medical procedures	
	Hospital-based play and recreation services	
Chaplain	Spiritual assessment of patients and families	
	Psychosocial and religious support for patient and family	
Case management	Liaison with insurance companies for authorization of medical services	

Source. Adapted from Fritz 1993.

treatment. It might include work with terminally ill children where feelings of guilt and hopelessness may result in avoidance on the part of the staff. Referrals for consultation can carry an implied request that the consultant assist in sharing the emotional burden in the management of the child with a chronic physical illness.

Education

Another role of the consultant is education of the pediatric team on issues including the recognition of psychiatric comorbidity. One of the goals is to help the medical team interpret the behavior of the patient and to provide guidance on how best to work with the patient and family. Education also serves to raise awareness of the psychological issues of the hospitalized child and to encourage early and appropriate referrals. Advising the staff about countertransference reactions can help reduce the risk of responding adversely to difficult patients.

Staffing of Pediatric Psychosomatic Medicine Services

National data on pediatric consultation-liaison psychiatry services suggest a relatively low staff-to-patient ratio (Shaw et al. 2006). The average full-time equivalent (FTE) in a national survey of pediatric consultation-liaison services was 0.44 FTE psychiatrists and 0.44 FTE child psychiatry residents, significantly lower than the FTE in a survey of adult consultation-liaison fellowship programs that reported an average 2.4 FTE psychiatrists and 1.6 FTE fellows (Strain et al. 1995). The ratio of pediatric attending consultation-liaison staff to number of hospital beds is still relatively low (1:675), significantly lower than the ratio of 1:300 recommended by Fink and Oken (1976). Inadequate staff to meet clinical need is reported by 43% of the nation's pediatric consultation-liaison programs, a common finding that is related to the national shortage of pediatric psychiatrists. It should also be noted that psychiatric consultation in pediatric settings often includes nonintegrated and sometimes competitive services provided by other disciplines. Nonintegrated mental health services provided by pediatric psychiatrists, psychologists, and social workers may lead to duplication of effort and potential confusion related to the referral process.

Funding of Pediatric Psychosomatic Medicine Services

Funding issues have been cited as a major problem for pediatric psychosomatic medicine services, and there is a long-standing disagreement over who should be financially responsible for psychiatric consultation services in the pediatric setting. Recent surveys suggest that the largest proportion of pediatric consultation-liaison funding (40%) comes from psychiatry departments (Shaw et al. 2006). Although funding from patient fees appears to have increased in recent years, reimbursement rates for psychiatric consultation services average only 30%, limiting the extent to which hospital-based pediatric psychosomatic medicine services can be financially self-sufficient. Many program directors have commented on the difficulty of negotiating with managed care companies to obtain reimbursement for psychiatric services. Pressure to generate billing income by seeing more patients potentially reduces time available for non-billable liaison activities. There is often confusion as to whether psychiatric services for hospitalized medical patients should be paid by the medical part of the patient's health care plan or by the psychiatric benefits, which are often carved-out to paneled providers who may not be credentialed by the hospital. Frequently neither side is willing to pick up the payment, and the consultant is left with the dilemma of whether to provide services that will not be reimbursed (Goldberg and Stoudemire 1995). These complicated payment arrangements also interfere with continuity of care for patients after discharge from the hospital. In addition, it should be noted that psychologists providing inpatient mental health consultations are often limited in their ability to bill for their services because they cannot use traditional evaluation management codes.

Referral Questions

One way to organize the classification of psychiatric issues in physically ill children and adolescents is to consider the issue of comorbidity (Figure 1–1). The term *coincidental comorbidity* describes patients with unrelated psychiatric and physical illnesses, whereas *causal comorbidity* refers to instances in which the psychiatric disorder is a direct result of physical illness or has a significant impact on the course or severity of the illness. Causal comorbidity also captures psychological symptoms that develop as a direct result of the stress of the illness or its treatment.

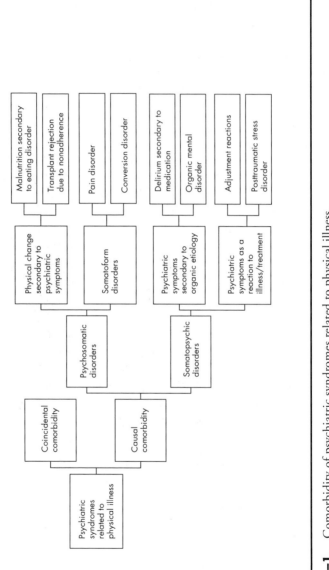

Figure 1–1.   Comorbidity of psychiatric syndromes related to physical illness.

Coincidental Comorbidity

Coincidental comorbidity refers to cases in which an emotional disorder that developed before or after the onset of the physical illness is related to factors other than the illness itself. Estimates of the prevalence of psychiatric disorders in the general pediatric population range from 10% to 20%, whereas studies suggest that up to 20% of pediatric patients in primary care clinics may have a diagnosable psychiatric disorder (Briggs-Gowan et al. 2003). In the inpatient setting, Lewis (1994) suggested that up to two-thirds of children admitted to pediatric wards would benefit from psychiatric consultation. The failure to recognize psychiatric issues in physically ill children and adolescents creates a potential for poor longer-term outcomes in a variety of areas, including psychological, educational, and social functioning.

Causal Comorbidity

Causal comorbidity refers to instances in which psychiatric symptoms either contribute to or result from the onset of physical illness. Disorders may be classified as psychosomatic or somatopsychic.

Psychosomatic Illness

Psychosomatic disorders are diagnosed when physical symptoms are caused by psychiatric illness. Examples include patients with eating disorders who develop medical complications as a result of malnutrition or patients who develop medical complications as a result of the failure to adhere to their medical treatment. Similarly, patients with somatoform or factitious disorders have physical symptoms that are primarily a manifestation of underlying psychiatric issues with no organic etiology.

Somatopsychic Illness

It is always important to consider the possibility that psychiatric symptoms are a direct consequence of either the illness or its treatment. Doctors should be particularly alert to this possibility when psychiatric symptoms develop suddenly, worsen or persist over time, are unresponsive to treatment, or have atypical clinical features. One category of somatopsychic illness includes those patients who develop psychiatric symptoms for which the underlying etiology is medical or medication-related. This includes patients with delirium or a mood disorder due to a general medical condition. A second category of somatopsychic illness includes those who develop symptoms of an adjustment disorder or medically related posttraumatic stress disorder as a result of the stress of the illness or its treatment.

Referral Patterns

Studies of pediatric patients suggest that referral rates for psychiatric consultation average only 2% of the hospital population and indicate that psychiatric illness in many physically ill children and adolescents goes unrecognized (Frank and Schäfert 2001). In the group of patients that are referred for consultation, school-age children and adolescents tend to be overrepresented, whereas preschool children are commonly underrepresented. Physicians initiate most referrals, with a smaller number of referrals coming from nurses, social workers, child life specialists, and family members (Ramchandani et al. 1997).

Most pediatric consultation-liaison services report a high frequency of referrals for the assessment of suicide attempts and adjustment to illness (Shaw et al. 2006). Burket and Hodgin (1993) reported that the major reasons for psychiatric consultation are behavior problems, suicide evaluation, depression, and reaction to illness. There is also a high frequency of requests for consultations regarding parental adjustment to their child's illness, suggesting that recognition of the effect of the child's illness on parental adaptation is increasing. Table 1–3 lists the most common reasons for pediatric psychiatric consultation in approximate order of frequency.

Practice Patterns

Hospital-based treatment interventions are often limited by the lack of time and staff available for their implementation, in addition to the challenge of coordinating the child's care with the large number of staff involved. In many cases the consultation is limited to triage and referral to outside agencies. Ramchandani et al. (1997) reported that the three most common treatment interventions are supportive psychotherapy, the use of psychoactive medications, and assistance with discharge planning by referral or transfer to another facility. Pediatric consultation often involves family therapy, preparation for procedures, and behavioral modification (Ramchandani et al. 1997). Liaison

Table 1–3.   Common pediatric psychiatry consultation requests

Adjustment to illness
Delirium
Differential diagnosis of somatoform disorder
Disposition and referral
Disruptive behavior
Medication consult
Nonadherence with treatment
Pain management
Parental adjustment to illness
Procedural anxiety
Protocol assessment
Suicide assessment

Source.   Adapted from Shaw et al. 2006.

with the pediatric team, in the form of helping interpret the patient's behavior and resolving physician–patient conflicts, also takes up a significant proportion of time.

Many pediatric psychosomatic medicine programs have reported a decline in the time available for liaison work and approximately two-thirds of pediatric consultation-liaison activity is dedicated to the direct provision of clinical service (Shaw et al. 2006). This finding appears to be related to increased demands of clinical work as well as increased financial constraints.

Education of the Family

One function of the consultant is to educate the family about what to expect from the child's emotional reaction to his or her illness. Hospitalization is often a stressful time in which the family experiences feelings of loss and a lack of control. Education may include information about regression as well as about how the child's level of cognitive development affects his or her understanding of the illness.

Psychopharmacology

The psychiatric consultant must have a strong grounding in the use of psychotropic medications, including potential drug interactions and the need to adjust dosages in patients with physical illnesses (Brown et al. 2000). Common consultation requests include the management of delirium, acute symptoms of anxiety or agitation, insomnia, and the use of adjunctive pain medications (see Chapter 5, "Delirium"; Chapter 6, "Mood Disorders"; Chapter 9, "Pediatric Pain"; and Chapter 15, "Psychopharmacological Approaches and Considerations").

Psychotherapy

Psychotherapy with physically ill patients is affected by the realities of the patient's situation (O'Dowd and Gomez 2001). Other constraints are the frequent interruptions in the hospital and the lack of privacy. Inpatient psychotherapy is generally supportive in nature. Family therapy may also be useful for parents and siblings and to help resolve conflicts that arise between family members (see Chapter 13, "Individual Psychotherapy in the Pediatric Setting," and Chapter 14, "Family Therapy"). It is important to clarify with the patient the limits of confidentiality in the inpatient setting.

Behavior Modification

Hospital-based behavior modification can be a simple yet effective treatment intervention. Examples include programs to facilitate cooperation with medical procedures, feeding issues, and activities of daily living. Patients with chronic pain or physical disabilities may respond to behavior modification programs that are presented as part of inpatient rehabilitation treatment. General principles of behavior modification include positive reinforcement of desired behaviors, ignoring negative behaviors, and consistency in the implementation of the program.

Guided Imagery/Relaxation/Hypnosis

Guided imagery and relaxation are potentially useful in the treatment of pain, anxiety, and insomnia. Patients who are admitted for stressful procedures such as bone marrow transplantation may benefit from early referral for these services. Hypnosis may be useful for patients with refractory issues of procedural anxiety or pain management (see Chapter 16, "Preparation for Procedures").

References

Briggs-Gowan MJ, Owens PL, Schwab-Stone ME, et al: Persistence of psychiatric disorders in pediatric settings. J Am Acad Child Adolesc Psychiatry 42:1360–1369, 2003

Bronheim HE, Fulop G, Kunkel EJ, et al: The Academy of Psychosomatic Medicine practice guidelines for psychiatric consultation in the general medical setting. Psychosomatics 39:8–30, 1998

Brown TM, Stoudemire A, Fogel BS, et al: Psychopharmacology in the medical patient, in Psychiatric Care of the Medical Patient, 2nd Edition. Edited by Stoudemire A, Fogel BS, Greenberg DB. Oxford, England, Oxford University Press, 2000, pp 373–394

Burket RC, Hodgin JD: Pediatricians' perceptions of child psychiatry consultations. Psychosomatics 34:402–408, 1993

DeMaso DR, Meyer EC: A psychiatric consultant's survival guide to the pediatric intensive care unit. J Am Acad Child Adolesc Psychiatry 34:1411–1413, 1996

Fink PA, Oken D: The role of general psychiatry as a primary care specialty. Arch Gen Psychiatry 33:998–1003, 1976

Frank R, Schäfert R: Child and adolescent psychiatric consultation in a pediatric hospital, in Basic Psychosomatic Care for Children and Adolescents. Edited by Frank R, Mangold B. Stuttgart, Germany, Kohlhammer, 2001, pp 150–164

Fritz GK: The hospital: an approach to consultation, in Child and Adolescent Mental Health Consultation in Hospitals, Schools, and Courts. Edited by Fritz GK, Mattison RE, Nurcombe B, et al. Washington, DC, American Psychiatric Press, 1993, pp 7–24

Goldberg RJ, Stoudemire A: The future of consultation-liaison psychiatry and medical-psychiatric units in the era of managed care. Gen Hosp Psychiatry 17:268–277, 1995

Herzog T, Stein B: Konsiliar-/Liaisonpsychosomatik (Consultation and liaison psychosomatics), in Psychosomatik am Beginn des 21. Jahrhunderts: Chancen einer biopsychosozialen Medizin. Edited by Deter H. Bern, Switzerland, Hans Huber, 2001, pp 243–251

Kathol RG, Mutgi A, Williams J, et al: Diagnosis of major depression in cancer patients according to four sets of criteria. Am J Psychiatry 147:1021–1024, 1990

Lewis M: Consultation process in child and adolescent psychiatric consultation-liaison in pediatrics. Child Adolesc Psychiatr Clin North Am 3:439–448, 1994

Lipowski Z: Review of consultation psychiatry and psychosomatic medicine. Psychosom Med 29:153–171, 1967

O'Dowd MA, Gomez MF: Psychotherapy in consultation-liaison psychiatry. Am J Psychother 55:122–132, 2001

Ramchandani D, Lamdan RM, O'Dowd MA, et al: What, why, and how of consultation-liaison psychiatry: an analysis of the consultation process in the 1990s at five urban teaching hospitals. Psychosomatics 39:349–355, 1997

Shaw RJ, Wamboldt M, Bursch B, et al: Practice patterns in pediatric consultation-liaison psychiatry: a national survey. Psychosomatics 47:43–49, 2006

Smith GC: From consultation-liaison psychiatry to psychosocial advocacy: maintaining psychiatry's scope. Aust N Z J Psychiatry 32:753–761, 1998

Strain JJ, Easton M, Fulop G: Composition and funding: consultation-liaison psychiatry services. Psychosomatics 36:113–121, 1995

2

Coping and Adaptation in Physically Ill Children

Between 10 and 20 million American children have a chronic health condition. Most of these conditions are relatively mild and interfere little with normal activities, but approximately 1%–2% of children have conditions that affect their daily lives (Perrin 1985). Chronic illnesses have been defined as conditions that last for a substantial period of time and which have persistent and debilitating sequelae. More specifically, chronic illnesses are conditions that interfere with daily functioning for more than 3 months in a year, or cause hospitalization for more than 1 month in a year, or are likely to do either of these at the time of diagnosis (Perrin 1985).

Categorical approaches to illness group pediatric illnesses in terms of specific diseases such as inflammatory bowel disease or asthma (Thompson and Gustafson 1996). These approaches consider the different rates and presentation of psychological problems in childhood within each category. Noncategorical approaches classify pediatric medical conditions along general dimensions that are considered common to the illness experience regardless of the specific condition a child has, such as visible/invisible, fatal/nonfatal, and stable/unpre-

15

dictable. Noncategorical approaches have become more common in recent years. They view the stressors that physically ill children and families experience as being due to a variety of environmental factors not related to the child's condition or to the experience of the illness. In this chapter we have chosen a noncategorical approach to consider aspects of physical illness related to both the direct experience of the hospitalization or procedure as well as long-term adaptation.

The impact of childhood illnesses includes the direct medical effects of the illness, such as restrictions on physical development and on the ability to engage in accustomed and expected activities. It also includes emotional and behavioral responses to the illness, including maladaptive coping strategies, which may last hours, days, months, or years. Physical illnesses can impinge on a child's health-related quality of life as a direct result of the disease state or as a result of a change in functional status or psychosocial functioning. These illnesses and their treatments may also involve physical pain and discomfort.

In addition, pediatric physical illnesses affect the family, because parents or other primary caregivers play central roles in the day-to-day management of these illnesses and may face related financial burdens (Perrin 1985). These caretakers experience stress as a result of the need to respond to and live with their child's condition. In some cases, they also face great uncertainty as to the prognosis and course of the child's illness, which is accompanied by a separate set of stressors (Cohen 1993). Siblings, relatives, friends, and teachers are also affected, to varying degrees, by a child's illness. Studies of chronic illness populations have shown that illness-specific and normal parenting tasks associated with developmental stages potentially alter the performance of key family roles, leading to role strain in both marital relationships and parents' relationships with their other children (Quittner et al. 1992).

Models of Adaptation and Coping

The trend in the coping literature has been toward developing integrative models of adaptation to pediatric illnesses that are inclusive rather than reductionist (Thompson and Gustafson 1996). Wallander and Varni (1992) and Thompson (1985) have developed such models, which display the interconnectedness of child and parent adjustment (Figures 2–1 and 2–2).

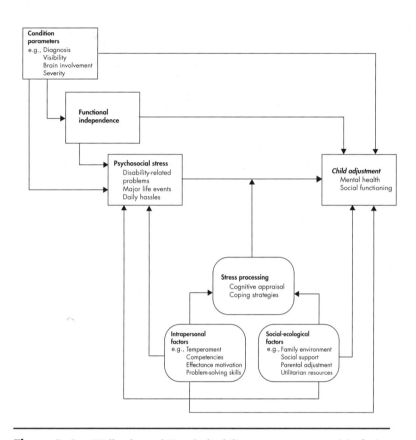

Figure 2–1. Wallander and Varni's disability-stress-coping model of adjustment.

Source. Reprinted from Wallander JL, Thompson RJ, Alriksson-Schmidt A: "Psychosocial adjustment of children with chronic physical conditions," in *Handbook of Pediatric Psychology*, 3rd Edition. Edited by Roberts MC. New York, Guilford, 2003, p. 152. Used with permission.

Wallander and Varni's model builds on simpler models of factors influencing child coping with chronic illnesses (Pless and Pinkerton 1975) and on a more general understanding of adjustment (Masten and Garmezy 1985). Their model presents a risk and resistance framework of responses to stress. In this model, children with chronic illnesses display adjustment problems because

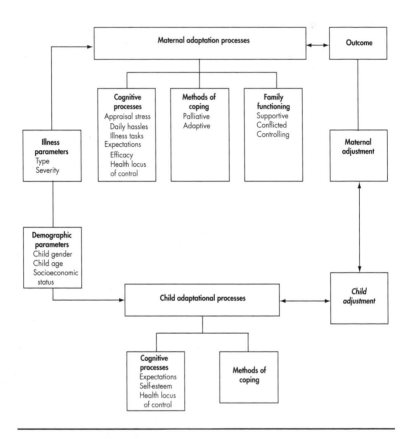

Figure 2–2.   Thompson's stress and coping model of adjustment.
Source.   Reprinted from Wallander JL, Thompson RJ, Alriksson-Schmidt A: "Psychosocial adjustment of children with chronic physical conditions," in *Handbook of Pediatric Psychology,* 3rd edition. Edited by Roberts MC. New York, Guilford, 2003, p. 153. Used with permission.

they are exposed to negative life events. These negative events stem from both their physical illness and from other general stressors in their lives that may or may not be related to the illness (Wallander and Thompson 1995). This model has guided a number of research studies (e.g., Varni et al. 1989), but because of its complexity, some aspects of it have yet to be evaluated.

Thompson (1985) used an ecological-systems theory perspective to develop a transactional model of stress and coping. Childhood chronic illness is seen as a stressor to which the child and family must adapt, and the relationship between illness and adjustment depends on biomedical, developmental, and psychosocial processes (Wallander and Thompson 1995). The model focuses on child and parental adaptational processes rather than on biomedical or demographic factors, partly because of the importance of the former in intervention efforts. Several studies have been conducted to test relationships within this model, particularly with regard to child health locus of control and self-esteem (e.g., Gil et al. 1991).

Coping During Hospitalization and Procedures

Acute medical distress is a common problem among children that has been associated with behavior management and adherence problems. Prevalence estimates for medical anxiety are as high as 7% in the pediatric population, and estimates of behavior management problems range from 9% to 11% (Van Horn et al. 2001). Overt emotional and behavioral distress often reflects children's efforts to avoid frightening and unpleasant situations that serve as a protective response to an external threat. Such reactions can range from verbal expressions of discomfort to resistance, physical protest, and refusal to cooperate. Negative medical experiences also increase the likelihood of behavioral distress during subsequent health care encounters. Contributors to acute medical distress include coping style, developmental level, history of illness and medical experience, temperament, and interactions with parents.

Contributors to Acute Medical Distress

Coping Style

A child's coping style is defined as the set of his or her cognitive, emotional, and behavioral responses to stressors (Van Horn et al. 2001). Coping involves a child's consistent use of particular strategies for managing stressors across contexts. The style a child adopts depends on the coping resources available to him or her, including problem-solving skills, social skills, social support, health and energy level, positive beliefs, and material resources (Rudolph et al. 1995). It is also dependent on the child's temperament, developmental level, and family coping patterns.

Children's coping styles have been categorized in a number of ways. *Approach-oriented coping* refers to behaviors and thoughts directed at addressing or managing the stressor or the feelings it elicits. This style includes asking questions, displaying interest in medical play and equipment, and seeking emotional and social support prior to procedures. *Avoidance-oriented coping* refers to thoughts and behaviors designed to avoid experiencing the stressor at the physical, cognitive, or emotional level. Examples of this coping style include going to sleep, daydreaming, and refusing to ask or answer questions (Rudolph et al. 1995).

Another method of categorizing coping responses identifies children's strategies as problem-focused versus emotion-focused (Folkman and Lazarus 1988). Problem-focused strategies are directed at altering the stressor or associated external circumstances. Emotion-focused strategies are aimed at regulating emotional responses to the stressor. For acute medical stressors, emotion-focused coping strategies tend to be more adaptive, primarily because the stressor (i.e., medical treatment) is unavoidable (Brown et al. 1986).

Many studies have examined associations between particular coping styles and outcomes based on hypotheses that specific coping styles and behaviors would be reliably associated with better adaptation (Rudolph et al. 1995). The results of this research have been inconsistent, perhaps due in part to variations in the conceptualizations of children's coping styles and the times at which they are assessed (e.g., prior to vs. during a procedure). The critical dimension appears to be whether a child has a coping plan for dealing with a procedure. Children characterized as having a plan prior to undergoing medical encounters have lower rates of procedural distress (Siegel 1983). Examples of such behaviors associated with adaptation include active seeking of information and exploration of medical equipment and toys or "deliberate" avoidance for those who become overwhelmed by medical information and encounters.

Developmental Level

Developmental factors have a profound effect on adaptation, affecting not only the coping resources available to the child but also his or her ability to process and benefit from health-related information, to reason about causality and responsibility for the disorder, and to adhere to medical regimens (Thompson and Gustafson 1996).

Preschool age.   The developmental characteristics of preschoolers can compromise their adjustment to medical stressors. Young children fail to understand why their parents do not protect them from the perceived threat of medical procedures and may feel threatened by forced separations during procedures because of normative anxieties about physical safety, separation from parents, and encounters with unfamiliar people. Preschoolers may also have difficulty due to normative constraints on their cognitive abilities. The cognition of preschool-age children is characterized by magical thinking, associative logic, and concrete thought processes and is qualitatively different from that of older children. These children often attribute events in their lives to their own thoughts, feelings, and behaviors and infer causal links between events that occur in close physical or temporal proximity. Medical procedures can easily be misinterpreted as "punishment" for bad behavior or other transgressions. As concrete thinkers, preschool-age children have difficulty comprehending abstract concepts such as quantity and duration (e.g., "It will only last a minute" or "This will only hurt a little bit"). Additionally, because of their limited verbal and attentional abilities, they are less likely to be able to recall and comprehend information designed to prepare them for procedures and less likely to seek out such information. Because these children are not able to use self-generated coping strategies, they are more likely to engage in avoidant behaviors when faced with procedural stressors.

School age.   Shifts in the emotional tasks of school-age children appear to be linked to changes in their reactions to medical stressors. The primary developmental tasks of this age group involve a need for mastery and control. The loss of control experienced during procedures challenges these basic emotional needs and can elicit feelings of anxiety and helplessness. Similarly, advances in cognitive skills can sensitize them to new aspects of medical encounters. They may become focused on the effects of interventions on their bodies and begin to display fears of bodily harm and death. With increased imagination, they are prone to misinterpretations and worries about painful procedures. Fortunately, children's coping repertoires tend to expand during this developmental period, which may be the reason that overall levels of medical fear decrease with age. The adaptive use of coping cognitions (particularly positive self-talk) and emotion-focused coping strategies increases and has been associated with declines in negative emotional and behavioral responses to procedures.

Adolescence.   Adolescents face the task of developing a sense of autonomy from family, often through the formation of close peer relationships that foster a sense of identity and belonging. Rapid physical changes associated with puberty engender heightened self-awareness and preoccupation with appearance. Procedures can impinge on the adolescent's emerging sense of autonomy and bodily integrity, particularly when the procedures involve a potential loss of functioning or alteration in appearance. The acceptance of authority and relinquishing of control required to undergo procedures can be difficult for this age group and may foster feelings of helplessness and dependence. Adolescents may become resistant and nonadherent with medical procedures if their need for control and independence is challenged. Cognitive advances during adolescence are both an asset and a liability in terms of medical interventions. Because they are capable of abstract thinking, adolescents may experience greater fears about potential outcomes and implications of medical conditions and procedures. However, their cognitive skills allow them to draw upon a wider range of coping strategies to address these fears, including positive self-talk, relaxing imagery, and cognitive reframing.

History of Illness and Medical Experience

Studies suggest that children who have had prior experiences of hospitalization display more anxiety during subsequent procedures (Dahlquist et al. 1986). By contrast, some investigators have found that children with prior experiences use more information-seeking strategies to cope with medical stressors (Smith et al. 1990). Knowledge of prior medical experiences may suggest which interventions are helpful to children in coping with medical anxiety. For example, preparation programs that emphasize information-giving, modeling, and demonstration may not have the same protective benefits for children who have previous experience with the procedure as they do for those without previous experience.

Temperament

Child temperament can affect children's adjustment to medical stressors directly, or it may moderate their preferences for particular styles of coping (Rudolph et al. 1995). More anxious children may choose techniques to avoid experiencing the stressor, such as distraction, whereas less anxious children may be more likely to seek information about the stressor. These factors may be quite significant, because there is evidence suggesting that the fit between child temperament and environmental influences may be important in determining adjustment.

Interactions With Parents

Parental trait anxiety has been associated with parental distress during procedures (Melamed 1993). Parental distress can interfere with parents' ability to respond to the emotional needs of their children, with their ability to help their child generate effective coping strategies, and with both immediate and long-term outcomes. Children who have highly anxious mothers often exhibit lower levels of distress when their mothers are absent during a procedure (Fishman et al. 1989). Several investigations have examined specific parent behaviors associated with increased child distress. Distress-promoting behaviors tend to involve criticism of the child's emotional reactions or behaviors, threats, and punitiveness (Dolgin and Katz 1988). Excessive parental attention to a child's distress through reassurance, empathy, apologies, and/or relinquishing control to the child is also associated with increased behavioral distress (Blount et al. 1989).

Long-Term Adaptation to Childhood Illness

Psychosocial adjustment can be defined as an umbrella term that encompasses psychological adjustment, social adjustment, and school performance (Perrin 1985). Studies have shown that children and their families are remarkably resilient in adapting to the challenges presented by a physical illness. The majority of chronically ill children and parents do not have identifiable mental health, behavioral, or educational difficulties (Wallander and Thompson 1995). However, children with chronic physical illnesses have an increased risk of subthreshold or subclinical mental health problems. The rate of emotional disorders in children younger than age 18 with medical illnesses has been found to be approximately 25%, as compared with 18%–20% in medically healthy children (Wallander and Thompson 1995). Moreover, research suggests that children with chronic physical illness primarily have internalizing syndromes (Thompson et al. 1990). In addition, research suggests that psychiatric problems, when they are present in chronically ill children, persist over time; one study found that nearly two-thirds of children with chronic physical illnesses who had been classified as "severely psychiatrically impaired" were still impaired 5 years later (Breslau and Marshall 1985).

Contributors to Medical Distress

Coping Style

It was previously noted that problem-focused coping is not usually adaptive in the context of acute medical stressors, because in these situations the stressor itself is largely uncontrollable. However, it may be that the opposite is true about long-term adaptation to chronic illness. Studies have found that in juvenile diabetes, primary control (or problem-focused coping) predicted better adjustment (Band and Weisz 1988). The relative adaptiveness of problem-focused and emotion-focused coping over the course of an illness that is characterized by relapses and remissions is an area for further research, because it may be that different coping strategies are effective during relapses and remissions. Research has also looked at the concept of locus of control. Patients with an internal locus of control often have better rates of long-term adjustment, whereas those who believe that their outcome is influenced by fate are more likely to be nonadherent or experience depressed mood (Williams and Koocher 1998). Health locus of control interacts with other dimensions, such as developmental level (younger children rely heavily on caregivers), family background and cultural beliefs, and child temperament (Williams and Koocher 1998).

Developmental Level

In contrast to the literature on acute illness, studies of chronically ill children have consistently failed to show that age affects child behavior problems or self-esteem in physically ill populations (Wallander and Thompson 1995). However, there remains a need to assess the influences of child age on developmental adjustment, particularly in terms of the effects of developmental transitions such as school entry and high school graduation.

Preschool age.   Preschoolers with chronic illnesses experience their parents' anxiety and watchfulness but simultaneously make efforts to explore the environment and separate from them. Parents of chronically ill preschoolers may experience shock, mourning, and anger after diagnosis of the medical condition and may experience denial related to their child's symptoms (Donovan

1989). These parental feelings and behaviors may result in an anxious or hypervigilant parenting style, which may affect the young child's later development (Miles et al. 1998).

School age.   School-age children often feel anxiety and dread as they become more aware of the implications of their illness. Potential difficulties with motor skills, separation from the primary caregiver, fear, and anger are common in this age group, and the introduction of significant peer relationships during this developmental period can be problematic and difficult (Donovan 1989).

Adolescence.   Adolescents also experience feelings of sadness, anger, and loss as a result of their physical illnesses. Chronic medical problems may affect the adolescent's functioning in new normative roles, affecting areas of his or her life, such as dating. As a result, some of these children may begin to be seen by their peers as loners. These adolescents may fear death and may withdraw from their environment, leading to further isolation. Parents of this age group may become increasingly concerned about the child's psychosocial adjustment but may be fatigued by their challenging parenting role. Separation issues can be as complex and confusing for parents as they are for adolescents, and some parents may feel torn and ambivalent about letting go. This ambivalence can have an impact on the extent to which the adolescent separates and engages with his or her peer group (Donovan 1989).

History of Illness and Medical Experience

Few studies have examined the relationship between illness duration and adjustment in chronically ill children. Some investigators have reported that children with chronic illnesses that require strict disease management, such as juvenile diabetes, perceive their illness as increasingly difficult to manage over time (Kovacs et al. 1990). Additionally, age at illness onset may play a role; one study found that boys with early-onset diabetes had more behavioral problems than either girls with early-onset diabetes or youngsters of either gender with late-onset illness (Rovet et al. 1987). Disease severity, however, does not appear to play a significant role in child adjustment and behavioral problems. Numerous studies have found that among conditions that do not involve the brain, such as congenital heart disease, cystic fibrosis, diabetes, and asthma, there is generally little relationship between disease severity and psychosocial adjustment (DeMaso et al. 1990).

Temperament

Temperamental difficulties have been found to predict poorer behavioral and emotional adjustment in children with chronic physical illnesses. Studies have found a relationship between dimensions such as child activity level, child reactivity, child behavioral difficulty, and child distractibility on the one hand and mother-reported behavior problems on the other (Wallander et al. 2003).

Interactions With Parents

Maternal depression and anxiety play important roles in child adjustment to chronic illnesses, just as they do in child behavior during procedures (Wallander and Thompson 1995). Maternal anxiety plays an important role in mother-reported behavior problems and in child-reported psychiatric symptoms. One longitudinal study of children with cystic fibrosis found this to be the case even after controlling for demographic parameters (Thompson et al. 1992). The same study also found that at follow-up, maternal anxiety was related to increases in child self-reported psychiatric symptoms while controlling for baseline child psychological functioning (Thompson et al. 1994). A parallel study of children with sickle cell anemia yielded similar findings (Thompson et al. 1993).

Guidelines for Assessing Medical Distress

Given the complexity of the factors influencing medical distress, early recognition of the psychosocial aspects of general health conditions is critical. Consultants should consider the socioeconomic risks faced by the child and family, assess for parent and family distress, and screen for academic, social, and behavioral problems in the child, particularly if the illness involves the central nervous system. A solution-focused or target symptom approach is often useful when intervention is required. The ultimate goals of many interventions are to 1) minimize the impact of the illness, 2) build parent and child social skills, 3) improve adherence, and 4) manage chronic and acute pain (Thompson and Gustafson 1996). These issues, including specific ways to reduce procedural anxiety and distress, are explored in subsequent chapters.

References

Band EB, Weisz JR: How to feel better when it feels bad: children's perspectives on coping with everyday stress. Dev Psychol 24:247–253, 1988

Blount R, Corbin SM, Sturges JW, et al: The relationship between adults' behavior and child coping and distress during BMA/LP procedures: a sequential analysis. Behav Ther 20:585–601, 1989

Breslau N, Marshall IA: Psychological disturbance in children with physical disabilities: continuity and change in a 5-year follow-up. J Abnorm Child Psychol 13:199–216, 1985

Brown JM, O'Keeffe J, Sanders SH, et al: Developmental changes in children's cognition to stressful and painful situations. J Pediatr Psychol 11:343–357, 1986

Cohen MH: Diagnostic closure and the spread of uncertainty. Issues Compr Pediatr Nurs 16:135–146, 1993

Dahlquist L, Gil K, Armstrong D, et al: Preparing children for medical examinations: the importance of previous medical experience. Health Psychol 5:249–259, 1986

DeMaso DR, Beardslee WR, Silbert AR, et al: Psychosocial functioning in children with cyanotic heart defects. J Dev Behav Pediatr 11:289–294, 1990

Dolgin MJ, Katz ER: Conditioned aversions in pediatric cancer patients receiving chemotherapy. J Dev Behav Pediatrics 9:82–85, 1988

Donovan EF: Psychosocial considerations in congenital heart disease, in Moss Heart Disease in Infants, Children, and Adolescents. Edited by Adams FH, Emmanouilides GC, Riemenschneider TA. Baltimore, MD, Williams & Wilkins, 1989, pp 984–991

Fishman B, Cook E, Hammock S, et al: Familial transmission of fear: effects of maternal anxiety and presence on children's response to dental treatment. Paper presented at the Florida Conference on Child Health Psychology, Gainesville, FL, April 1989

Folkman S, Lazarus RS: The relationship between coping and emotion: implications for theory and research. Soc Sci Med 26:309–317, 1988

Gil KM, Williams DA, Thompson RJ, et al: Sickle cell disease in children and adolescents: the relation of child and parent pain coping strategies to adjustment. J Pediatr Psychol 16:643–664, 1991

Kovacs M, Iyengar S, Goldston D, et al: Psychological functioning of children with insulin-dependent diabetes mellitus: a longitudinal study. J Pediatr Psychol 15:619–632, 1990

Masten AS, Garmezy N: Risk, vulnerability and protective factors in developmental psychopathology, in Advances in Clinical Child Psychology. Edited by Lahey BB, Kazdin AE. New York, Plenum, 1985, pp 1–512

Melamed BG: Putting the family back in the child. Behav Res Ther 31:239–247, 1993

Miles MS, Holditch-Davis D, Shepherd H: Maternal concerns about parenting: prematurely born children. Am J Matern Child Nurs 23:70–75, 1998

Perrin JM: Introduction, in Issues in the Care of Children With Chronic Illness. Edited by Hobbs N, Perrin JM. San Francisco, CA, Jossey-Bass, 1985, pp 1–10

Pless IB, Pinkterton P: Chronic Childhood Disorder: Promoting Patterns of Adjustment. London, Henry Kimpton Publishers, 1975

Quittner AL, Opipari LC, Regoli MJ, et al: The impact of caregiving and role strain on family life: comparisons between mothers of children with cystic fibrosis and matched controls. Rehabil Psychol 37:275–290, 1992

Rovet JF, Ehrlich RM, Hoppe M: Behavior problems in children with diabetes as a function of sex and age of onset of disease. J Child Psychol Psychiatry 28:477–491, 1987

Rudolph KD, Dennig MD, Weisz JR: Determinants and consequences of children's coping in the medical setting: conceptualization, review, and critique. Psychol Bull 118:328–357, 1995

Siegel LJ: Hospitalization and medical care of children, in Handbook of Clinical Child Psychology. Edited by Walker E, Roberts M. New York, Wiley, 1983, pp 1089–1108

Smith KE, Ackerson JP, Blotcky AD, et al: Preferred coping styles of pediatric cancer patients during invasive medical procedures. J Psychosoc Oncol 8:59–70, 1990

Thompson RJ: Coping with the stress of chronic childhood illness, in Management of Chronic Disorders of Childhood. Edited by O'Quinn AN. Boston, MA, GK Hall, 1985, pp 11–41

Thompson RJ, Gustafson KE: Adaptation to Chronic Childhood Illness. Washington, DC, American Psychological Association, 1996

Thompson RJ, Hodges K, Hamlett KW: A matched comparison of adjustment in children with cystic fibrosis and psychiatrically referred and nonreferred children. J Pediatr Psychol 15:745–759, 1990

Thompson RJ, Gustafson KE, Hamlett KW, et al: Psychological adjustment of children with cystic fibrosis: the role of child cognitive processes and parental adjustment. J Pediatr Psychol 17:741–755, 1992

Thompson RJ, Gil KM, Burbach DJ, et al: The role of child and maternal processes in the psychological adjustment of children with sickle cell disease. J Consult Clin Psychol 61:468–474, 1993

Thompson RJ, Gustafson KE, George LK, et al: Change over a 12-month period in the psychological adjustment of children and adolescents with cystic fibrosis. J Pediatr Psychol 19:189–204, 1994

Van Horn M, Campis LB, DeMaso DR: Reducing distress and promoting coping for the pediatric patient, in OMS Knowledge Update: Self-Study Program, Vol 3; Pediatric Surgery Section. Edited by Piecuch JF. Alpharetta, GA, American Association of Oral and Maxillofacial Surgeons, 2001, pp 5–18

Varni JW, Rubenfeld LA, Talbot D, et al: Family functioning, temperament, and psychological adaptation in children with congenital or acquired limb deficiencies. Pediatrics 84:323–330, 1989

Wallander JL, Thompson RJ: Psychosocial adjustment of children with chronic physical conditions, in Handbook of Pediatric Psychology, 2nd Edition. Edited by Roberts MC. New York, Guilford, 1995, pp 124–141

Wallander JL, Varni JW: Adjustment in children with chronic physical disorders: programmatic research on a disability-stress-coping model, in Stress and Coping in Child Health. Edited by La Greca AM, Siegel LJ, Wallander JL, et al. New York, Guilford, 1992, pp 279–297

Wallander JL, Thompson RJ, Alriksson-Schmidt A: Psychosocial adjustment of children with chronic physical conditions, in Handbook of Pediatric Psychology, 3rd Edition. Edited by Roberts MC. New York, Guilford, 2003, pp 141–158

Williams J, Koocher GP: Addressing loss of control in chronic illness: theory and practice. Psychotherapy 35:325–335, 1998

3

Pediatric Consultation Psychiatry Assessment

The goal of the psychiatric assessment of the physically ill child is to develop a developmentally based biopsychosocial formulation that leads to a comprehensive treatment approach with the patient, the family, and their health care providers. The assessment should determine where the child falls along the continuum from "normal" to "developmental variation" to "problem" to a "disorder" (Wolraich et al. 1996). This assessment is also the basis by which working alliances with the patients, family, and health care providers are established and should facilitate acceptance of the consultant's formulation and treatment recommendations.

This chapter outlines the critical steps in the psychiatric consultation process to guide the consultant in understanding and approaching the assessment in the pediatric hospital setting (Table 3–1).

Table 3–1. The consultation process: critical steps in pediatric consultation psychiatry assessments

1. Set up a responsive intake system
2. Establish the referral question
3. Obtain multiple sources of information
4. Prepare the patient and the family for the psychiatric assessment
5. Meet initially with the parent(s) or caretaker(s)
6. Interview the child or adolescent
7. Observe behavior and play
8. Be alert to developmental issues in the assessment
9. Develop a biopsychosocial formulation
10. Communicate findings and recommendations to the medical team and family
11. Consider standardized assessment instruments

The Consultation Process

Set Up a Responsive Intake System

Ideally, it is best to have an intake worker with a dedicated phone line as the first point of contact with the referring medical team. This person should respond quickly to routine (within 24 hours) and emergency requests as well as those that occur after hours or on weekends. The intake worker should obtain the following information: patient's name, birth date, hospital record number, hospital location, referring physician contact information, reason for request, level of urgency, and insurance information. This individual should also find out if the patient and family have been informed of the consultation request. Given the inherent time required by the consultant for liaison work (i.e., speaking with physicians or nurses), it is critical that billing for direct patient care be maximized. In this regard, the service should establish policies regarding billing uninsured or out-of-managed-care-network patients and obtaining medical copayments. Finally, there should be clear policies regarding the assessments of adults hospitalized in pediatric settings and parents of hospitalized children.

Establish the Referral Question

There is considerable variability among pediatric settings regarding the reasons and regularity with which psychiatric consultants are used and the expectations for the consultations (Drotar 1995). Nevertheless, consultation requests generally fall into three overlapping types: diagnostic, management, and disposition. The effective consultant will identify which of these referral types is primarily being requested. He or she may need to tolerate some level of ambiguity regarding the referral questions and assist the referring physician in more clearly identifying the problem (DeMaso and Meyer 1996). The consultant should attempt to delineate the circumstances, frequency, intensity, and duration of the problematic behaviors as well as factors that may precipitate, worsen, or ameliorate the problem. The consultant should acknowledge the explicit referral concerns but also be attentive to potential unspoken issues that may need to be addressed. For example, the referring clinician may be unaware of conflicts between the patient and the medical staff or of underlying emotional stresses that may be directly influencing the patient's current behavior. It is also important to be aware of the referrer's expectations based on previous consultations. The consultant should be alert to identifying unrealistic expectations or a lack of knowledge regarding the role of the consultant that may adversely affect the consultation process.

Obtain Multiple Sources of Information

The current and past medical record should be reviewed prior to beginning the consultation; this review should include nursing notes, which can often be important sources of information. The consultant should supplement this chart review by obtaining additional information from available pediatric staff (i.e., nurses, specialists, social workers, or child life specialists) who have had significant contact with the patient or family. Records of relevant outside psychiatric, psychological, or special educational evaluations should be reviewed when available, and in some cases information should be obtained from the school. When children are involved with child welfare agencies or the juvenile justice system, or are in institutional care, it may be important to obtain records and current information from those sources.

Prepare the Patient and Family for the Psychiatric Assessment

Involving the patient and family in a psychiatric assessment can present special challenges. Psychiatric assessment in the pediatric setting is unique in that the referring physician is in fact the consultee, in contrast to the more typical psychiatric assessment where the parents are the referring agents. It is not unusual for the family to be unaware that a referral has been made. Under these circumstances, many families may interpret the consultation request as a communication from their medical team that they are not coping adequately. In addition, the stress of the child's physical illness may make the family much less receptive to meeting with a representative from a service that they do not perceive as necessary for their child's care.

As with consultation from other medical specialties, it is important that the referring physician inform the patient and family about the referral and its purpose prior to the consultation. Most families will respond to the idea that hospitalizations are stressful and that their children may benefit from the added support provided by meeting with the consultant. Parents are usually open to concepts such as the use of relaxation or biofeedback to reduce anticipatory anxiety or assist with pain management. In high-stress procedures such as bone marrow transplantation it is useful to present psychiatric consultation as a routine part of the care of all children to help normalize the process.

Meet Initially With the Parent(s) or Caretaker(s)

The initial meeting with the family should begin in most cases by speaking separately with the parents or the child's primary caretakers. Given the importance of establishing a working relationship with the family, the consultant should begin by eliciting their understanding of the reason for the referral. It is important to keep in mind that this may be the family's first experience with a mental health professional and that they may be focused solely on medical causes for their child's problem and not have considered the impact of emotional factors. One approach that may be helpful in engaging the family is to start with an inquiry about the child's medical history and its impact in the different domains of the child's life. A psychoeducational approach may be used to explain to the parents the developmental issues and typical reactions of children to illness and hospitalization. It may also be necessary to explain some of the psychiatric concepts that may be unfamiliar to parents, such as the need to meet separately with the child and the importance of confidentiality regarding sensitive information. Parents may have suggestions as to how to introduce the consultant to the child and may be useful allies in the therapeutic process.

The consultant should let the family know that the findings of the psychiatric assessment will be communicated to the medical team. As indicated by the referral concerns, the consultant may also inform the family of situations in which confidentiality cannot be maintained beyond the hospital setting (e.g., allegations of physical or sexual abuse).

Interview the Child

The child or adolescent should be seen routinely as part of each consultation. It may be necessary to meet with the patient together with the parents if either the child or the parents are reluctant to meet alone. Subsequent meetings may occur alone with the child when there is greater familiarity and comfort with the consultant. Attention should be paid to concerns about confidentiality, particularly if the child is sharing a room with another patient. If possible, younger children should be taken to a playroom, but if the child is too ill to leave the bed, the consultant should have a selection of toys and accessories to help engage the child in the assessment.

Establishing the therapeutic alliance with the patient is one of the keys to an effective consultation. The consultant should explain in simple terms the concerns of the medical team and help normalize the assessment. It may be helpful to start with a review of the child's medical problems, because the child will generally be more familiar and comfortable giving this history. It is often easier to transition to an inquiry about the emotional impact of the illness and its treatment after obtaining the medical history. Inquiry about nonmedical issues, such as the child's school and social functioning, the child's strengths and interests, and his or her life outside the hospital is an alternative starting point for the interview. The techniques that follow can be used to help establish rapport (Hobday and Ollier 1999).

Draw-a-Person Test

The standard draw-a-person projective test is modified for the hospitalized child. The child is asked to draw a picture of him- or herself prior to the illness or injury and then, in a second drawing, a picture of him- or herself after the illness or hospitalization. This exercise can also be expanded by asking the child to draw a picture of the family both before and after the illness or hospitalization in order to examine the impact of the illness on the family relationships. The child may be asked to comment on the feelings of the individuals represented in the artwork.

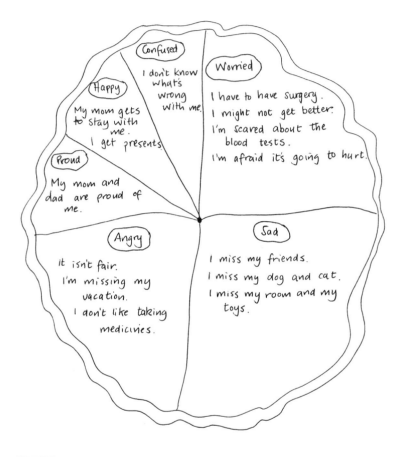

Figure 3–1.   Feelings pie.

Feelings Pie Project

In the feelings pie exercise, the consultant draws a large circle representing a pie and divides the circle into sections of different sizes. The consultant then designates specific feelings for each section of the circle and labels each section (Figure 3–1). The consultant gives examples of things that make him or her have the feeling represented in each section. After completing this part of the exercise, the consultant asks the child to draw a similar circle and pick a number of feelings that they discuss together. The size of each section may designate the relative importance of each feeling. If this exercise is too threatening, the child may be asked to comment on the feelings of the pie rather than on his or her own feelings. Another variation of this exercise can be used in which the child is told that the pie is about to have an operation and that the consultant and the child are going to come up with some of the feelings that it might have.

Feelings Mandala Project

For the feelings mandala exercise, the consultant draws a large circle on a piece of paper. The consultant then chooses four or five feelings—happy, sad, angry, worried, excited—and matches each of the feelings with a colored crayon. The consultant then colors in the circle with the crayons to designate each feeling (Figure 3–2). The consultant then asks the child to create a similar mandala and comment on the drawing after its completion.

Mood Scales

With mood scales, the child is asked to rate his or her feelings on a scale from 1 to 10 after the consultant has specified the specific feelings that are to be rated. This may be done verbally, as part of an interview, or using a visual scale similar to that used to rate pain (Figure 3–3). The exercise may be modified using certain prompts, for example, "This is the way I feel on my birthday" or "When I come into the hospital, this is how I feel." Feelings may need to be modified based on the age of the child.

Feelings Words Exercise

In the feelings words exercise, the consultant and the child write down a number of different feelings on small pieces of paper. These pieces of paper are placed in a "feelings box" or container, which can be created as an art project as part of the exercise. The consultant and child then take turns taking out pieces of paper and discussing the feeling that has been chosen. There are many variations to which questions may be asked. For example, the prompt can be, "I feel… (happy, sad, excited) whenever…" or "Whenever I feel…, I like to…" The consultant may need to model responses to the questions, depending on the age and ability of the child.

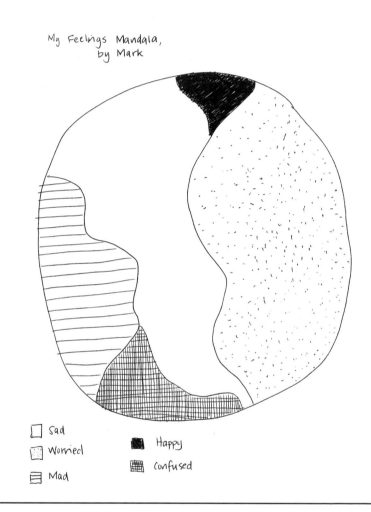

Figure 3–2.   Feelings mandala.

Road Map of Life

For the road map of life, the consultant models how to draw a "road map" of his or her life (Figure 3–4). The map starts with birth and progresses through various stages of life, which are illustrated with pictures. When the child draws his or her own road map, he or she should be prompted to put in the onset of

NAME: _____ DATE: _____

These are my feelings when _____

	Not at all								Most ever	
Happy	1	2	3	4	5	6	7	8	9	10
Sad	1	2	3	4	5	6	7	8	9	10
Angry	1	2	3	4	5	6	7	8	9	10
Excited	1	2	3	4	5	6	7	8	9	10
Worried	1	2	3	4	5	6	7	8	9	10
Scared	1	2	3	4	5	6	7	8	9	10
Disappointed	1	2	3	4	5	6	7	8	9	10

Figure 3–3.   Mood scale.

their illness or injury. In a variation of this exercise, the child can be asked to draw a future road map that designates the important obstacles that have to be overcome for the child to get through a particular problem or difficulty.

Complete-a-Sentence

In the complete-a-sentence exercise, the consultant and the child take turns completing sentences that start with simple, nonthreatening prompts but can then be modified depending on the ability of the child to engage in the discussion (Figure 3–5). It is also possible to introduce medical prompts toward

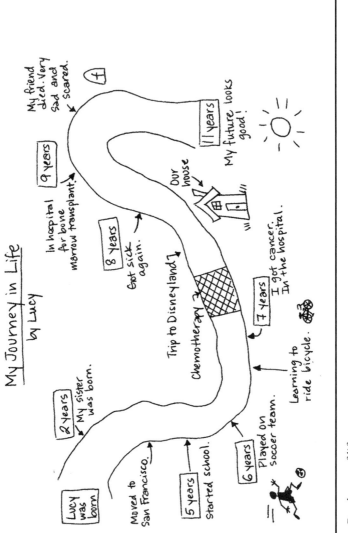

Figure 3–4. Road map of life.

My favorite food is..........

My favorite television show is ....

My favorite place to go on vacation is ....

My favorite time of the year is ....

I don't like it when my mother ....

I don't like it when my doctor ....

The best thing about missing school is ....

The worst thing about missing school is ....

The worst thing about being in the hospital is ....

The best thing about being in the hospital is ....

If I could have three magic wishes, they would be ....

Figure 3–5. Complete-a-sentence.

the end of the exercise. To initiate this exercise, the consultant may want to introduce some humorous sentence completions.

Psychiatric Assessment Protocol

The components of the "Practice Parameters for the Psychiatric Assessment of Children and Adolescents" (American Academy of Child and Adolescent Psychiatry 1997) are applicable to hospitalized children and adolescents. The consultant should use the child interview, supplemented by information from multiple other sources, to generate a comprehensive biopsychosocial history that includes the chief complaint, history of presenting illness, current medications, and psychosocial stressors as well as medical, psychiatric, developmental, social, and substance abuse histories. A full mental status examination should be completed if possible, but there may be times during the initial interview in which the comprehensive and detailed mental status examination is not possible. Serial mental status examinations may be indicated in consult requests for concerns such as delirium.

In the interview with both pediatric patients and their parents, it is important for the consultant to explore the following interrelated domains: illness factors, illness understanding, emotional impact, family functioning, siblings, social relationships, academic functioning, coping mechanisms, spirituality, and relationship with the pediatric team (Table 3–2).

Illness Factors

The impact of the illness on the child will vary depending on the stage of the illness. Reactions after the new diagnosis of a life-threatening illness will be different from those in a patient who has been struggling with a chronic illness for many years or those of a child who has just relapsed after a period of remission. Also significant is the nature of the illness, in terms of whether it is a chronic progressive illness, one with the potential for normal functioning and recovery between episodes, or one with a terminal prognosis. It is important to collect information regarding treatment history, including the frequency of hospitalizations, difficulties related to the treatment regimen, and experiences with traumatic and painful procedures.

Understanding of Illness

Both the child and parents should be assessed regarding their understanding of the illness, including its prognosis and treatment. It is helpful to know how fully the illness was explained to the child at the time of diagnosis and whether the child has received further age-appropriate explanations as his or her level of cognitive development. If there are cognitive issues that may affect the ability of the parents or child to understand the illness, these should be noted. There may be cultural and religious factors that influence the way the family interprets and understands medical illness.

Emotional Impact

It is important to assess the emotional impact of the illness on the child. This should start with an account of the child's level of emotional functioning prior to the diagnosis of the illness. The child's reaction to the illness at the time of diagnosis should be reviewed, as well as his or her current psycholog-

Table 3–2.   Protocol for the psychiatric assessment of the physically ill child

What are the illness factors?

1. Stage of illness
    New diagnosis of illness
    Relapse following a period of recovery
    Chronic phase of illness

2. Course of illness
    Relapsing (e.g., cancer)
    Single event with incomplete recovery (e.g., stroke, head trauma)
    Inter-interval recovery with normal functioning between episodes (e.g., sickle cell disease)
    Chronic deteriorating course (e.g., cystic fibrosis)

3. Prognosis
    Preservation of functioning with adequate treatment (e.g., diabetes, organ transplant)
    Decline in functioning over time (e.g., rheumatoid arthritis)
    Terminal illness (e.g., cystic fibrosis)

4. Treatment history
    Number of hospitalizations
    Frequency of outpatient appointments
    Treatment regimen
    Medication side effects (e.g., cosmetic, cognitive, energy, nausea)
    Difficulties with treatment adherence
    History of traumatic procedures
    Presence of pain

What is the understanding of the illness by the child and parent?

1. How was the illness explained to the child (e.g., full vs. partial explanation)?

2. Is there a realistic comprehension of the illness and its prognosis?

3. Is there an adequate understanding of the treatment?

4. Are there cognitive factors affecting the comprehension of the illness and its treatment?

5. Are there cultural issues affecting the assimilation of medical information?

What is the emotional impact of the illness on the child?

1. How was the child's emotional functioning prior to the diagnosis of the illness?

Table 3–2. Protocol for the psychiatric assessment of the physically ill child (continued)

2. What are the child's current emotional reactions to the illness?

Depression (e.g., understandable reaction vs. futility and hopelessness)

Anxiety (e.g., fear of recurrence, posttraumatic stress disorder symptoms)

Impact on self-esteem (e.g., body image, medication side effects, restriction on functioning)

Anger (e.g., acting out, regressed behavior)

3. What is the child's current degree of acceptance of the illness?

Denial

Acceptance and integration

What is the impact of the illness on family functioning?

1. Family functioning

What was the nature of the family functioning prior to the illness?

What has been the impact of the illness on home life (e.g., demands of treatment, decreased time for recreational activities, lack of availability of parent, increased dependency of ill child, increased levels of family conflict)?

2. Marital relationship

Has the illness resulted in decreased time for the marital relationship?

Have there been increased levels of conflict related to the illness (e.g., division of labor, disagreement regarding treatment, blaming of spouse)?

What has been the impact of the illness on the quality of the marital relationship (e.g., estrangement vs. increased feelings of closeness)?

3. Occupational functioning

Has there been a need to miss work for appointments, hospitalizations, or supervision of the treatment?

Have the parents had difficulties functioning at work due to emotional factors?

Is there a need for one of the parents to work to maintain health insurance?

4. Financial issues

What has been the financial burden of the treatment (e.g., lost income, transportation, increased need for childcare, need for special home accommodations, medical expenses)?

What is the impact of the illness on the healthy siblings?

1. What has been the impact of the illness on the healthy siblings?

Has there been decreased availability of parents (e.g., absence at important events and functions)?

Has there been an inequitable distribution of parental and financial resources?

Table 3–2. Protocol for the psychiatric assessment of the physically ill child *(continued)*

2. What have been the emotional reactions of the healthy siblings?
    Anger and resentment
    Anxiety about health of affected sibling
    Embarrassment regarding affected sibling (e.g., physical appearance, stigma of illness)

What is the impact of the illness on social and peer relationships?

1. What has been the impact of the illness on peer relationships?
    Stigma of illness (e.g., teasing, exclusion from social group)
    Increased closeness with specific peers

2. Has there been a decreased ability for social and recreational activities?

3. What has been the impact of the illness on dating and sexuality?
    Insecurity about physical appearance
    Delays in growth and puberty

What is the impact of the illness on academic functioning?

1. What was the level of academic functioning prior to the illness?

2. What has been the impact of the illness on academic functioning?
    Missed school days due to illness
    Academic difficulties due to illness or treatment
    Necessity for home schooling

3. Have there been difficulties with school reintegration?

4. Are there appropriate educational resources, including special education services?

What are the child's habitual coping mechanisms?

1. Turning to support from family members and friends

2. Religious or spiritual resources

3. Social withdrawal and isolation

4. Denial and avoidance

5. Maladaptive coping patterns (e.g., alcohol or substance abuse)

What is the role of religion and spirituality?

1. What is the family's religious affiliation?

2. What are the family's religious beliefs regarding illness and death?

3. What is the role of religion and spirituality as a source of support for the family?

What is the relationship of the family with the medical team?

1. Is the family able to trust members of the medical team?

2. What is the quality of communication with the medical team?

3. What is the family's desire for involvement in medical decision making?

ical status. Symptoms of depression may be an appropriate response to the diagnosis of an illness or reflect a more serious underlying mood disorder (see Chapter 6). For example, there may be symptoms of anxiety related to fear about recurrence of an illness, as well as symptoms of posttraumatic stress disorder related either to the news of the diagnosis of the illness or to aspects of the treatment (see Chapter 7). Self-esteem may be strongly affected because of limitations in the child's level of functioning or related to factors such as cosmetic side effects of medications and body image. Illness may interfere with important developmental milestones including driving, dating, and leaving home. Adolescent patients are particularly prone to feelings of anger and resentment about the illness and its impact on their lives and may act out in several ways, including nonadherence with the treatment (see Chapter 11).

Family Functioning

Medical illness may have a significant effect on family functioning. Demands of treatment may interfere with the normal routine that had been established prior to the illness, and there may be decreased time available for other activities. The medical illness may also change the dynamics in the family. In addition to the logistical demands of treatment, a previously healthy child may become more physically and emotionally dependent on his or her parents. The parents' marital relationship may be affected. A child's illness may result in there being less time for marital intimacy, and there is the potential for conflict related to such issues as division of labor related to the illness and how to manage the affected child. Illness may have a significant effect on the parents' occupations. Parents may have to take additional time off work or put career aspirations on hold. Conversely, there may be pressure on one of the parents to maintain their employment in order to continue necessary health insurance. Finally, there are often considerable financial implications, not only in terms of lost income if one of the parents has to miss work but also due to the costs of additional childcare and medical expenses.

It is common for the consultant to receive requests to evaluate parents of medically ill children (Shaw et al. 2006). In these situations, it may be helpful to meet individually with the parent in question to conduct a more formal psychiatric assessment. In other situations it may be more productive to conduct the assessment in the form of a family assessment with both parents present. Parental reactions include expected reactions of anxiety, anger, and depression as well as symptoms of acute stress reaction and posttraumatic stress disorder (see Chapter 7). Specific instruments have been developed to assess parental stress in the hospital setting, including those for parents who have children or infants hospitalized in the pediatric or neonatal intensive care units (Carter and Miles 1989; Miles et al. 1993).

Siblings

Although siblings are often overlooked following the initial diagnosis of a new illness, they commonly experience symptoms of anxiety about the affected sibling in addition to feelings of sadness and loss. Siblings may also have feelings of resentment about the lack of availability of their parents, whose attention is focused on the ill child, as well as the disruption to their daily routine. Parents may need to miss important school and social events in the healthy siblings' lives, and there may be a diversion of financial and other resources. Siblings may have feelings of embarrassment about the stigma of the illness and be reluctant to have friends over to their home.

Social Relationships

The diagnosis of the medical illness is likely to have a significant impact on the child's peer relationships. The illness may interfere with their ability to participate in desired social functions and activities and lead to isolation from their peer group. The child may experience feelings of being stigmatized by the illness, being teased at school, and being further excluded from the peer group. In some cases there may be a deepening of some close personal relationships as well as a reappraisal of other relationships. Adolescents may face additional issues related to sexuality and dating. Many illnesses, for example, result in delays in growth or delays in the onset of puberty that further sets the child apart from his or her peers.

Academic Functioning

The onset of a major medical illness is likely to have an important effect on the child's academic functioning. The need to miss periods of schooling over the course of a chronic illness may result in difficulty keeping abreast of the academic work. In addition, many illnesses and associated treatments may affect cognitive and academic functioning, resulting in lower academic performance. There should be a determination as to whether the child needs referral for neuropsychological assessment. School reintegration after the initial period of treatment is another consideration for the consultant. There may be a need for periods of home schooling during specific phases of the illness. It is important to ensure that the child has adequate support from the school district, including (where appropriate) an up-to-date educational program to address specific health and learning disabilities.

Coping Mechanisms

It is helpful to understand the characteristic or habitual coping mechanisms used by the child at times of stress, including those used after the diagnosis of a major illness. Knowledge of these mechanisms may assist in formulating the treatment plan. Children who are helped by talking about their illness may benefit from a referral for psychotherapy. However, it is more common for children to have periods of denial, especially during periods of remission from their illness, when they are quite reluctant to engage in any discussion about potential future implications. It is also important to know about potential maladaptive coping mechanisms, including alcohol and substance abuse and risk-taking behaviors.

Spirituality and Religion

An assessment of the family's religious and faith traditions may identify potential sources of support for the child. There may also be specific religious factors that interfere with the treatment of the illness—for example, if the family has strong religious or cultural beliefs that are at odds with the treatment recommendations being made by the medical team. Table 3–3 outlines a list of questions that may be relevant in the assessment of the child's religion and spirituality (Barnes et al. 2000; Moncher and Josephson 2004; Sexton 2004).

Relationship With the Medical Team

It is often illuminating to explore the feelings of the patient and family in relation to the medical team. It is common to identify problems with communication as well as the potential for lack of trust in the medical team. It is important to raise these issues, because there is the potential for them to interfere with the child's treatment.

Table 3–3.   Questions related to religious and spiritual assessment

1. Is the family affiliated with a specific faith background?
2. What is the level of activity within the family's religious community?
3. To what extent does the family receive support from their religious community?
4. What are the particular religious rituals that are important to the family?
5. To what degree is the child involved in these religious activities?
6. What is the family's approach to religious or spiritual questions that arise in the context of a serious medical illness?
    - How does the family understand life's purpose and meaning?
    - How does the family explain illness and suffering?
    - What are the family's beliefs regarding the afterlife?
    - How do religious beliefs intersect with feelings of fairness and blame?
    - How does the family view the person in the context of body, mind, soul, and spirit?

Source.   Adapted from Barnes et al. 2000; Moncher and Josephson 2004; Sexton 2004.

Observation of Behavior and Play

After the initial psychiatric assessment, it is important to collect further data based on observations of the child and family members both informally and, for younger children, in the format of a structured play assessment.

Hospital Behavior

It is important to evaluate the behavioral changes of the child in different hospital contexts—for example, during visits or absences of family members or , during participation in hospital-based activities with physical therapists or child life specialists. In patients with somatoform disorders, it may be possible to observe changes in the child's symptoms that reflect aspects of the child's relationship with his or her parents. Reinforcement of behavior and symptoms may be observed by both family members and staff and may suggest potential treatment interventions.

Play Observation

In younger or preverbal children, the play session is the primary instrument to assess the child's mental status and may involve a direct observation of the child's interactions with the parents—for example, when there are questions about parenting, feeding disorders, or disorders of attachment. Play observation can be used to assess the developmental stage of the child's play and whether it is appropriate to his or her chronological age (American Academy of Child and Adolescent Psychiatry 1997). The clinician should invite the parents to interact as they usually would at home for approximately 15–20 minutes. Unstructured parent–child or family play provides the best opportunity for observation of the interaction. The role of the consultant during the family play session should be clearly explained to the family, including the degree to which he or she will be involved in the interaction. It is important to observe the parent's ability to attend to and read the child's cues as well as the child's response to separation from the parent. Observations should also be made regarding the child's ability to engage in symbolic and age-appropriate play and the child's reactions to the ending of the session.

Specific issues observed during the session include the parents' level of affection expressed toward the child, the willingness and ability to engage the child both verbally and nonverbally, the parents' level of attunement, and their ability to both regulate the child's emotional responses and set appropriate limits. The consultant should also assess the child's capacity for and interest in interpersonal relatedness, the amount and extent of physical and eye contact, the degree to which the child engages in or initiates play with the parents, and the quality and quantity of verbal exchange. Observations should be made regarding the child's capacity for affective involvement with the parents, their capacity for imaginative play, and the thematic content of the play.

Developing a Biopsychosocial Formulation

The consultant's formulation must prioritize and integrate the information obtained regarding the child and family into a brief summary that describes the patient's problems and places them in the context of their current life situation and developmental history. A good formulation must organize the clinical material into a format that is helpful for the patient, family, and referring team. It should foster increased understanding and empathy toward the patient. Biological, psychiatric, and social dimensions need to be evaluated both separately and in relation to each other in the consultant's formulation (Richtesmeier and Aschkenasy 1988). The formulation is a summary of what the consultant "thinks is going on" from a developmental biopsychosocial standpoint that makes meaning of the patient's current circumstances.

Various systems for the formulation have been proposed, including the use of headings—for example, the "three Ps" that include predisposing, precipitating, and perpetuating factors (Kline and Cameron 1978). The precipitating event—in this case, the onset of the medical illness or hospitalization—should be interpreted based on its specific meaning to the patient. This may include issues related to the loss of omnipotence regarding the child's physical health, concerns about abandonment and loss, or reenactments of past traumatic medical events. The formulation should include special strengths of the child and relevant protective factors in addition to the more conventional description of symptoms, risks, and vulnerabilities. The formulation includes a careful weighing of those factors in the patient's life that promote development and allow for recovery.

The biopsychosocial approach to the formulation lists the relevant biological, psychological, and social factor. It has the advantage of being more accessible to the pediatrician who does not generally have a detailed understanding of psychodynamic concepts. The components of the biopsychosocial approach are noted in the following sections.

Biological

Biological factors include family and genetic history; the child's inborn temperament; developmental stage, including height, weight, physical ability, age, and stage of maturity; and intelligence. Physical health and intrauterine drug exposure as well as family psychiatric histories of depression and substance abuse are also relevant.

Psychological

Psychological factors include the child and family's emotional development, personality styles, primary defenses and weaknesses, and history of emotional trauma. The child's developmental stage and relevant developmental issues should be highlighted. Psychological issues should include habitual ways of managing anger, reaction to loss, self-esteem, and functioning in the major areas of daily life.

Social

Social factors include an assessment of the child's functioning within the larger social unit, which includes community, ethnic background, economic status, and spiritual and cultural traditions. It is important to comment on the presence of social isolation or support in the context of the family as well as consider the concept of the child as the *identified patient*, or the individual who is expressing the conflicts of the family and bringing the family into treatment (see Chapter 14).

Communicating Findings to the Medical Team and Family

Once the biopsychosocial formulation is developed, the consultant should begin by communicating this understanding to the referring physician. The consultant aims to frame the presenting problem into a biopsychosocial understanding as opposed to the limited (but common) medical model framework in which psychosocial factors have little role in the patient's presentation. In so doing, the consultant should be alert to the frustration engendered in physicians by patients with emotional and behavior presentations (DeMaso and Beasley 2005).

With acceptance of the formulation by the pediatrician, the next step is an *informing conference* that includes both the physician and family (DeMaso and Beasley 2005). The consultant may or may not attend this meeting, depending on the comfort and expertise of the pediatrician. In a supportive and nonjudgmental manner, the pediatrician (and consultant) should present the patient and the family with both the medical and psychosocial findings. Williams and DeMaso (2000) classified the types of team meetings that commonly occur in the pediatric setting. The *traditional medical team meeting* is focused on gathering medical information used to make a medical diagnosis and formulate the treatment plan and usually does not include the family. The *psychosocial team meeting* predominantly assesses psychosocial issues, for example, treatment adherence or child abuse, and has the goal of reviewing psychosocial issues and formulating a treatment plan that addresses coping and emotional adjustment. The *family conference* is called to provide medical and psychosocial information to the family and generally to establish a consensus with the family about the treatment plan. The *staff-centered meeting* commonly addresses ethical issues that may arise in the context of the child's treatment. The role of the psychiatric consultant in these respective meetings may involve giving advice to the medical team, advocating for the family, providing psychosocial support for team members, and educating the team about the developmental and mental health needs of the child.

Following acceptance of a new biopsychosocial formulation of the problem, the consultant, together with the patient, family, and referring physician, can develop and implement an integrated medical and psychiatric treatment program that is responsive to the presenting problem (Table 3–4).

Writing the Report

A summary of the consultant's opinion should be documented in a written report (Garrick and Stotland 1982). The consultation note is a unique medical document. Like the medical record, it records the history and examination as well as the physician's assessment of the patient, but it also functions as an official document for doctor-to-doctor communication. It is important to keep in mind that the consultation note may be available to the patient and family for review. Although the consultation report contains treatment recommendations, it does not constitute an official order for the nursing or house staff. It is important always to leave a note after every contact with the patient or family, even if it is not possible to give a full, definitive report. Short notes that indicate that the consultation is in process are helpful to the medical team. These notes are also important for billing and medical legal purposes. The report should be clear and concise and should generally avoid including personal details that are inappropriate or not required by the medical team.

Title

The written consultation note should be given a title that indicates the involvement of the psychiatry service as well as the service provided (e.g., initial evaluation, individual psychotherapy, family therapy, team conference, discharge note). The title may also include the position of the person responsible for providing the service.

Table 3–4.   Treatment recommendations

Category of recommendation	Examples
Clarification of diagnosis	Further review of medical records
	Discussion with outside providers
	Additional laboratory tests or diagnostic procedures
	Additional subspecialty consultation
	Neuropsychological testing
Management by psychiatry team	Psychopharmacology interventions
	Specific dosages and timing of doses
	Highlight potential drug interactions
	Highlight common side effects
	Individual psychotherapy
	Family therapy
	Behavior modification programs
	Specific instructions on how to set limits or deemphasize attention being paid to problematic behaviors
	Clarification of roles of staff members and parents in implementation of the program
	Outlining specific approaches to behavior management
	Medical hypnosis
Legal issues	Referrals to child protective services or police department
	Ascertaining the need to obtain and document informed consent for specific treatments
	Providing assistance with steps necessary for involuntary psychiatric hospitalization and transfer
Involvement of other services	Childlife/Recreation therapy for therapeutic play and recreation
	Social work for assistance with resources and family support
	Chaplaincy for spiritual and religious support
	Occupational therapy for activities of daily living, including feeding issues
	Physical therapy for rehabilitation and biofeedback
	Speech and language for evaluation and assistance with communication needs

Table 3–4.   Treatment recommendations *(continued)*

Category of recommendation	Examples

Outpatient recommendations	Referral for outpatient mental health follow-up
	    Specify model, frequency, duration, and potential location of therapy
	    Specify the need for substance abuse treatment if relevant
	    Outlining specific approaches to behavior management
	Referral to school district for educational testing or evaluation for specific school-based resources

Source.   Adapted from Spirito and Fritz 1993.

Date, Time, and Sources

The note should always be dated and timed and include a list of the sources of information used by the consultant. This informs the referring team about the process by which information has been obtained and records the database used in the preparation of the report. The frequency of contact and the time of each session should also be recorded to facilitate billing and insurance issues.

Reason for Consultation

The note should include a brief summary of the original request for consultation in addition to any clarification or amplification obtained after further discussion with the staff. This helps focus the perception of the patient's problems. The opening sentence of the note should attempt to distill the information about the patient into a succinctly worded summary of the patient's presenting condition as well as help clarify the reasons for the psychiatric consultation.

History

There should be a brief review of the history, without unnecessary duplication of history that is already available in the chart. Summary statements may be helpful (e.g., on academic failure or behavioral issues) for sections of the history. The written history should include a chronologically organized presentation of the medical, social, developmental, and interpersonal issues that have led to the consultation request. Issues of confidentiality must be carefully considered. The history should also include a review of recent stresses; academic, family, and social issues; habitual coping mechanisms; and previous psychiatric treatment, including psychopharmacology.

Mental Status Examination

The mental status examination should be clear and comprehensive and include significant negative findings, particularly with regard to suicidality and other risk behaviors. The mental status examination also provides a clinical baseline for comparison in subsequent evaluations. Serial mental status examinations can also help document changes in the patient's clinical course. It is helpful to spell out specific tests that are carried out, particularly with regard to cognitive testing (e.g., subtests of the Mini-Mental State Examination) (see Chapter 5).

Biopsychosocial Formulation

A clearly worded formulation should be included that summarizes the salient details of the case and provides a review of the pertinent factors that may be relevant in the patient's presentation. The formulation can be used to outline the differential diagnosis that is being considered as well as the steps that are needed before a definitive diagnosis can be made.

Diagnoses

Standardized psychiatric diagnoses should be included to help communication with subsequent mental health care providers and to assist with billing issues.

Treatment Recommendations

Detailed and practical recommendations should be made, organized in terms of priority, and should indicate whether further evaluation is necessary prior to the implementation of specific recommendations, such as those for pharmacological interventions. There should be details of who will be responsible for specific interventions (Table 3–4).

Legible Signature

Finally, the report should be signed with a clear and legible name and a pager or telephone number so that the consultant can be easily contacted by the referring team.

References

American Academy of Child and Adolescent Psychiatry: Practice Parameters for the Psychiatric Assessment of Children and Adolescents. J Am Acad Child Adolesc Psychiatry 36 (suppl 10):4S–20S, 1997

Barnes LP, Plotnikoff GA, Fox K, et al: Spirituality, religion, and pediatrics: intersecting worlds of healing. Pediatrics 104:899–908, 2000

Carter MC, Miles MS: The Parental Stressor Scale: Pediatric Intensive Care Unit. Matern Child Nurs J 18:187–198, 1989

DeMaso DR, Beasley PJ: The somatoform disorders, in Clinical Child Psychiatry. Edited by Klykylo WM, Kay JL. Indianapolis, IN, John Wiley and Sons, 2005, 471–486, 1998

DeMaso DR, Meyer EC: A psychiatric consultant's survival guide to the pediatric intensive care unit. J Am Acad Child Adolesc Psychiatry 34:1411–1413, 1996

Drotar D: Consulting With Pediatricians: Psychological Perspectives. New York, Plenum, 1995

Garrick TR, Stotland NL: How to write a psychiatric consultation. Am J Psychiatry 139:849–855, 1982

Hobday A, Ollier K: Creative Therapy With Children and Adolescents. Atascadero, CA, Impact Publishers, 1999

Kline S, Cameron PM: Formulation. Can Psychiatr Assoc J 23:39–42, 1978

Miles MS, Funk SG, Carlson J: Parental Stressor Scale: Neonatal Intensive Care Unit. Nurs Res 42:148–152, 1993

Moncher FJ, Josephson AM: Religious and spiritual aspects of family assessment. Child Adolesc Psychiatr Clin North Am 13:49–70, 2004

Richtesmeier AJ, Aschkenasy JR: Psychological consultation and psychosomatic diagnosis. Psychosomatics 29:338–341, 1988

Sexton SB: Religious and spiritual assessment of the child and adolescent. Child Adolesc Psychiatric Clin North Am 13:35–47, 2004

Shaw RJ, Wamboldt M, Bursch B, et al: Practice patterns in pediatric consultation-liaison psychiatry: a national survey. Psychosomatics, 47:43–49, 2006

Spirito A, Fritz GK: Psychological interventions for pediatric patients, in Child and Mental Health Consultation in Hospitals, Schools, and Courts. Edited by Fritz Gk, Mattison RE, Nurcombe B, et al. Washington, DC, American Psychiatric Publishing, 1993, 67–90

Williams J, DeMaso DR: Pediatric team meetings: the mental health consultant's role. Clin Child Psychol Psychiatry 5:105–113, 2000

Wolraich ML, Felice ME, Drotar D (eds): The Classification of Child and Adolescent Mental Diagnoses in Primary Care: Child and Adolescent Version. Elk Grove Village, IL, American Academy of Pediatrics, 1996

4

Legal and Forensic Issues

The psychiatry consultant faces a number of challenging legal and forensic issues in the pediatric setting. It is critical that the consultant have a solid working understanding of these issues. Consultants must be knowledgeable about the specific statutes in their particular jurisdictions because these rules have a significant impact on patients, the medical team, and even the consultants themselves. Consultants must be open to looking for legal assistance if they have questions. It is advisable that consultants establish an ongoing working relationship with the lawyer or legal service responsible for the pediatric setting in which they practice. Together they can effectively advise and coach the pediatric team in its responses to the legal and forensic issues presented by patients and their families. This chapter offers a general orientation to treatment consent and confidentiality with children and adolescents and an overview regarding the consultant's role in the assessment of parental capacity and medical neglect in the pediatric setting.

Consent for Treatment

Consent and authorization are required for all medical treatments except in unusual circumstances, and any health care provider who provides treatment without proper consent would be open to a charge of battery and could be subject to a civil action for damages for performing a procedure or investigation without consent of the individual concerned (Macbeth 2002). *Informed consent* requires that patients or legal guardians (if the patient is a minor) receive a full and reasonable explanation of the risks and benefits of treatment, including no treatment, and possible alternative treatments from their health care providers (Kuther 2003). The consent must be voluntary; it must also be volitional and not reflect mere acquiescence to consequence. It must be rational, implying that it is rendered by an intellectually competent and mature individual (Kuther 2003). Clinicians should obtain written consent, particularly for complicated treatments, even though statutes do not always require this.

Issues regarding consent are more complicated with children and adolescents because the doctrine of informed consent has only a limited direct application in pediatrics. Only those with legal entitlement and decisional capacity can give informed consent. If a patient does not meet those criteria, a parent or guardian must provide permission. Minors are generally considered to be incompetent to make decisions regarding their medical treatment. Instead, consent must be obtained from the parent or legal guardian who is assumed to act in the best interest of the child. Consent issues with minors are complicated partially because the best interests of the child are hard to define, and they often are subjective (Kuther 2003).

There is an increasing recognition that most adolescents have the capacity to participate in decisions about their health care and a greater willingness by parents and health care providers to include them in decision making (Kuther 2003). The American Academy of Pediatrics Committee on Bioethics (1995) has taken a developmental perspective toward informed consent and recognizes that as minors approach and progress through adolescence, they need a more independent relationship with their health care givers. Pediatricians have been advised that they have an ethical duty to promote the autonomy of minor patients by involving them in the medical decision-making process to a degree commensurate with their abilities.

Assent is a means of involving minors in treatment decisions. It is an interactive process between a minor and a health care provider that involves developmentally appropriate disclosure about the illness and solicitation of the minor's willingness and preferences regarding treatment (American Academy of Pediatrics Committee on Bioethics 1995; Kunin 1997). This commonly accepted definition of assent—a minor's agreement to participate—sets a lower standard of competence than informed consent because it does not require the depth of understanding or the demonstration of reasoning ability required for informed consent (Kuther 2003). The consultant can serve an invaluable role in helping the pediatric team navigate the developmental issues involved in medical decision making. Assent is a means of empowering children and adolescents to their full abilities (Kuther 2003).

Treatment Without Parental Consent

There are some important exceptions to the rule requiring parental consent prior to treatment.

Emergency Treatment

Consent is generally not required when the child needs emergency treatment, but the consultant (when involved) should make every attempt to contact and inform the parent or legal guardian and should document such efforts in the patient's medical record. This exception is based on the assumption that the parent would agree to allow emergency treatment if there were sufficient time to obtain consent. Courts are especially willing to allow this exception if delay in treatment caused by efforts to obtain legal consent would endanger the child's health. Physicians are also generally permitted to carry out diagnostic tests, including skeletal X rays, to diagnose child abuse or neglect without parental consent. Physicians must be aware of the statutes and their legal implications in the jurisdictions in which they practice.

Emancipated Minors

Emancipated minors have the authority to make their own decisions regarding treatment, and parental consent is not required to treat these patients. Children become emancipated minors through marriage, military service, or parenthood, or by demonstrating their ability to financially manage their own affairs. Homeless minors, defined as children under age 18 years who are living apart from their parents in a supervised shelter or temporary accommodation, also have authority to give consent. Although financial independence is an important issue, a child may be an emancipated minor even if he or she is still obtaining financial support from his or her parents, provided the minor is independently managing his or her own financial affairs. Children under the age of 18 may also receive a declaration of emancipation through the courts.

Mature Minor Exception

Older children who do not meet the criteria for being emancipated minors may still have authority to give consent for treatment in limited situations. One such situation occurs when the child is capable of appreciating the nature, extent, and consequences of the medical treatment. This exception is designed to cover situations in which the parents are not available to give consent for low-risk treatments. This exception requires an assessment by the pediatric team of the maturity and judgment of the child and the nature of the treatment in question. For example, treatments that involve psychiatric medications may be of higher risk than treatments with psychotherapy. It is important to document the rationale used to justify the belief that the child is competent to give his or her own consent.

Reproductive Health

Under the statutes of some jurisdictions, parental consent is not required for treatment of sexually transmitted diseases in minors. Similarly, minors may be able to give consent for HIV testing without notification of their parents or legal guardians. Minors can generally consent to medical care related to the prevention or treatment of pregnancy, including prenatal care, but not sterilization. Consent issues regarding abortion are complex, with individual jurisdictions having different laws governing the authorization for an abortion without parental consent. Children of any age are usually entitled to free contraception services without parental consent. Obviously, the age of the patient and his or her partner and the nature of the activity and relationship may trigger other clinical and legal obligations. Finally, victims of sexual assault can be evaluated and treated without parental consent, but local statutes may require the physician to inform the parent or legal guardian unless it is believed that the parent or legal guardian committed the assault.

Alcohol and Substance Abuse Treatment

Many jurisdictions allow emergency treatment of intoxicated minors or minors at risk of complications from withdrawal from alcohol or substances without parental consent. Minors can often consent to medical care and counseling related to the diagnosis and treatment of alcohol and substance abuse–related problems. However, minors cannot receive replacement narcotic abuse treatment without parental consent. Federally funded substance abuse treatment programs are bound by federal confidentiality laws that prohibit disclosure of any information to the parents unless the consultant believes that the minor's situation poses a substantial threat to the life or physical well-being of the minor or another person and that the threat may be reduced by communicating with the minor's parents.

Mental Health Treatment

In some jurisdictions, minors can give consent for mental health treatment or for residential shelter services if a doctor or clinician decides that they are mature enough to participate in these treatment services and that there is potential risk of physical or mental harm without the treatment. Many jurisdictions stipulate that the treating therapist should try to open lines of communication between the child and the parents or to involve the parents in treatment unless the provider decides that such involvement is inappropriate. Shelter services are generally expected to notify the parent or guardian about the minor's request for help, although they may not be permitted to release the minor's medical records.

Limits of Parental Authority

Situations sometimes arise in which the child wishes to refuse a treatment that the parent or legal guardian has requested. In most cases, depending on age and maturity, courts do not allow children to refuse medical treatment if the treatment is necessary to save the child's life or preserve the child's health. Some jurisdictions have similar stipulations regarding alcohol or substance abuse treatment. These issues may be pertinent when a child has religious beliefs that influence his or her opinions about medical treatment or when a child with an eating disorder wants to refuse food and yet is at acute medical risk. As always the consultant must be aware of the relevant statutes in his or her jurisdiction.

Consent for Children of Divorced or Separated Parents

The consultant should be aware that one of the parents may not have the legal right to make decisions regarding the child's treatment. Health care providers are not obligated to raise this question unless there are reasonable grounds that suggest that a parent may not have legal custody. If the physician becomes aware of questions regarding legal guardianship or if parents with equal legal rights differ on treatment options, he or she must take immediate steps to clarify the custody situation, including obtaining a copy of the custody decree. It may then be necessary to get legal informed consent from the authorized parent or for the parents to return to court for judicial clarification. If parents separate or divorce during their child's treatment, the physician may need to obtain parental consent again in order to continue treatment.

Payment for Treatment

There are complications regarding payment for treatment for minors who can legally give their own consent for treatment. In emergency situations the health care providers may look to the parent or legal guardian for payment, but in situations where the purpose of allowing the minor to give consent is to protect confidentiality, the physician must look to the minor for payment. However, most jurisdictions do not allow health care givers to demand payment from the minor until he or she turns 18 years of age, and minors cannot be held liable for payment until they do so. Minors who do not have the financial means to pay for health care services may be eligible for free or low-cost programs that reimburse confidential health services provided to the young. Providers may have to be enrolled in these programs to be reimbursed.

Confidentiality and Privilege

Physicians and health care givers are legally and ethically mandated to protect the confidentiality of information they obtain through their clinical work. Privilege rules govern the disclosure of information in legal and administrative proceedings. Information revealed to a mental health practitioner in the course of treatment is regarded as *privileged,* which means that no one else is generally entitled to see the information shared between the practitioner and the patient. *Confidentiality* rules are broader and govern the disclosure of personal information to anyone not involved in the patient's care.

Confidentiality

Elements of confidentiality that are taken for granted in work with adult patients are more complicated in work with children. The parents or legal guardians of the child are entitled to access to some personal information to help them make treatment decisions, but the child has some independent rights to confidentiality that must be considered. Many jurisdictions have statutes that govern the handling and protection of medical information and records. Violations of these rules place the treating clinician and institution at risk of lawsuit or fine. Parents or legal guardians who authorize treatment are generally also authorized to waive confidentiality and to give permission for release of information.

In the hospital setting, issues are further complicated by the fact that the consultant has a professional relationship with the pediatric team and is expected to share information and opinions with other individuals involved in the patient's care. This relationship should be explicitly defined so that there is a clear understanding of how information obtained in the psychiatric consultation will be used, including potential limits on confidentiality in the hospital setting. The team relationship does not exempt the psychiatric consultant from protecting confidential information that does not need to be disclosed and that is not immediately relevant to the patient's medical care.

Release of Information to Parents

Parents often expect full access to information regarding their child's treatment. This expectation is usually met with regard to medical treatment except in cases where there is investigation of possible child abuse. In addition, information obtained by a mental health practitioner may be of a delicate nature, and disclosure to parents may complicate the relationship between the child and the therapist and potentially jeopardize the child's treatment. Clinicians should discuss these issues with both the child and the parents prior to treatment and stipulate which types of information may be released and which will be protected. This type of conversation can clarify expectations and inform all parties about the terms of the treatment.

Adolescents have greater authority regarding the release of information, particularly regarding issues of sexual behavior and substance abuse. Many jurisdictions link the ability to consent to treatment with the authority to release information, so that the adolescent who is competent to consent to treatment has the right to protect information that emerges in the course of that treatment. Other jurisdictions require the consent of both the parent and the adolescent to disclose confidential information once the adolescent has reached a certain age. If the adolescent cannot consent to treatment, it is important to discuss the disclosure rules with both the patient and the parents. The mental health practitioner is also bound by legal and ethical codes. The consultant who fails to disclose information that would allow the parents to protect the child may be held liable if the child is harmed. Some jurisdictions require disclosure if the child's safety is at risk. The consultant should always attempt to work therapeutically to encourage the child to disclose relevant information to his or her parents.

Further issues arise when the parents of the patient are divorced or separated. Generally the parent with legal custody retains the legal rights regarding access to information and authority to disclose this information. However, many jurisdictions have granted similar rights to the noncustodial parent. In situations in which the noncustodial parent has visitation rights, it is important that the physician provide this parent with any information regarding the treatment necessary to ensure the child's safety. The doctor may have to obtain consent for the release of this information from the parent who has legal custody.

Release of Information to Third Parties

Authority for release of information to schools, insurance companies, and researchers normally lies with the custodial parents, but each jurisdiction has its own statutes that may be relevant. Certain jurisdictions permit the disclosure of information for the purposes of continuity of care. The consultant carefully monitors the information that is released to ensure that the disclosure does not harm the child.

Child Abuse Reporting

Consultants who identify or have reasonable cause to suspect child abuse are mandated to report this information to the appropriate child protection agencies. Each jurisdiction or state has a list of professionals (e.g., physicians, mental health practitioners) who must disclose child abuse. Child abuse reports from "mandated reporters" usually need to be made within 24–48 hours. In all jurisdictions there are statutes in place to provide immunity from civil liability for clinicians who are required to report concerns. Consultants should generally inform patients and families that they have no discretion over whether to report child abuse before starting an assessment or treatment. Consultants must be familiar with the definition of abuse or neglect in his or her jurisdiction.

Corporal punishment may be viewed differently depending on the jurisdiction. There may also be variations based on who perpetrated the abuse; some jurisdictions require the report only if a parent, legal guardian, or person with caretaking authority perpetrated or tolerated the abuse. Different statutes demand different levels of confidence in the suspicion of abuse before mandatory reporting is triggered. Some states require reporting when there is any suspicion of abuse or neglect, whereas others allow the clinician some discretion. The reporting obligation can also be limited to those health care providers who have had professional or clinical interactions with the child. If abuse is suspected but a report is not made, it is important to document the reasons for this decision. In most jurisdictions, because there is a sanction for not reporting and immunity for a false allegation, it is legally prudent to report to protective services if one is in doubt about the mandate to do so.

Sexual Activity

The consultant may be required to report consensual sexual activity if he or she learns that there is an age disparity between the two individuals concerned or if the minor is below the legal age of consent. Each jurisdiction has specific regulations regarding permissible age disparities, statutory rape, and what circumstances trigger a mandatory report to the child abuse authorities. Usually "lewd and lascivious acts" must be reported if the minor is under 14 or if there is an age gap of 10 or more years between the individuals, even if the minor says that the sexual activity was consensual. Clinicians are normally not required to ask about the age of the sexual partner. Sexual activity by a minor may also need to be reported if the doctor believes that the patient was coerced or intimidated into the activity, regardless of whether the minor describes the activity as consensual.

Health-Related Statutes

Jurisdictions may have reporting requirements that include notification regarding infectious diseases or disorders that could impair driving. These statutes may include emotional disorders and substance abuse that can potentially impair motor skills. Some laws authorize or require health care givers to breach confidentiality to issue warnings about certain dangers posed by a patient. Physicians may be required to disclose information that suggests that a patient may endanger the life or safety of another person and can be held legally liable for failure to do so. Similarly, patients who disclose thoughts or plans regarding suicidality lose their right to confidentiality and may face civil commitment procedures.

Custody Disputes

When the parents of a patient separate or divorce during the child's treatment, one or both parents may request a consultant's assistance in the custody hearing as well as access to confidential or privileged information. Legal rules may prevent this testimony from being admitted in court, but even when legally allowable, it is advisable for the consultant to avoid allying with one of the parents because it could jeopardize the child's mental health treatment. Independent custody evaluations are preferable in these situations.

Authorization to Release Information

Once it is clear who has the authority to consent to release information, any such consent should be obtained in writing. Consultants must ensure that the consent form qualifies the extent of the information that may be released and that it complies with state statutes. Specific sections of the consent form may describe how the information can be used and may allow the consenting party to examine any disclosed information. Before information is released, consultants should establish that the child and the parents have given fully informed consent by describing the nature of information that has been requested and what information will be released. If a consultant believes that the patient or parents would not have consented to the release of information to third parties such as schools or insurance companies if they were aware of the nature of information involved, it may be necessary for the consultant to obtain a new consent from the family. It is generally recommended that the patient and parent be provided with a copy of the information intended for release.

Privilege

Privilege rules govern the disclosure of confidential information in judicial and administrative proceedings. Statutes protect certain types of relationships at the expense of full disclosure to encourage open communication in these relationships. One type of privilege exists between a patient and the physician or psychotherapist, and this includes child and adolescent patients. Federal regulations protect information disclosed in the course of psychotherapy based on the assumption that effective treatment would be impossible without patient confidence in a confidential discourse. In work with children and adolescents, some important issues of privilege may arise. Information disclosed in the presence of a third person such as a parent has traditionally not been regarded as privileged, but this rule is under review in many jurisdictions. Another issue is whether information that a physician receives from family members or other third parties about a child's treatment is protected by privilege. Consultants need to be aware of the specific rulings on these questions in their own jurisdictions.

Exceptions to Privilege

There are several exceptions to the general rule of privilege that apply to commitment proceedings, will contests, and criminal matters. In work with minors, exceptions are also made regarding information about child abuse or neglect. In some jurisdictions, privilege can be lost in child custody cases, even if the child and parents object.

Waiver

Physician–patient privileges may be waived at the discretion of the patient or the person authorized to act on the patient's behalf. In some court hearings, a guardian *ad litem* is appointed to decide whether an incompetent child would choose to waive privilege if he or she were competent to do so. Children and adolescents may decline to exercise their right to privilege, and in some jurisdictions, parents or legal guardians can waive privilege on behalf of their child. When parents are divorced or separated, it is important to establish whether this authorization to waive privilege needs to be obtained from both parents. In custody disputes there is often disagreement between the parents about disclosure of confidential information. Privilege may also be waived when the patient has already testified about his or her treatment. The consultant should be particularly cautious about releasing information to lawyers or legal representatives unless he or she has a signed release from the patient or parents. This caution extends to subpoenaed requests for information.

Assessment for Parenting Capacity and Medical Neglect

Issues of parental competence frequently arise in the hospital, often with regard to the parents' ability to manage their child's treatment regimen. It is not uncommon to encounter parental neglect and abuse of physically ill children. Child protective service agencies often become involved during the inpatient admission and are ultimately responsible for decisions regarding placement, although the consultant can be asked to give an opinion about parental capacity.

Parental Capacity

Barnum (2002) noted that socialization, advocacy, and protection are important aspects of parental capacity.

Socialization

Parents are responsible for the socialization of their child. Effective parents support the cognitive development of their child by imparting knowledge and fostering the development of abilities such as language, self-care, academic functioning, and social skills. Parents also have a responsibility to promote positive and social behavior by providing adequate and consistent supervision and by setting developmentally appropriate limits on negative or antisocial behavior. It is important for parents to foster the emotional development of the child by providing support, guidance, and direction. Parents whose coping style is characterized by anger, conflict, or criticism are likely to undermine their child's development, whereas overly protective parental behavior may result in insecurity and lack of confidence in the child.

Advocacy and Protection

Parents are expected to provide a safe and secure environment and protection from physical harm or exposure to emotional trauma such as domestic violence and sexual or emotional abuse. This expectation includes the parental responsibility to provide appropriate medical care for children with medical illnesses and to ensure that their child maintains satisfactory school attendance. Parents must also recognize and assist children with mental or physical disabilities. Parents who cannot provide these basic functions may be guilty of medical, emotional, or educational neglect.

Medical Neglect

Medical neglect is the failure of parents or legal guardians to provide appropriate health care, including psychological treatment, for their child even though they have the financial means to do so. Medical neglect can result in adverse health consequences, such as the worsening of the child's existing physical illness. According to data from the National Clearinghouse on Child Abuse and Neglect Information, medical neglect affected 45,300 children in 2003, accounting for 2.3% of substantiated cases of child maltreatment in the United States (U.S. Department of Health and Human Services 2003). Concern is warranted when a parent refuses medical care for a child in an emergency or for one with an acute illness and when a parent ignores medical recommendations for a child who has a treatable chronic disease or disability, resulting in frequent hospitalizations or significant medical deterioration. Cases in which parents withhold medical care based on their religious beliefs do not fall under the definition of medical neglect, but most jurisdictions are moving toward eliminating these religious exemptions. Parents may also fail to provide medical care because of cultural norms, insufficient information, or lack of financial resources.

Child protective services agencies generally will intervene when a child needs emergency medical treatment or when a child has a life-threatening or chronic illness that may result in disability or disfigurement if left untreated. Most jurisdictions issue court orders to permit appropriate medical treatment in these situations. Social and financial assistance may be available when poverty rather than neglect limits parents' resources to provide adequate medical treatment for their child.

Assessment

At some point, all consultants will be asked to help assess parenting competence and medical neglect. As in the assessment of violence, it is important that the consultant clarify the expectations underlying the request. The consultant must be clear that he or she can provide a psychiatric assessment that includes parental psychopathology and a sense of the parent–child relationship but that he or she is not a detective able to determine who abused or neglected whom. In the hospital setting, the source of these referrals may be a child abuse protection team that consults with the pediatric team on all cases of suspected neglect or abuse. The consultant should not begin an assessment until the patient and family have been told of the consultation and its purposes. If the parents refuse appropriate assessment, the refusal itself may constitute neglect. The consultant should explicitly state to the family that the information and findings obtained in this assessment are not confidential or privileged and must be communicated to the pediatric team.

Table 4–1 is a summary of parental qualities that should be assessed in the determination of parental capacity and are particularly relevant to the treatment of physically ill children and adolescents.

Termination of Parental Rights

Child protective services agencies can petition for temporary or permanent termination of parental rights if the parents are found to be unfit, unwilling, or unable to competently manage their child's medical care. These agencies may temporarily place the child in foster care during a period of intensive medical treatment, with the goal of reunification after the treatment. Temporary foster care placement or other substitute care can also be used to give parents the opportunity to correct issues that are interfering with their ability to provide competent medical treatment. Parental rights may be permanently terminated in more extreme circumstances when the parents are found to be unlikely to be able to change their parenting behaviors within the foreseeable future or when conditions such as Munchausen syndrome by proxy are present.

Table 4–1.   Assessment of parental capacity

Parental strengths	Parental deficits
Cognitive understanding of the child's physical, medical, and emotional needs	Cognitive limitations or mental retardation interfering with understanding of the child's physical or medical needs
Presence of adequate organizational skills and ability to supervise the child's treatment	
Consistency	Inadequate financial resources to support the child's physical and emotional needs
Presence of extended family and social support	Inability to enforce discipline or set limits in an appropriate manner
Capacity for emotional warmth and nurturance	Parental psychopathology
	Parental alcohol or substance abuse
	Parental history of abuse or neglect

Source.   Adapted from Barnum 2002.

The consultant may be asked to assist in these evaluations and to make recommendations regarding the mental health needs of children placed in foster care. Children who are removed from their parents may experience the separation as unexpected and traumatic, because removal frequently occurs without preparation or adequate explanation to the child. Placement may disrupt the child's social support network and can entail a change in schools. In making these decisions, it is important to consider data that suggests that foster children are at greater risk for maltreatment and physical abuse than the general population. Despite the deficiencies of foster care and out-of-home placement, they may be necessary in order to lessen the likelihood of reinjury by parents or legal guardians.

Conclusion

We end by returning to the points made at the beginning of this chapter and reemphasizing the importance that consultants have a solid foundation in legal and forensic issues in the pediatric setting. This means understanding the specific statutes in their own jurisdictions that are most germane to their work setting. Consultants should establish a consulting relationship with a lawyer familiar with the pediatric setting. This partnership can have enormous impact on advancing patient care. Consultants should never hesitate to call for legal assistance.

References

American Academy of Pediatrics Committee on Bioethics: Informed consent, parental permission, and assent in pediatric practice. Pediatrics 95:314–317, 1995

Barnum R: Parenting assessment in cases of neglect and abuse, in Principles and Practice of Child and Adolescent Forensic Psychiatry. Edited by Schetky DH, Benedek EP. Washington, DC, American Psychiatric Publishing, 2002, pp 81–96

Kunin H: Ethical issues in pediatric life-threatening illness: dilemmas of consent, assent, and communication. Ethics Behav 7:43–57, 1997

Kuther TL: Medical decision-making and minors: issues of consent and assent. Adolescence 38:343–358, 2003

Macbeth JD: Legal issues in the treatment of minors, in Principles and Practice of Child and Adolescent Forensic Psychiatry. Edited by Schetky DH, Benedek EP. Washington, DC, American Psychiatric Publishing, 2002, pp 309–323

U. S. Department of Health and Human Services: Administration for Children and Families, National Clearinghouse on Child Abuse and Neglect Information, 2003. Available at http://nccanch.acf.hhs.gov. Accessed June 7, 2005.

5

Delirium

Delirium involves a global dysfunction in cerebral metabolism that is due to the direct physiological consequences of a general medical condition. It presents with a wide array of neuropsychiatric abnormalities, including disturbances of attention, consciousness, psychomotor activity, perception, and sleep (American Psychiatric Association 2000). Many different labels have been used to describe delirium, including acute brain syndrome, encephalopathy, confusional state, and intensive care unit (ICU) psychosis. Delirium has been associated with rates of morbidity and mortality that surpass those of all other psychiatric diagnoses (Wise and Trzepacz 1996).

The DSM classification for delirium underwent many versions prior to the current DSM-IV-TR criteria that emphasize a core disturbance of consciousness (i.e., reduced awareness of the environment) with reduced ability to focus, sustain, and shift attention (American Psychiatric Association 2000). The criteria involve a change in cognition (e.g., memory deficit, disorientation, language disturbance) or a perceptual disturbance that develops over a short period of time (usually hours to days) and tends to fluctuate during the course of the day (American Psychiatric Association 2000). It is common for psychiatric consultants to be asked to assess and help manage children with acute mental status changes in the pediatric setting. Yet the study of delirium has been neglected in pediatrics, with no published studies between 1980 and 2003. It has only recently been established that the DSM-IV-TR diagnostic criteria are clinically relevant and applicable in pediatric patients (Turkel and Tavaré 2003). This chapter outlines the clinical characteristics, epidemiology, and differential diagnosis of delirium and describes evaluation and management approaches to pediatric delirium.

Clinical Characteristics

Patients with delirium have characteristic changes in several domains of functioning, reflecting the diffuse nature of the central nervous system pathology (Table 5–1). The clinical presentation of delirium in children and adolescents is similar to that of adults, with some minor differences in specific symptoms as described later (Prugh et al. 1980; Turkel and Tavaré 2003; Turkel et al. 2004).

Table 5–1. Clinical characteristics of delirium

Prodrome (anxiety, irritability, restlessness, or sleep disturbance)

Rapid fluctuating course (lucid intervals may occur)

Disorientation (time and place, rarely to person)

Impaired memory (cannot remember recent events)

Attention decreased (easily distractible)

Sleep-wake disturbance (reversal of sleep-wake cycle)

Perceptual disturbances (misperceptions, illusions, delusions [poorly formed], hallucinations [visual or tactile])

Arousal disturbance and psychomotor abnormalities (hyperactive, hypoactive, or mixed)

Thinking and speech disorganized

Neurological abnormalities (dysgraphia, constructional apraxia, dysnomic aphasia)

Motor abnormalities (asterixis, myoclonus, reflex and tone changes, intention tremor

Electroencephalographic abnormalities (global slowing)

Source. Adapted from Wise MG, Brandt G: "Delirium," in American Psychiatric Press Textbook of Neuropsychiatry, 2nd Edition. Edited by Hales RE, Yudofsky SC. Washington, DC, American Psychiatric Press, 1992, p 295.

Prodrome

During the prodromal phase patients may exhibit nonspecific symptoms, such as restlessness, anxiety, irritability, sleep disturbances (e.g., nightmares), and even transient illusions or hallucinations. These symptoms may be noted for hours to days prior to the more florid manifestations of an acute delirium.

Temporal Course

Delirium can have abrupt or acute onset, particularly after surgery or when sedative and hypnotic medications are being withdrawn. There is often a stepwise decline or alteration in behavior associated with a characteristic waxing and waning of symptoms with lucid intervals (fluctuating consciousness). However, if closely examined, cognitive impairment persists even during the apparent lucid intervals. Symptoms are often worse at night, a phenomenon referred to as *sundowning*. Patients may make a full recovery if the underlying etiology is identified and found to be reversible, but a significant number of patients may progress to stupor, coma, or even death. Although overall mortality rates are generally lower in pediatric patients compared with adults, mortality rates as high as 20% have been reported in specific pediatric subgroups (i.e., transplantation and autoimmune diseases; Turkel and Tavaré 2003). In those children who do recover, perceptual and motor deficiencies can persist for several weeks (Prugh et al. 1980).

Cognitive Impairment

Attention

Patients with delirium characteristically present with difficulties in sustained attention—a review of delirium studies found inattention in nearly 100% of cases (Turkel et al. 2004). In young children, impaired attention may be most apparent in an inability to interpersonally engage with the clinician, whereas in older children and adolescents the nature of the attention difficulties is very similar to those in adults (i.e., difficulties in concentration and focus; Turkel and Tavaré 2003). Reductions in attention are likely based on a combination of prefrontal, parietal, and subcortical dysfunction (Wise and Trzepacz 1996).

Memory

Immediate and recent event memory is frequently impaired. Patients have trouble with registration, retention, and recall. Although long-term declarative memory is generally intact, there may be problems with procedural memory. After successful recovery, patients often have amnesia for the entire delirium episode or limited recollection of events (generally of negative ones). Problems with memory in younger children are not as common as those experienced by adolescents (Turkel and Tavaré 2003).

Disorientation

Patients are usually disoriented to time and place but rarely to person. There may be some fluctuation in levels of orientation during lucid periods. Although disorientation may be difficult to assess in younger children who developmentally may have a limited conception of time, a review of pediatric delirium suggested that disorientation is present in approximately 77% of cases (Turkel et al. 2004). Children who have developed verbal skills are usually able to cooperate with questions regarding orientation.

Visuoconstructional Impairment

Patients with delirium may be unable to copy simple geometric designs or complex figures (dysgraphia and constructional apraxia). The ability to draw a clock face is a useful test because it assesses functioning in three different neuroanatomical regions: the nondominant parietal cortex (overall spatial proportions and relations), the dominant parietal cortex (details such as numbers and hands), and the prefrontal cortex (understanding the concept of time).

Prefrontal Executive Functions

Delirium is often associated with an impaired ability to process information, reason, solve problems, anticipate consequences of actions, and grasp the meanings of abstract words. These deficits are thought to develop as a result of impaired functioning of the dorsolateral region of the prefrontal cortex. Patients show symptoms of perseveration, concrete thinking, and impaired performance on the Trail Making Tests (Trzepacz et al. 1988b; Wise and Trzepacz 1996).

Thought and Language Disturbance

Thought processes are often disorganized and inaccurate, with tangentiality and loosening of associations. Severe cases may resemble a fluent aphasia (Wise and Trzepacz 1996). Patients may develop poorly systematized and mood-incongruent paranoid delusions that can lead to violent behavior. Speech can be characterized by incoherence, rambling, mild dysarthria, mumbling, muteness, and word-finding difficulties.

Perceptual Disturbance

Illusions (misperceptions of real objects) and hallucinations (false perceptions) are common. Visual hallucinations or visual combined with auditory hallucinations are common, occurring in up to 43% of cases, whereas tactile, gustatory, and olfactory hallucinations occur less frequently (Turkel et al. 2004). Organized delusions are rare. Patients have a reduced ability to discriminate and integrate perceptions, resulting in their confusion of images, dreams, and hallucinations. Confusion and misidentification are present in pediatric delirium, as opposed to the perceptional disturbances of derealization and depersonalization. Younger children may be less likely to report perceptual disturbances.

Psychomotor Disturbance

Impaired psychomotor activity is common in pediatric delirium, with symptoms of apathy or agitation occurring with equal frequency. Traditionally this has led to the classification of delirium based on the nature of the psychomotor disturbance (Liptzin and Levkoff 1992). A *hyperactive* delirium classically presents with confusion, psychosis, disorientation, psychomotor agitation, hypervigilance, hyperalertness, fast or loud speech, combativeness, and behavioral problems (e.g., pulling out catheters and lines). A *hypoactive* or silent delirium presents with somnolence, decreased activity, slow or decreased speech, psychomotor slowing, apathy, and confusion. Patients with this latter presentation are less likely to be diagnosed or may be misdiagnosed with depression. *Mixed type* delirium describes patients who fluctuate between hyperactive and hypoactive states. Review of pediatric delirium suggests that rates of presentation of hyperactive and hypoactive states are similar in child and adolescent patients (Turkel et al. 2004).

Sleep-Wake Cycle Disruptions

Delirium classically presents with disruptions to the sleep-wake cycle. There is often a reversal in the diurnal rhythm, with lethargy during the day and arousal, disorientation, and agitation at night.

Affective Lability

Patients with delirium may have rapid fluctuations in their emotional state, with symptoms of anxiety, fear, anger, sadness, apathy, and less commonly euphoria (e.g., steroid-induced delirium). Affective lability, anxiety, and irritability are found in the majority of children with delirium (Turkel and Tavaré 2003).

Neurological Abnormalities

Physical Examination

Findings on physical examination include tremor, myoclonus, and asterixis, particularly in those patients with metabolic uremia and hepatic insufficiency. The nature of the tremor varies according to etiology but is more commonly an intention tremor. Symmetric reflex and muscle tone changes may be seen in myxedema, carbon monoxide poisoning, and neuroleptic malignant syndrome. Nystagmus and ataxia may occur in drug intoxications. Patients with lithium toxicity may present with cerebellar signs.

Electroencephalograms

Patients with delirium classically have a generalized nonspecific slowing on their electroencephalograms, with the degree of slowing correlating with the severity of their deliriums (Pro and Wells 1977). Less typically, there may be excess activity (e.g., the low-voltage fast activity beta waves seen in delirium tremens).

Epidemiology

Epidemiological data on pediatric delirium is not well described, although children and adolescents may be more susceptible than adults to delirium, especially in the context of febrile illness and certain medications (e.g., anticholinergic medications) (American Psychiatric Association 2000; Wise and Trzepacz 1996). Based on adult studies, the following categories of patients are thought to be at increased risk of delirium: 1) preexisting brain abnormalities; 2) burn injuries; 3) postanesthesia; 4) postsurgery (especially postcardiotomy and posttransplant); 5) multiple medications (particularly narcotic medication); 6) visual and hearing impairments; 7) dehydration; 8) substance dependence; 9) infections; and 10) low serum albumen resulting in reduced protein-bound drug carrying capacity (i.e., malnutrition, nephrotic syndrome, and hepatic insufficiency) (Wise and Trzepacz 1996).

Although there are few data in pediatric settings, delirium has been reported in 15%–18% of patients on acute medical and surgical wards, with higher rates in specific population groups (Wise and Trzepacz 1996). For example, immediately prior to death, delirium rates of 68%–88% have been reported in adult oncology patients (Liptzin 2000; Morita et al. 2001). Delirium has been related to increased utilization of hospital resources, increased lengths of stay, increased postsurgical complications, and poor functional recovery (Kane et al. 1993; Marcantonio et al. 1994).

Differential Diagnosis

There is an extensive range of general medical etiologies that cause pediatric delirium (Wise and Trzepacz 1996). Virtually any physical condition and its treatment have the ability to induce the disabling cognitive disturbances seen in delirium. It is important to note that delirium is often multifactorial in nature. Table 5–2 outlines a differential diagnosis of pediatric delirium that uses the mnemonic "I WATCH DEATH".

Turkel and Tavaré (2003) found that the most common etiology for pediatric delirium was infection with central nervous system involvement (e.g., bacterial meningitis), closely followed by medication-related causes. Head trauma after bicycle or motor vehicle accidents is also a common etiology for pediatric delirium, in contrast to falls, which are more frequently seen in geriatric patients. Table 5–3 is a list of selected medications that have been etiologic agents in delirium. Opioids and medications with anticholinergic side effects are commonly incriminated in delirium. The following well-known medications have little-known anticholinergic side effects: captopril, cimetidine, codeine, digoxin, furosemide, prednisolone, ranitidine, theophylline, and warfarin.

Assessment

The evaluation of delirium includes an interview with parents to obtain a thorough medical history. The consultant should review the medical chart, including laboratory and imaging test results (see Table 5–4). Nursing staff

Table 5–2.   Differential diagnosis of pediatric delirium: the "I WATCH DEATH" mnemonic

Infection	Encephalitis*, meningitis*, syphilis, HIV, or sepsis*
Withdrawal	Alcohol, barbiturates, or sedative-hypnotics*
Acute metabolic	Acidosis, alkalosis, electrolyte disturbance*, hepatic failure, or renal failure
Trauma	Closed-head injury*, heatstroke, postoperative*, or severe burns*
Central nervous system pathology	Abscess, hemorrhage, hydrocephalus, subdural hematoma, infection*, seizures*, stroke, tumors, metastases, or vasculitis*
Hypoxia	Anemia, carbon monoxide poisoning, hypotension, pulmonary failure, or cardiac failure
Deficiencies	Vitamin B_{12}, folate, niacin, or thiamine
Endocrinopathies	Hyper/hypoadrenocorticism, hyper/hypoglycemia, myxedema, or hyperparathyroidism
Acute vascular	Hypertensive encephalopathy, stroke, arrhythmia, or shock*
Toxins or drugs	Medications*, illicit drugs, pesticides, or solvents
Heavy metals	Lead, manganese, or mercury*

*More commonly seen in pediatric delirium.
Source.   Reprinted from Wise and Brandt 1992, pp 302.

observations should be obtained at different points in time to capture fluctuations in levels of consciousness.

The direct examination of the delirious patient is dictated by the nature of the cognitive disturbances described earlier in this chapter. Depending on the patient's mental status functioning, the consultant's questioning can range from basic orientation questions (i.e., time, person, place, and circumstances) to specific questions about cognitive and perceptual disturbances (i.e., hearing and seeing things). In moments of lucidity, patients will often acknowledge that their thinking is "confused or mixed up." The consultant can often spend a few minutes outside a patient's bedspace and readily observe the presence or absence of psychomotor agitation.

Rating Scales for Delirium

Rating scales are useful in the evaluation of delirium and to assess treatment response. With the exception of the Pediatric Anesthesia Emergence Delirium

Scale (Sikich and Lerman 2004) and the Children's Delirium Scale (Martini et al. 2002), there are few instruments specifically developed for pediatric patients. However, the very commonly used Delirium Rating Scale–Revised–98 has been utilized in studies of pediatric delirium (Trzepacz et al. 2001; Turkel et al. 2004).

Mini-Mental State Examination

The Mini-Mental State Examination (MMSE) is a widely used screening instrument primarily used in adults, although it can be given to older children and adolescents (Folstein et al. 1975). It assesses orientation, attention, immediate and short-term recall, language, and the ability to follow simple verbal and written commands to provide a total score of cognitive functioning. It has been used to detect impairment, follow the course of an illness, and monitor response to treatment. MMSE scores below 24 indicate possible organic cognitive component, whereas MMSE scores below 20 indicate severe cognitive decline.

Delirium Rating Scale-Revised-98

The Delirium Rating Scale, used to assess symptoms of delirium, has shown good reliability and validity (Trzepacz et al. 1988a). It has been found to be applicable in children with delirium, with scores comparable with those reported of adults. Available in English, French, Spanish, Portuguese, Dutch, Japanese, Italian, and Mandarin Chinese, its threshold score of 10 or greater identifies delirium (Turkel et al. 2003). The Delirium Rating Scale–Revised–98 (see Appendix) was developed to address limitations in the original scale (Trzepacz et al. 2001). The revised version is a 16-item clinician-rated scale divided into a 13-item severity section and a 3-item diagnostic section; their sum constitutes the total scale score. The severity scale can be used to provide repeated measurement of the patient's clinical status within an episode of delirium. The total scale can be scored initially to enhance differential diagnosis by capturing characteristic features of delirium, such as acute onset and fluctuation of symptom severity.

Management

Efforts should be made wherever possible to prevent the onset of delirium by identifying those patients at high risk and proactively treating their underlying

Table 5–3.   Selected drugs associated with delirium

Analgesic	Opiates	Salicylates
Antibiotic	Aminoglycosides	Cephalexin
	Ethambutol	Cephalosporins
	Rifampin	Chloramphenicol
	Tetracycline	Chloroquine
	Vancomycin	Gentamicin
		Isoniazid
		Sulfonamides
		Ticarcillin
Anticonvulsant	Phenobarbital	Valproic acid
	Phenytoin	
Anti-inflammatory	Adrenocorticotropic	Corticosteroids
	hormone	Indomethacin
	Ibuprofen	Phenylbutazone
	Naproxen	
	Steroids	
Antineoplastic	Aminoglutethimide	Asparaginase
	Dacarbazine (DTIC)	5-Fluorouracil
	Tamoxifen	Methotrexate (at high dose)
	Vinblastine	Vincristine
Antiparkinsonian	Amantadine	Carbidopa
	Benztropine	Levodopa
	Biperiden	Trihexyphenidyl
	Bromocriptine	
Antiviral	Acyclovir	Interferon
	Ganciclovir	
Antituberculous	Isoniazid	Rifampin
Cardiac	Beta blockers	Captopril
	Clonidine	Disopyramide
	Digoxin	Lidocaine
	Methyldopa	Mexiletine
	Tocainide	Quinidine
	Isosorbide	Procainamide
	Dyazide	Furosemide
Drugs withdrawal	Alcohol	Barbiturates
	Benzodiazepines	
Sedative-hypnotics	Barbiturates	Benzodiazepines

Table 5–3. Selected drugs associated with delirium *(continued)*

Sympathomimetics	Aminophylline	Amphetamines
	Cocaine	Ephedrine
	Epinephrine	Phenylephrine
	Phenylpropanolamine	Theophylline
Miscellaneous	Amphotericin B	Metrizamide
	Antihistamines	Metronidazole
	Antispasmodics	Phenothiazines
	Atropine	Phenelzine
	Baclofen	Podophyllin
	Belladonna alkaloids	Procarbazine
	Bromides	Promethazine
	Chlorpropamide	Propylthiouracil
	Cimetidine	Quinacrine
	Diphenhydramine	Ranitidine
	Disulfiram	Scopolamine
	Ergotamine	Timolol ophthalmic
	Lithium	Tricyclic antidepressants

Source.   Adapted from Wise MG, Brandt G: "Delirium," in *American Psychiatric Press Textbook of Neuropsychiatry,* 2nd Edition. Edited by Hales RE, Yudofsky SC. Washington DC, American Psychiatric Press, 1992, pp 301. Copyright 1992, American Psychiatric Press. Used with permission.

physical conditions. Prevention of perioperative hypotension and hypoxemia, as well as attention to choice of anesthetic and pain agents, may help reduce the incidence of delirium. Appropriate tapering of sedative-hypnotic agents used in the ICU to prevent withdrawal delirium is important and frequently overlooked. Steps to reduce the anticholinergic load of medications, such as using benzodiazepines rather than diphenhydramine for anxiety, may be helpful.

When called about a mental status change consistent with delirium, the psychiatric consultant must remember that cognitive dysfunction is due to the direct physiological consequences of a physical condition or its treatment. The consultant may need to advocate for the patient with the pediatric service to continue investigating and treating potential medical etiologies for delirium. It is important to note that delirium may have multiple etiologies within the same patient.

Environmental Interventions

Practical interventions include placing the patient near the nursing station, preferably in a private room, with a family member or staff person present to

Table 5–4. Laboratory tests in delirium

Basic laboratory tests	Additional laboratory tests
Complete blood count	Heavy metals screening
Blood chemistry	Serum B_{12} and folate
Liver function tests	Lupus erythematosus prep
Magnesium	Antinuclear antibody
Phosphorus	Urinary porphyrins
Venereal Disease Research Laboratory (VDRL) test	Ammonia levels
	Erythrocyte sedimentation rate
Serum drug levels	HIV
lithium	Electroencephalogram
cyclosporin	Head magnetic resonance imaging scan
tricyclic antidepressants	Computed tomography scan
digoxin	Lumbar puncture
anticonvulsants	
quinidine	
Arterial blood gases	
Urine analysis	
Electrocardiogram	
Chest X ray	
Urine toxicology screen	

Source. From Wise MG, Trzepacz PT: "Delirium (Confusional States)," in the *American Psychiatric Press Textbook of Consultation-Liaison Psychiatry.* Edited by Rundell JR, Wise MG. Washington, DC, American Psychiatric Press, 1996, pp 258–275. Copyright 1996, American Psychiatric Press, Inc. Used with permission.

provide one-to-one observation to ensure the patient's safety. Efforts to restore the normal sleep-wake cycle should be made by having room lights on during the day and off at night, but with sufficient nighttime illumination to decrease the likelihood of illusions. The presence of familiar objects from home, a calendar, and a clock may help to reassure and reorient the patient. Vital signs should be checked frequently, and it is important to ensure good oxygenation and fluid intake. Patients who are significantly out of control (e.g., agitation, pulling intravenous lines) may require physical restraint for their own safety as well as that of others. Physical restraints may be necessary to prevent the patient from causing harm to him- or herself or to staff members and to avoid intravenous lines and catheters being inadvertently pulled out by the patient. In these situations, established hospital protocols for the use of mechanical restraints should be closely followed.

The consultant can be helpful to family members by providing education and support for the acute mental status changes that they are witnessing. Helping parents understand the confusion that their child is experiencing may allow them to more effectively implement supportive interpersonal techniques with their child (e.g., simple and repeated words of reassurance and reorientation).

Pharmacological Interventions

The consultant should conduct a thorough review of all of the patient's current and recent medications. This review may suggest that the patient is overmedicated or responding adversely to the current regimen, leading to suggestions to discontinue rather than add medications. Opioids are particularly notorious for their adverse impact on a patient's mental status, whereas benzodiazepines may disinhibit the child rather than relieve anxiety. By contrast, the consultant may identify situations in which medications are being withdrawn too rapidly, resulting in a withdrawal syndrome (e.g., opioids or benzodiazepines). The latter likely will involve reinstitution of the medication with a more gradual taper being designed or other medications being added (i.e., methadone)

There are situations in the pediatric setting in which a patient's agitation and distress cannot await resolution of their physical illness or change in its treatment. At these junctures, it is critical to the patient's care and safety that these behaviors be rapidly contained. Chemical restraint generally plays a much more important role than mechanical restraint in managing a patient with delirium.

Use of Antipsychotic Agents

Most patients with severe delirium will respond fairly rapidly to haloperidol (Wise and Trzepacz 1996). This high-potency agent is preferred over the low-potency agents because of the lower likelihood of hypotensive and anticholinergic effects, and it has been found to be safe and effective in managing cases of pediatric delirium (Brown et al. 1996) and in targeting agitation seen in delirium. Pediatric dosages range from 0.25–10 mg/day to 0.05–0.15 mg/kg/day (Williams 2002). Clinically, many cases of delirium will respond to even low dosages of haloperidol given once or twice a day. The consultant is advised to follow the medication on a daily basis given the transient nature of delirium and to help titrate the dosage. Although not approved for use in this form by the U.S. Food and Drug Administration, haloperidol is often given intravenously, either by bolus injection or continuous infusion. Intravenous use results in more reliable absorption and a decreased incidence of extrapyramidal reactions and has minimal effect on blood pressure, respiration, and heart rate (Beliles 2000; Menza et al. 1987). The intravenous dosage is twice as potent as oral administration. The incidence of *torsades de pointes* or ventricular tachycardia is only 0%–0.01%, although there may be an elevated risk in cardiomyopathy (Hunt and Stern 1995). Cardiac monitoring is recommended, and, if the QT_c is greater than 450 msec or greater than 25% over baseline, it is prudent to obtain a cardiology consultation and consider stopping the medication.

The newer atypical antipsychotic agents, including olanzapine, risperidone, and quetiapine have also been reported to be useful in the pharmacological management of delirium (Han and Kim 2004). Olanzapine, for example, has been used effectively in studies of adult patients, whereas risperidone may also be a good alternative to haloperidol, with the potential for fewer side effects (Sipahimalani and Masand 1997, 1998; Zimnitzky et al. 1996). Use of the atypical antipsychotic agents is limited by the lack of availability of parenteral formulations and data regarding appropriate dosages and specific treatment protocols in pediatric patients.

Although adult patients with delirium are commonly treated with combinations of haloperidol and lorazepam, benzodiazepines are generally not recommended in the treatment of pediatric delirium except in cases of withdrawal delirium. There is concern about the potential for disinhibition in children treated with benzodiazepines, and to date, no studies support their use in pediatric delirium. In addition, there have been studies of adult patients that have not supported the use of lorazepam and in fact suggested a greater incidence of treatment-limiting adverse effects related to benzodiazepine use (Breitbart et al. 1996). However, combined neuroleptic-benzodiazepine protocols are described for adult patients and justified on the basis that addition of lorazepam allows lower dosages of haloperidol and may minimize side effects (Maldonado et al. 2003).

**Addiction Research Foundation Clinical Institute Withdrawal
Assessment for Alcohol (CIWA-Ar)**

For each section, ask the prompts and/or observe behavior.
1. Time: *24 hour clock, midnight=00:00* <div align="right">_ _:_ _</div>
2. Pulse or heart rate, taken for one minute <div align="right">_ _ _ bpm</div>
3. Blood pressure <div align="right">_ _ _/_ _ _ mm/Hg</div>
4. Nausea and vomiting Do you feel sick to your stomach? Have you vomited? No nausea and no vomiting ☐0 Mild nausea with no vomiting ☐1 ☐2 ☐3 Intermittent nausea with dry heaves ☐4 ☐5 ☐6 Constant nausea, frequent dry heaves and vomiting ☐7
5. Tactile disturbances Have you any itching, pins and needles sensations, any burning, any numbness, or do you feel bugs crawling on or under your skin? None ☐0 Very mild itching, pins and needles, burning or numbness ☐1 Mild itching, pins and needles, burning or numbness ☐2 Moderate itching, pins and needles, burning or numbness ☐3 Moderately severe hallucinations ☐4 Severe hallucinations ☐5 Extremely severe hallucinations ☐6 Continuous hallucinations ☐7
6. Tremor *Arms extended and fingers spread apart.* No tremor ☐0 Not visible, but can be felt fingertip to fingertip ☐1 ☐2 ☐3 Moderate, with patient's arms extended ☐4 ☐5 ☐6 Severe, even with arms not extended ☐7

Figure 5–1.   Addiction Research Foundation Clinical Institute Withdrawal Assessment for Alcohol (CIWA-Ar).
Source.   From Sullivan et al. 1989.

7. Auditory disturbances
Are you more aware of sounds around you? Are they harsh? Do they frighten you? Are you hearing anything that is disturbing to you? Are you hearing things you know are not there?

Not present ☐ 0
Very mild harshness or ability to frighten ☐ 1
Mild harshness or ability to frighten ☐ 2
Moderate harshness or ability to frighten ☐ 3
Moderately severe hallucinations ☐ 4
Severe hallucinations ☐ 5
Extremely severe hallucinations ☐ 6
Continuous hallucinations ☐ 7

8. Paroxysmal sweats

No sweat visible ☐ 0
Barely perceptible sweating, palms moist ☐ 1
☐ 2
☐ 3
Beads of sweat obvious on forehead ☐ 4
☐ 5
☐ 6
Drenching sweats ☐ 7

9. Visual disturbances
Does the light appear to be too bright? Is its color different? Does it hurt your eyes? Are you seeing anything that is disturbing to you? Are you seeing things you know are not there?

Not present ☐ 0
Very mild sensitivity ☐ 1
Mild sensitivity ☐ 2
Moderate sensitivity ☐ 3
Moderately severe hallucinations ☐ 4
Severe hallucinations ☐ 5
Extremely severe hallucinations ☐ 6
Continuous hallucinations ☐ 7

10. Anxiety
Do you feel nervous?

No anxiety, at ease ☐ 0
Mild anxious ☐ 1
☐ 2
☐ 3
Moderately anxious, or guarded, so anxiety is inferred ☐ 4
☐ 5
☐ 6
Equivalent to acute panic states as seen in severe delirium or acute schizophrenic reactions ☐ 7

Figure 5–1. Addiction Research Foundation Clinical Institute Withdrawal Assessment for Alcohol (CIWA-Ar). *(continued)*

---

11. Headache, fullness in head
Does your head feel different? Does it feel like there is a band around your head?
Do not rate for dizziness or lightheadedness. Otherwise, rate severity.

Not present ☐ 0
Very mild ☐ 1
Mild ☐ 2
Moderate ☐ 3
Moderately severe ☐ 4
Severe ☐ 5
Very severe ☐ 6
Extremely severe ☐ 7

12. Agitation

Normal activity ☐ 0
Somewhat more than normal activity ☐ 1
☐ 2
☐ 3
Moderately fidgety and restless ☐ 4
☐ 5
☐ 6
Paces back and forth during most of the interview or constantly thrashes about ☐ 7

13. Orientation and clouding of sensorium
What day is this? Where are you? Who am I?

Oriented and can do serial additions ☐ 0
Cannot do serial additions or is uncertain about date ☐ 1
Disoriented for date by no more than 2 calendar days ☐ 2
Disoriented for date by more than 2 calendar days ☐ 3
Disoriented for place/or person ☐ 4

14. Total score: __ __
Maximum possible score=67
Patients scoring less than 10 do not usually need additional medication for withdrawal.

Figure 5–1. Addiction Research Foundation Clinical Institute Withdrawal Assessment for Alcohol (CIWA-Ar). *(continued)*

Alcohol Withdrawal Protocol

Although seen less commonly than in adult patients, consultants will encounter adolescents with signs and symptoms of alcohol withdrawal. Signs of early withdrawal may be detected during the first day, peaking at 24–48 hours and lasting 5–7 days. Treatment involves abstinence from alcohol, adequate nutrition, potential use of restraints, maintenance of the correct fluid and electrolyte balance, and careful monitoring of vital signs. Thiamine, folate, and multivitamins are routinely given with the addition of vitamin K if the international normalized ratio (INR) is greater than 1.3.

Pharmacological management of alcohol withdrawal involves the use of long-acting benzodiazepines, which result in reduced severity of withdrawal, incidence of delirium, and incidence of seizures (Mayo-Smith 1997). In practice, diazepam or chlordiazepoxide are the most widely used benzodiazepines, although it may be necessary to add haloperidol for severe agitation. The patient is given a loading dose of benzodiazepines to achieve a reduction in the vital signs, although dosing is stopped if the patient becomes somnolent or difficult to rouse or has signs of respiratory depression with a respiratory rate of less than 10 per minute. The Clinical Institute Withdrawal Assessment for Alcohol, revised by Sullivan et al. (1989) can used to assess the severity of withdrawal and guide the assessment protocol (Figure 5–1). Patients with a score of less than 10 can be treated with nonpharmacological therapy. If the score is 8–15 and there are moderate symptoms, the patient may benefit from medications. If the score is greater than 15, the patient will definitely require benzodiazepines for control of his or her symptoms (Liptzin 2000). In patients with hepatic insufficiency, benzodiazepines that are metabolized by glucuronidation, such as lorazepam or oxazepam, may be preferred.

References

American Psychiatric Association: Diagnostic and Statistical Manual of Mental Disorders, 4th Edition, Text Revision. Washington, DC, American Psychiatric Association, 2000

Beliles KE: Alternative routes of administration of psychotropic medications, in Psychiatric Care of the Medical Patient, 2nd Edition. Edited by Stoudemire A, Fogel BS, Greenberg DB. Oxford, England, Oxford University Press, 2000, pp 395–405

Breitbart W, Marotta R, Platt MM, et al: A double-blind trial of haloperidol, chlorpromazine, and lorazepam in the treatment of delirium in hospitalized AIDS patients. Am J Psychiatry 153:231–237, 1996

Brown RL, Henke A, Greenhalgh et al: The use of haloperidol in the agitated, critically ill pediatric patient with burns. J Burn Care Rehabil 17:34–8, 1996

Folstein MF, Folstein SE, McHugh PR: "Mini-mental state." A practical method for grading the cognitive state of patients for the clinician. J Psychiatr Res 12:189–198, 1975

Han C-S, Kim Y-K: A double-blind trial of risperidone and haloperidol for the treatment of delirium. Psychosomatics 45:297–301, 2004

Hunt N, Stern TA: The association between intravenous haloperidol and torsades de pointes. Psychosomatics 36:541–549, 1995

Kane FJ Jr, Remmel R, Moody S: Recognizing and treating delirium in patients admitted to general hospitals. South Med J 86:985–988, 1993

Liptzin B: Clinical diagnosis and management of delirium, in Psychiatric Care of the Medical Patient, 2nd Edition. Edited by Stoudemire A, Fogel BS, Greenberg DB. Oxford, England, Oxford University Press, 2000, pp 581–596

Liptzin B, Levkoff SE: An empirical study of delirium subtypes. Br J Psychiatry 161:843–845, 1992

Maldonado JR, Dhami N, Wise L: Clinical implication of the recognition and management of delirium in general medical wards. Psychosomatics 22:157–158, 2003

Marcantonio ER, Goldman L, Mangione CM, et al: A clinical prediction rule for delirium after elective noncardiac surgery. JAMA 271:134–139, 1994

Martini DR, Mazurek AJ, Przybylo HJ, et al: Postoperative delirium in children following administration of inhalation anesthetics. Psychosomatics 43:144–145, 2002

Mayo-Smith MF: Pharmacological management of alcohol withdrawal: the meta-analysis and evidence-based practice guidelines. JAMA 278:144–151, 1997

Menza MA, Murray GB, Holmes VF, et al: Decreased extrapyramidal symptoms with intravenous haloperidol. J Clin Psychiatry 48:278–280, 1987

Morita T, Tei Y, Tsunoda J, et al: Underlying pathologies and their associations with clinical features in terminal delirium of cancer patients. J Pain Symptom Manage 22:997–1006, 2001

Pro JD, Wells CE: The use of the electroencephalogram in the diagnosis of delirium. Dis Nerv Syst 38:804–808, 1977

Prugh DC, Wagonfield, Metcalf D, et al: A clinical study of delirium in children and adolescents. Psychosom Med 42 (suppl 1):177–195, 1980

Sikich N, Lerman J: Development and psychometric evaluation of Pediatric Anesthesia Emergence Delirium Scale. Anesthesiology 100:1138–1145, 2004

Sipahimalani A, Masand PS: Use of risperidone in the delirium: case reports. Ann Clin Psychiatry 9:105–107, 1997

Sipahimalani A, Masand PS: Olanzapine in the treatment of delirium. Psychosomatics 39:422–430, 1998

Sullivan JT, Sykora K, Schneiderman J, et al: Assessment of alcohol withdrawal: the revised Clinical Institute Withdrawal Assessment for Alcohol Scale (CIWA-Ar). Br J Addict 84:1353–1357, 1989

Trzepacz PT, Baker RW, Greenhouse J: A symptom rating scale for delirium. Psychiatry Res 23:89–97, 1988a

Trzepacz PT, Brenner R, Coffman G, et al: Delirium in liver transplantation candidates: discriminate analysis of multiple test variables. Biol Psychiatry 24:3–14, 1988b

Trzepacz PT, Mittal D, Torres R, et al: Validation of the Delirium Rating Scale-Revised-98: comparison with the Delirium Rating Scale and the Cognitive Test for Delirium. J Neuropsychiatry Clin Neurosci 13:229–242, 2001

Turkel SB, Tavaré CJ: Delirium in children and adolescents. J Neuropsychiatry Clin Neurosci 15:431–435, 2003

Turkel SB, Braslow K, Tavaré CJ, et al: The Delirium Rating Scale in children and adolescents. Psychosomatics 44:126–129, 2003

Turkel SB, Trzepacz PT, Tavare J: Comparison of delirium symptoms across the life cycle. Psychosomatics 45:162, 2004

Williams DT: Neuropsychiatric signs, symptoms, and syndromes, in Child and Adolescent Psychiatry: A Comprehensive Textbook, 3rd Edition. Edited by Lewis M. Philadelphia, PA, Lippincott Williams & Wilkins, 2002, pp 399–404

Wise MG, Brandt G: Delirium, in American Psychiatry Press Textbook of Neuropsychiatry, 2nd Edition. Edited by Hales RE, Yudofsky SC. Washington DC, American Psychiatric Press, 1992, pp   –

Wise MG, Trzepacz PT: Delirium (confusional states), in Textbook of Consultation-Liaison Psychiatry. Edited by Rundell JR, Wise MG. Washington, DC, American Psychiatric Press, 1996, pp 258–275

Zimnitzky B, DeMaso DR, Steingard RJ: Use of risperidone in psychotic disorder following ischemic brain damage. J Child Adolesc Psychopharmacol 6:75–78, 1996

6

Mood Disorders

Mood disorders are a critical health care problem affecting individuals across the life span. Approximately 20% of children and adolescents will experience the onset of a depressive episode before the age of 18 years (Lewisohn et al. 1993). Mood disorders not only place individuals at risk for suicide but often result in poor academic performance, impairments in social functioning, and an increased risk of substance abuse that persists into adulthood. Children and adolescents with medical illnesses have rates of depression nearly double those seen in the community, along with adverse medical outcomes and decreased quality of life (McDaniel et al. 2000). When compared with community samples, estimates of the prevalence of major depression in physically ill patients range from 0% to 54%, depending on the population sample and the methodology used. The pediatric patient who presents with a depressive episode will generally fall into one of the following categories: 1) a primary mood disorder; 2) mood disorder as a psychological reaction to medical illness (adjustment disorder or situational depression syndrome); or 3) mood disorder secondary to an organic etiology (Waller and Rush 1983). Although these categories often overlap, this framework provides the psychiatric consultant with a pragmatic approach to the diagnosis of depression in physically ill children (Figure 6–1).

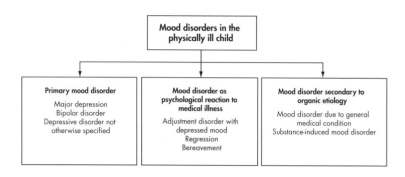

Figure 6–1. Classification of mood disorders in the physically ill child.

Definition

Major Depressive Episode

DSM-IV-TR (American Psychiatric Association 2000) diagnostic criteria for major depressive episode are given in Table 6–1. Five out of nine specific symptoms in a 2-week period are required, including persistent depressed mood or pervasive anhedonia.

Manic Episode

DSM-IV-TR manic episodes are characterized as a distinct period lasting at least 1 week, during which there is abnormally and persistently elevated, expansive, or irritable mood (Table 6–2). Hypomania is a manic episode in which the disturbance is not severe enough to cause marked impairment in social or occupational functioning or to require hospitalization and in which there are no psychotic symptoms. Manic episodes may be part of a primary bipolar disorder, but also secondary to a medical or toxic etiology. *Secondary mania* is the term sometimes given to manic or hypomanic episodes that are secondary to a medical condition or are induced by exposure to medications or toxic factors.

Table 6–1. DSM-IV-TR diagnostic criteria for major depressive episode

A. Five (or more) of the following symptoms have been present during the same 2-week period and represent a change from previous functioning; at least one of the symptoms is either (1) depressed mood or (2) loss of interest or pleasure.

Note: Do not include symptoms that are clearly due to a general medical condition, or mood-incongruent delusions or hallucinations.

(1) depressed mood most of the day, nearly every day, as indicated by either subjective report (e.g., feels sad or empty) or observation made by others (e.g., appears tearful). Note: In children and adolescents, can be irritable mood.

(2) markedly diminished interest or pleasure in all, or almost all, activities most of the day, nearly every day (as indicated by either subjective account or observation made by others)

(3) significant weight loss when not dieting or weight gain (e.g., a change of more than 5% of body weight in a month), or decrease or increase in appetite nearly every day. Note: In children, consider failure to make expected weight gains.

(4) insomnia or hypersomnia nearly every day

(5) psychomotor agitation or retardation nearly every day (observable by others, not merely subjective feelings of restlessness or being slowed down)

(6) fatigue or loss of energy nearly every day

(7) feelings of worthlessness or excessive or inappropriate guilt (which may be delusional) nearly every day (not merely self-reproach or guilt about being sick)

(8) diminished ability to think or concentrate, or indecisiveness, nearly every day (either by subjective account or as observed by others)

(9) recurrent thoughts of death (not just fear of dying), recurrent suicidal ideation without a specific plan, or a suicide attempt or a specific plan for committing suicide

B. The symptoms do not meet criteria for a mixed episode.

C. The symptoms cause clinically significant distress or impairment in social, occupational, or other important areas of functioning.

D. The symptoms are not due to the direct physiological effects of a substance (e.g., a drug of abuse, a medication) or a general medical condition (e.g., hypothyroidism).

E. The symptoms are not better accounted for by bereavement, i.e., after the loss of a loved one, the symptoms persist for longer than 2 months or are characterized by marked functional impairment, morbid preoccupation with worthlessness, suicidal ideation, psychotic symptoms, or psychomotor retardation.

Source. Reprinted from *Diagnostic and Statistical Manual of Mental Disorders,* 4th Edition, Text Revision. Washington, DC, American Psychiatric Association, 2000. Used with permission.

Diagnosis of Depression in the Physically Ill

Although depression is common in the physically ill patient, it is frequently underdiagnosed. Some studies suggest that pediatricians identify less than 20% of children who have mental health issues (Wells et al. 2001). A variety of interrelated reasons likely underlie the missed diagnosis of depression in physically ill patients. For example, children and adolescents are more likely to present with irritability or somatic complaints rather than classic complaints of sadness. In the medical setting, patients and their families are also more likely to emphasize somatic complaints rather than mood or cognitive symptoms. In addition, pediatricians tend to focus on physical signs and symptoms and may be reluctant to stigmatize patients with a psychiatric diagnosis. One commonly held belief is that depression is an understandable reaction to the stress of a physical illness and therefore does not warrant treatment. In addition, many of the neurovegetative symptoms used to diagnose depression such as insomnia, fatigue, weight loss, and change in appetite can also be secondary effects of the illness or treatment (Table 6–3). Nevertheless, concern about depression in the physically ill child or adolescent remains one of the most frequent reasons for psychiatric consultation.

Clinical Considerations in the Physically Ill Child

The following clinical considerations are important in approaching the assessment and management of depressive disorders in the medical setting.

Depression as a Continuum

In the medical setting the term *depression* is used with different meanings. It may refer to an array of clinical conditions ranging from a transient mood change requiring no treatment to a severe clinical disorder associated with thoughts of death that requires psychiatric hospitalization (Beasley and Beardslee 1998). Mental health classification systems have been of limited value to pediatricians in describing this range of behavioral and emotional symptoms because of their focus on severe pathology. To address this issue, *The Classification of Child and Adolescent Mental Diagnoses in Primary Care, Child and Adolescent Version* has been introduced to provide a system to identify and classify emotional disorders ranging on a continuum from "developmental variation" to "problem" to "disorder" (Wolraich et al. 1996).

Table 6–2. DSM-IV-TR diagnostic criteria for manic episode

A. A distinct period of abnormally and persistently elevated, expansive, or irritable mood, lasting at least 1 week (or any duration if hospitalization is necessary).

B. During the period of mood disturbance, three (or more) of the following symptoms have persisted (four if the mood is only irritable) and have been present to a significant degree:
   (1) inflated self-esteem or grandiosity
   (2) decreased need for sleep (e.g., feels rested after only 3 hours of sleep)
   (3) more talkative than usual or pressure to keep talking
   (4) flight of ideas or subjective experience that thoughts are racing
   (5) distractibility (i.e., attention too easily drawn to unimportant or irrelevant external stimuli)
   (6) increase in goal-directed activity (either socially, at work or school, or sexually) or psychomotor agitation
   (7) excessive involvement in pleasurable activities that have a high potential for painful consequences (e.g., engaging in unrestrained buying sprees, sexual indiscretions, or foolish business investments)

C. The symptoms do not meet criteria for a mixed episode.

D. The mood disturbance is sufficiently severe to cause marked impairment in occupational functioning or in usual social activities or relationships with others, or to necessitate hospitalization to prevent harm to self or others, or there are psychotic features.

E. The symptoms are not due to the direct physiological effects of a substance (e.g., a drug of abuse, a medication, or other treatment) or a general medical condition (e.g., hyperthyroidism).

Note: Manic-like episodes that are clearly caused by somatic antidepressant treatment (e.g., medication, electroconvulsive therapy, light therapy) should not count toward a diagnosis of bipolar I disorder.

Source. Reprinted from *Diagnostic and Statistical Manual of Mental Disorders,* 4th Edition, Text Revision. Washington, DC, American Psychiatric Association, 2000. Used with permission.

Depression and Physical Symptom Perception

Patients with symptoms of depression have more medically unexplained symptoms even when controlling for the severity of their medical illness (Katon et al. 2001). Patients with comorbid depressive and physical medical illnesses have a heightened awareness and tendency to focus on the physical symptoms of their illness as well as other organ symptoms (Walker et al. 1996). Common physical symptoms in depression include joint pain, limb pain, back pain, gastrointestinal problems, fatigue, weakness, and appetite changes. Chronic abdominal pain and headaches are particularly common

Table 6–3. Overlap between DSM-IV-TR symptoms of depression and physical illness symptoms and treatment

DSM-IV-TR diagnostic item	Physical illness confound	
Weight loss Decreased appetite	Cancer chemotherapy agents Chronic disease Cancer Cystic fibrosis Diabetes mellitus Inflammatory bowel disease Renal failure	Infection (e.g., HIV, tuberculosis) Malabsorption Vitamin deficiency
Weight gain Increased appetite	Anticonvulsant medications Antihistaminergic medications Corticosteroids Cushing's disease Hypogonadism	Hypothalamic lesions Hypothyroidism Insulinoma Polycystic ovary disease
Insomnia	Alcohol Asthma Caffeine Corticosteroids Duodenal ulcers Hyperthyroidism	Nocturia Pain Psychostimulant medications Restless legs syndrome Sleep apnea Sympathomimetic amines
Hypersomnia	Brain tumors Diabetic ketoacidosis Encephalitis Hypercapnia Hypothyroidism	Liver failure Opiates Sleep apnea (daytime hypersomnia) Uremia
Fatigue/Loss of energy	Addison's disease Anemia Anticonvulsant medications Chronic disease Endocarditis Guillain-Barré syndrome Heart failure Hepatitis Mononucleosis	Motor neuron disease Multiple sclerosis Muscular dystrophy Narcolepsy Poliomyelitis Rheumatoid arthritis Tumors Uremia Vitamin B_{12} deficiency

Table 6–3.   Overlap between DSM-IV-TR symptoms of depression and physical illness symptoms and treatment *(continued)*

DSM-IV-TR diagnostic item	Physical illness confound	
Difficulty with thinking/ concentration	Cirrhosis Dementia Huntington's disease Lead poisoning	Marijuana Metachromatic leukodystrophy Opiates
Loss of interest in sex	Cirrhosis Hemochromatosis	Hormonal disorder Substance abuse
Psychomotor agitation	Hypercalcemia Psychostimulant medications Reye's syndrome	Substance withdrawal or abuse Wernicke-Korsakoff syndrome

manifestations of depression in children, but other physical symptoms include diarrhea, insomnia, and nervousness.

Depression may go undiagnosed in patients seen in the primary care setting because the physical symptoms associated with depression may be interpreted as symptoms of a physical illness. These patients frequently deny having any emotional disturbance and may resist referrals to a psychiatrist or treatment with psychiatric medications. The term *alexithymia* has been used to describe patients with a tendency toward somatization and who have a reduced ability to express psychological distress directly. However, patients with a high number of physical symptoms are more likely to have a mood disorder. For example, a study of adult patients in primary care showed that the presence of any physical symptom doubled the likelihood that the patient had a mood disorder (Kroenke et al. 1994). Finally, it is important to consider that physical symptoms, in particular complaints of pain, tend to increase the duration of the patient's depressed mood. Treatment that does not address pain and other physical symptoms is likely to be associated with incomplete response to the treatment of their depression. By contrast, improvement in physical symptoms is correlated with improvement in symptoms of depression.

Depression and Functional Impairment

Studies of physically ill adult patients have suggested a strong relationship between depression and functional impairment. Depressed patients tend to have a poor perception of their physical health and more impairment in their social and academic functioning. For example, symptoms of depression and anxiety at the initial diagnosis of coronary artery disease have been shown to be more highly correlated with functional impairment at both 1- and 5-year follow-up than any physiological measure (Sullivan et al. 1997). In fact, the presence of depression may be more predictive of functional impairment over time than severity of physical illness. By contrast, as symptoms of depression improve, so do measures of functional impairment (Ormel et al. 1993).

Depression and Health Care Behaviors

The presence of a mood disorder may have economic implications. Children with internalizing symptoms such as depression and anxiety have been shown to have higher rates of health care utilization and higher health care costs (Bernal et al. 2000; Haaralsilta 2003). Katon (2003) has also shown that depression is associated with an approximately 50% increase in medical costs of chronic medical illness, even after controlling for severity of physical illness. Major depression has been associated with higher rates of adverse health-risk behaviors, including overeating, smoking, and a sedentary lifestyle (Goodman and Whitaker 2002). Depression and anxiety are risk factors for adolescent smoking and obesity in early adulthood. Mood disorders may affect the patient's motivation as well as adherence with the medical treatment. For example, depressed patients with diabetes mellitus have decreased adherence to the prescribed diet as well as poorer diabetic control (Ciechanowski et al. 2000).

Morbidity and Mortality

Depression and medical illness occurring together have a worse prognosis than when they occur in isolation. The presence of depression is associated with higher morbidity and mortality rates in adult patients with medical illnesses such as cancer, renal failure, and coronary artery disease. Studies of adult patients have shown that those who develop symptoms of depression after myocardial infarction are at significantly greater risk of death than those who are not depressed (Glassman and Shapiro 1998). Death rates are also increased in patients with diagnoses of stroke and those on renal dialysis. Patients with medical illnesses are at greater risk of relapse in their symptoms of depression. In a study of adults, Lustman et al. (1997) reported a 5-year depression recurrence rate of 92% in patients with comorbid depression and diabetes mellitus. In addition, the risk of suicide is greatly increased in physically ill patients, particularly adults with diagnoses of cancer or HIV and those on renal dialysis. Chronic pain in particular may be a risk factor for suicide.

Primary Mood Disorder

Patients with primary depression meet the full DSM-IV-TR criteria for major depressive episode (Table 6–1). They are more likely to have suicidal thoughts, feelings of helplessness, dysphoria, guilt, distractibility, and discouragement than patients experiencing mood symptoms directly related to or in reaction to their physical condition. The neurovegetative symptoms of depression may be less descriptive of depression in children because many medical conditions and treatment side effects are accompanied by lethargy, decreased appetite, and sleep difficulties. One factor that may help with the differential diagnosis is the past psychiatric history. Patients with a previous history of depressive episodes are more likely to have an underlying psychiatric disorder. By contrast, only 20% of patients with mood disorder due to a general medical condition are likely to have a past history of depression (Yates et al. 1991).

Mood Disorder as Reaction to Medical Illness

Adjustment Disorder

The stress of having a medical illness and receiving treatment may trigger feelings of helplessness and result in symptoms of depression, particularly in the early phases after the diagnosis. This dysphoric mood is a reactive or situational response to an aversive event. It tends to be milder in form and responsive to distraction. It is sometimes difficult to differentiate between depressed mood as an adjustment to the medical illness and the clinical syndrome of major depression. The essential feature of an adjustment disorder with depressed mood is the presence of symptoms of depression that do not meet criteria for major depression but are associated with an impairment in social or occupational functioning (Table 6–4). The DSM-IV-TR diagnostic criteria specifically exclude the diagnosis of adjustment disorders when a diagnosis of bereavement is present. Adjustment disorders differ from normal grief and demoralization based on the severity of impairment. Hinshaw et al. (2002) reported that only 5%–15% of adult patients with cancer met criteria for ma-

Table 6–4. DSM-IV-TR diagnostic criteria for adjustment disorder

A. The development of emotional or behavioral symptoms in response to an identifiable stressor(s) occurring within 3 months of the onset of the stressor(s).

B. These symptoms or behaviors are clinically significant as evidenced by either of the following:

  1) marked distress that is in excess of what would be expected from exposure to the stressor

  (2) significant impairment in social or occupational (academic) functioning

C. The stress-related disturbance does not meet the criteria for another specific Axis I disorder and is not merely an exacerbation of a preexisting Axis I or Axis II disorder.

D. The symptoms do not represent bereavement.

E. Once the stressor (or its consequences) has terminated, the symptoms do not persist for more than an additional 6 months.

Specify if:

  Acute: if the disturbance lasts less than 6 months

  Chronic: if the disturbance lasts for 6 months or longer

Adjustment disorders are coded based on the subtype, which is selected according to the predominant symptoms. The specific stressor(s) can be specified on Axis IV.

  309.0 With depressed mood

  309.24 With anxiety

  309.28 With mixed anxiety and depressed mood

  309.3 With disturbance of conduct

  309.4 With mixed disturbance of emotions and conduct

  309.9 Unspecified

Source. Reprinted from *Diagnostic and Statistical Manual of Mental Disorders,* 4th Edition, Text Revision. Washington, DC, American Psychiatric Association, 2000. Used with permission.

jor depression. Adjustment disorder with depressed mood, by contrast, is frequently seen at some point during the treatment of a patient with serious medical illness. For example, estimates of adjustment problems range from 36% to 60% in children with diabetes mellitus (LeBlanc et al. 2003).

Regression

Another issue to consider in the evaluation of the child with depression is the possibility that the stress of the illness has led to a behavioral regression. Pediatric patients commonly regress in the hospital in the face of overwhelming stress. It is common for children and adolescents to display types of emotional and behavior responses that are more commonly seen in younger children. Regressed behavior in a child or adolescent may manifest in several ways, including clinginess, social withdrawal, and tearfulness, and may mimic symptoms of depression. Symptoms of regressed behavior are particularly common during the inpatient phases of a child's treatment and generally resolve spontaneously when the stress of the illness or hospitalization is over.

Bereavement

Finally, it is important to differentiate major depression from depression that occurs as part of the normal bereavement process in children with a life-threatening illness (Table 6–5). Children in the terminal stages of their illness frequently cycle in and out of symptoms of depression, anger, anxiety, and fear. Feelings of sadness tend to be intermittent and often do not meet criteria for a major depression. Fleeting thoughts of suicide also are not uncommon in terminally ill patients. It is important for both the parents and the medical team to be able to tolerate the child's sadness and accept these feelings as part of the normal mourning process in the terminally ill child. It is not uncommon for the medical team to call in the psychiatric consultant in the terminal stages of the child's illness with a request for antidepressant medication, motivated by feelings of helplessness on the part of the staff. In these cases, it is important to help the child, the family, and the medical team work through their feelings of loss and to interpret the symptoms of depression as a normal and important part of the grieving process.

Mood Disorder Due to a General Medical Condition

DSM-IV-TR specifies criteria for the diagnosis of the mood disorder due to a medical condition (Table 6–6). The mood disturbance may involve depressed mood, elevated mood, or irritability. This diagnostic category is used when it is believed that the mood disorder is secondary to an underlying medical disorder. DSM-IV-TR does not list specific symptoms of depression that are needed to make this diagnosis.

Table 6–5. Comparison of grief with major depression in terminally ill patients

Characteristic of grief	Characteristic of depression
Patients experience feelings, emotions, and behaviors that result from a particular loss.	Patients experience feelings, emotions, and behaviors that fulfill criteria for major depression that is generalized in all facets of life.
Almost all terminally ill patients experience grief, but only a minority develop a mood disorder requiring treatment.	Major depression occurs in 1%–53% of terminally ill patients.
Patients usually cope with distress on their own.	Medical or psychiatric intervention is usually necessary.
Patients experience somatic distress, loss of usual patterns of behavior, agitation, sleep and appetite disturbances, decreased concentration, and social withdrawal.	Patients experience similar symptoms, plus hopelessness, helplessness, worthlessness, guilt, and suicidal ideation.
Grief is associated with disease progression.	Depression has increased prevalence in patients with advanced disease; pain is a major risk factor.
Patients retain the capacity for pleasure.	Patients enjoy nothing.
Grief comes in waves.	Depression is constant and unremitting.
Patients expresses passive wishes for death to come quickly.	Patients express intense and persistent suicidal ideation.
Patients are able to look forward to the future.	Patients have no sense of a positive future.

Source. Reprinted from Block S: "Assessing and Managing Depression in the Terminally Ill Patient." *Annals of Internal Medicine* 132:209–218, 2000. Copyright 2000, American College of Physicians. Used with permission.

Depressive Episodes

Depression may be one of the first symptoms of medical illnesses, such as pancreatic carcinoma, in which psychiatric symptoms may precede physical symptoms by as long as 3–4 years (Fras et al. 1967) (Table 6–7). Depression is also seen in patients with Cushing's disease, Addison's disease, hyperthyroidism, and hypothyroidism. Rundell and Wise (1989) reported that 3.5%

Table 6–6. DSM-IV-TR diagnostic criteria for mood disorder due to a general medical condition

A. A prominent and persistent disturbance in mood predominates in the clinical picture and is characterized by either (or both) of the following:
    (1) depressed mood or markedly diminished interest or pleasure in all, or almost all, activities
    (2) elevated, expansive, or irritable mood
B. There is evidence from the history, physical examination, or laboratory findings that the disturbance is the direct physiological consequence of a general medical condition.
C. The disturbance is not better accounted for by another mental disorder (e.g., adjustment disorder with depressed mood in response to the stress of having a general medical condition).
D. The disturbance does not occur exclusively during the course of a delirium.
E. The symptoms cause clinically significant distress or impairment in social, occupational, or other important areas of functioning.

Specify type:

With depressive features: if the predominant mood is depressed but the full criteria are not met for a major depressive episode
With major depressive–like episode: if the full criteria are met (except Criterion D) for a major depressive episode
With manic features: if the predominant mood is elevated, euphoric, or irritable
With mixed features: if the symptoms of both mania and depression are present but neither predominates
Coding note: Include the name of the general medical condition on Axis I, e.g., 293.83 mood disorder due to hypothyroidism, with depressive features; also code the general medical condition on Axis III (see Appendix G for codes).
Coding note: If depressive symptoms occur as part of a preexisting vascular dementia, indicate the depressive symptoms by coding the appropriate subtype, i.e., 290.43 vascular dementia, with depressed mood.

Source. Reprinted from *Diagnostic and Statistical Manual of Mental Disorders,* 4th Edition, Text Revision. Washington, DC, American Psychiatric Association, 2000. Used with permission.

of 775 consecutive psychiatric consultations met criteria for an organic mood disorder, representing one-third of all patients diagnosed with depression. Findings that suggest an underlying medical etiology include an atypical clinical picture, resistance to conventional treatment modalities, and unexplained personality changes (Goldman 1992). The patient's mood is often more flat or malaise-like in quality and has a temporal relationship to the physical con-

Table 6–7.   Physical illnesses etiologically related to episodes of depression and mania

Illness	Depressive episode	Manic episode
Neurological disorders		
Epilepsy	+	+
Huntington's disease	+	+
Multiple sclerosis	+	+
Postconcussion	+	+
Stroke	+	+
Parkinson's disease	+	+
Wilson's disease	+	+
Sleep apnea	+	–
Subarachnoid hemorrhage	+	–
Posttraumatic encephalopathy	–	+
Idiopathic calcification of basal ganglia	–	+
Endocrine disorders		
Cushing's syndrome	+	+
Hyperthyroidism	+	+
Hypothyroidism	+	+
Addison's disease	+	–
Hyperparathyroidism	+	–
Hypoparathyroidism	+	–
Infectious diseases		
AIDS	+	+
Encephalitis	+	+
Infectious mononucleosis	+	+
Influenza	+	+
Syphilis	+	+
Hepatitis	+	–
Pneumonia	+	–
Subacute bacterial endocarditis	+	–
Tuberculosis	+	–
Post-St. Louis type A encephalitis	–	+

Table 6–7. Physical illnesses etiologically related to episodes of depression and mania *(continued)*

Illness	Depressive episode	Manic episode
Viral meningoencephalitis	-	+
Cryptococcal meningoencephalitis	-	+
Tumors		
Central nervous system	+	-
Lung	+	-
Pancreas	+	-
Gliomas	-	+
Meningiomas	-	+
Thalamic	-	+
Miscellaneous		
Anemia	+	+
Uremia	+	+
Hemodialysis	+	+
Hypokalemia	+	-
Hyperkalemia	+	-
Failure to thrive	+	-
Porphyria	+	-
Carcinoid	-	+
Klinefelter's syndrome	-	+
Kleine-Levin syndrome	-	+
Niacin deficiency	-	+
Postoperative excitement	-	+
Vitamin B_{12} deficiency	-	+

Source. Adapted from Wise and Rundell 1988.

dition as well as significant physical examination (e.g., weight loss) or study findings (e.g., increased creatinine). Central nervous system lesions involving the frontal, limbic, and temporal lobes are more frequently associated with mood disorders. Left-sided lesions are reported to be correlated with an increased risk for depression, in contrast to right-sided lesions that are more likely to be associated with mania (Cummings 1986).

Table 6–8.   DSM-IV-TR diagnostic criteria for substance-induced mood disorder

A. A prominent and persistent disturbance in mood predominates in the clinical picture and is characterized by either (or both) of the following:

  (1) depressed mood or markedly diminished interest or pleasure in all, or almost all, activities

  (2) elevated, expansive, or irritable mood

B. There is evidence from the history, physical examination, or laboratory findings of either (1) or (2):

  (1) the symptoms in Criterion A developed during, or within a month of, substance intoxication or withdrawal

  (2) medication use is etiologically related to the disturbance

C. The disturbance is not better accounted for by a mood disorder that is not substance induced. Evidence that the symptoms are better accounted for by a mood disorder that is not substance induced might include the following: the symptoms precede the onset of the substance use (or medication use); the symptoms persist for a substantial period of time (e.g., about a month) after the cessation of acute withdrawal or severe intoxication or are substantially in excess of what would be expected given the type or amount of the substance used or the duration of use; or there is other evidence that suggests the existence of an independent non-substance-induced mood disorder (e.g., a history of recurrent major depressive episodes).

D. The disturbance does not occur exclusively during the course of a delirium.

E. The symptoms cause clinically significant distress or impairment in social, occupational, or other important areas of functioning.

Note: This diagnosis should be made instead of a diagnosis of substance intoxication or substance withdrawal only when the mood symptoms are in excess of those usually associated with the intoxication or withdrawal syndrome and when the symptoms are sufficiently severe to warrant independent clinical attention.

Code [Specific substance]–induced mood disorder:

  (291.89 Alcohol; 292.84 Amphetamine [or amphetamine-like substance]; 292.84 cocaine; 292.84 hallucinogen; 292.84 inhalant; 292.84 opioid; 292.84 phencyclidine [or phencyclidine-like substance]; 292.84 sedative, hypnotic, or anxiolytic; 292.84 other [or unknown] substance)

Specify type:

  With depressive features: if the predominant mood is depressed

  With manic features: if the predominant mood is elevated, euphoric, or irritable

  With mixed features: if symptoms of both mania and depression are present and neither predominates

Table 6–8. DSM-IV-TR diagnostic criteria for substance-induced mood disorder *(continued)*

Specify if:

    With onset during intoxication: if the criteria are met for intoxication with the substance and the symptoms develop during the intoxication syndrome

    With onset during withdrawal: if criteria are met for withdrawal from the substance and the symptoms develop during, or shortly after, a withdrawal syndrome

Source. Reprinted from *Diagnostic and Statistical Manual of Mental Disorders*, 4th Edition, Text Revision. Washington, DC, American Psychiatric Association, 2000. Used with permission.

Manic Episodes

Patients with a genetic predisposition to bipolar disorder are more likely to develop manic episodes in response to medical illness or medications such as corticosteroids (Table 6–7). Patients with brain atrophy are also more prone to develop secondary mania (Starkstein et al. 1987). Sleep deprivation may also play a role in predisposing patients to manic episodes. It is not uncommon to find precipitants to manic episodes in the patient with a primary bipolar disorder; however, in cases of secondary mania, the precipitation of symptoms is more directly related to the underlying medical condition or its treatment. Secondary manic episodes usually respond quickly to treatment of the underlying precipitating factor.

Substance-Induced Mood Disorder

DSM-IV-TR specifies diagnostic criteria for substance-induced mood disorders that are more commonly seen in adult patients (Table 6–8). Depression is more likely in patients who abuse drugs and alcohol. Although lower doses of alcohol may enhance mood, long-term or heavy use of alcohol is more likely to be associated with depression. More than 50% of patients with severe alcohol abuse have symptoms of depression that may be indistinguishable from a primary mood disorder (Schuckit 1983). Most alcohol-induced depressions resolve within 2 days to 2 weeks with abstinence. Patients who are going through withdrawal from cocaine may have symptoms of depression, irritability, and anxiety that begin shortly after abstinence and may last up to 3 days.

Table 6–9.   Selected medications associated with depression and mania

Associated with depression	Associated with mania
Analgesics (narcotics)	Androgens (anabolic steroids)
Methadone	Bronchodilators
Oxycodone	Albuterol
Cancer chemotherapy agents	Terbutaline
Vincristine	Cardiovascular
Vinblastine	Captopril
Procarbazine	Clonidine withdrawal
L-Asparaginase	Methyldopa
Amphotericin B	Corticosteroids
Interferon	Cancer chemotherapy agents
Cardiovascular	Procarbazine
Atenolol	Decongestants
Methyldopa	Histamine-2 receptor antagonists
Nadolol	Cimetidine
Procainamide	Psychiatric medications
Propafenone	Alprazolam
Propranolol	Antidepressants
Corticosteroids	Buspirone
Prednisone	Lorazepam
Histamine-2 receptor antagonists	Methylphenidate
Cimetidine	Triazolam
Immunosuppressants	Miscellaneous
Cyclosporine	Amantadine
Tacrolimus	Baclofen
Interferon	Carbamazepine
Oral contraceptives	Cyclobenzaprine
	Cyproheptadine
	Metoclopramide
	Thyroid preparations
	Tolmetin
	Zidovudine

Although many medications are listed as potential causes of depression, in practice very few of these are likely to be significant factors in physically ill patients presenting with symptoms of depression (Table 6–9). There have been no known controlled prospective studies that show an association of any medication with a DSM-IV-TR diagnosis of a major depression. It is impor-

Table 6–10. Mnemonic for diagnostic criteria for major depressive episode

SIG: E CAPS ("Prescribe energy capsules")

Sleep—insomnia or hypersomnia

Interests—loss of interests or pleasure

Guilt—excessive guilt, worthlessness, hopelessness

Energy—loss of energy or fatigue

Concentration—diminished concentration ability, indecisiveness

Appetite—decreased appetite, more than 5% weight loss or gain

Psychomotor—psychomotor retardation or agitation

Suicidality—suicidal thought, ideation, plan, or attempt; includes thoughts of death or preoccupation with death

Source. Reprinted from Wise MG, Rundell JR: "Depression and Mania," in *Concise Guide to Consultation Psychiatry*, 2nd Edition. Washington, DC, American Psychiatric Press, 1994, pp 56. Copyright 1988, American Psychiatric Press, Inc. Used with permission.

tant to note whether there is a temporal relationship between the onset of depression and the medication in question or with changes in the dosage of the medication. Diagnosis may also be supported by the finding that reintroduction of the suspected medication leads to a recurrence of the depression.

Assessment

History and Physical Examination

The diagnosis of depression in the physically ill child begins with an assessment as outlined in Chapter 3. The evaluation should include an assessment for the presence of psychological and somatic symptoms consistent with a DSM-IV-TR depressive episode (Table 6–1). The SIG: E CAPS mnemonic may be used as a memory aid for major depressive episode (Table 6–10). It is critical to explore the family psychiatric history for any genetic vulnerability for mood disorders as well as to obtain thorough medical and substance use histories. Table 6–11 outlines a working model in the differential diagnosis of depression in the medical setting.

Table 6–11. Working model for distinguishing between primary depression, organic mood disorder, and mood disorder as psychological reaction to medical illness

	Primary mood disorder	Organic mood syndrome	Adjustment disorder
DSM-III criteria depressive episode	++	+	±
Preoccupation with worthlessness	++	+	-
Family history of depression	++	-	±
Previous depressive episodes	+	±	±
Mood more flat or malaise quality	+	++	-
Weight loss of 25% or more	+	++	-
Abnormal neurological signs or studies	-	++	-
On medications that cause depression	-	+	-
Environmental stresses evident	±	±	++
Mood brightens when distracted	±	±	++
Expect antidepressant response	++	-	-
Response to supportive psychotherapy	±	±	++
Behavioral intervention maybe helpful	±	±	++

Source. Reprinted from Waller DA, Rush AJ: "Differentiating Primary Affective Disease, Organic Affective Syndromes, and Situational Depression on a Pediatric Service." *Journal of the American Academy of Child Psychiatry* 22:52–58, 1983. Copyright 1983, Lippincott Williams & and Wilkins. Used with permission.

Diagnostic Investigations

Routine laboratory tests that should be performed include a complete blood count, blood chemistries, thyroid function tests, and urine analysis with toxicology screening. If underlying medical conditions are suspected, a chest X ray, electrocardiogram, and cortisol levels should be obtained. Arterial blood gas or oxygen saturation measurements may help rule out respiratory causes of fatigue and weakness. Central nervous system scans (e.g., computed tomography, magnetic resonance imaging) and electroencephalography as well as lumbar puncture may be helpful. Tables 6–12 and 6–13 provide overviews of diagnostic investigations to consider in evaluating depression and mania respectively.

Table 6–12. Evaluation of depression

Medical-psychiatric history
    Current medical symptoms
    Recent infections
    Use of prescribed medications
Vital signs
Mental status examination, with emphasis on mood, psychotic symptoms, and
  cognition
Laboratory evaluation
    Blood glucose
    Electrolytes
    Renal/Hepatic function tests
    Complete blood count
    Thyroid function tests
Electrocardiogram
Computed tomography/Magnetic resonance imaging scan
Lumbar puncture
Electroencephalogram

Treatment

The management of depression in the pediatric setting begins with a biopsychosocial formulation that is presented to the patient, family, and health care providers. It is critical to emphasize to the primary physician that the active treatment of any underlying or accompanying physical illness may help alleviate symptoms of depression. This includes aggressive management of pain and exploring possible diagnostic entities that may be contributing to the patient's dysphoria.

There are a number of nonpharmacological interventions that can be instituted. The first step is to mobilize the patient within the constraints of his or her physical illness. These include changes to the hospital environment (e.g., making the room more familiar with pictures as well as making sure drapes are open) or having the patient take part in the hospital's child life or activity program. The psychiatric consultant can also see the child in supportive psychotherapy. Parents can be educated about the impact of hospitalization on their child and their importance in this process. Principles of individual and family therapy are outlined in Chapters 13 and 14.

Table 6–13. Evaluation of mania

Medical-psychiatric history

    Current medical symptoms

    Recent infections

    Use of prescribed medications

        Antidepressants

        Corticosteroids

    Use of drugs of abuse

        Amphetamine

        Cocaine

        Hallucinogens

        Phencyclidine

    History of psychiatric disorders, especially mood disorders

    Family history of psychiatric disorders, especially mood disorders

    Vital signs

Physical examination, with attention to focal neurological deficits

    Nondominant hemisphere

        Anosognosia

        Constructional dyspraxia

        Babinski sign

        Hemiparesis

        Hyperactive tendon reflexes

        Left-sided neglect

    Frontal lobe

        Basal ganglia

        Athetosis

        Chorea

        Parkinsonism

Mental status examination, with emphasis on mood, psychotic symptoms, and cognition

Laboratory evaluation

    Blood alcohol

    Blood glucose

    Complete blood count

    Electrolytes

    Pregnancy test

    Renal/Hepatic function tests

    Serum calcium

Table 6–13. Evaluation of mania *(continued)*

Serum cortisol

Serum lithium, valproic acid, or carbamazepine levels (if applicable)

Serum thyroxine

Toxicology screening

Vitamin B_{12}

Electrocardiogram

Computed tomography/Magnetic resonance imaging scan

Lumbar puncture

Electroencephalogram

Pharmacotherapy becomes a consideration when there is insufficient response to the psychosocial interventions, daily functioning is significantly impaired, the depression is sufficiently severe to interfere with hospital treatment, or there is a history of previous depressive episodes, manic episodes, or psychosis (see Chapter 15). Although there is little information in the literature pertaining to pharmacological treatment of comorbid depression and physical illness, clinical experience suggests that the target symptoms of depression in physical illnesses may respond to pharmacotherapy. The psychiatric consultant will generally target depression with one of the selective serotonin reuptake inhibitor antidepressants. Anticipated potential drug interactions and potential side effects need to be reviewed. The use of a stimulant medication is another consideration in the physically ill child with symptoms of fatigue and malaise due to a general medical condition.

References

American Psychiatric Association: Diagnostic and Statistical Manual of Mental Disorders, 4th Edition, Text Revision. Washington, DC, American Psychiatric Association, 2000

Beasley PJ, Beardslee WR: Depression in the adolescent patient. Adolesc Med 9:351–362, 1998

Bernal P, Estroff DB, Aboudarham JF, et al: Psychosocial morbidity: the economic burden in a pediatric health maintenance organization sample. Arch Pediatr Adolesc Med 154:261–266, 2000

Ciechanowski PS, Katon WJ, Russo JE: Depression and diabetes: impact of depressive symptoms on adherence, function, and costs. Arch Intern Med 160:3278–3285, 2000

Cummings JL: Organic psychoses: delusional disorders and secondary mania. Psychiatr Clin North Am 9:293–311, 1986

Fras L, Litin EM, Pearson JS: Comparison of psychiatric symptoms in carcinoma of the pancreas with those in some other intra-abdominal neoplasms. Am J Psychiatry 123:1553–1561, 1967

Glassman AH, Shapiro PA: Depression and the course of coronary artery disease. Am J Psychiatry 155:4–11, 1998

Goldman MB: Neuropsychiatric features of endocrine disorders, in Textbook of Neuropsychiatry, 2nd Edition. Edited by Yudofsky SC, Hales RE. Washington, DC, American Psychiatric Press, 1992, pp 519–540

Goodman E, Whitaker R: A prospective study of the role of depression in the development and persistence of adult obesity. Pediatrics 110:497–504, 2002

Haaralsilta L: Major depressive episode and health care use among adolescents and young adults. Soc Psychiatry Psychiatr Epidemiol 38:366–372, 2003

Hinshaw DB, Carnahan JM, Johnson DL: Depression, anxiety, and asthenia in advanced illness. J Am Coll Surg 195:271–277, 2002

Katon WJ: Clinical and health service relationships between major depression, depressive symptoms, and general medical illness. Biol Psychiatry 54:216–226, 2003

Katon W, Sullivan M, Walker E: Medical symptoms without identified pathology: relationship to psychiatric disorders, childhood and adult trauma, and personality traits. Ann Intern Med 134:917–925, 2001

Kroenke K, Spitzer RL, Williams JB, et al: Physical symptoms in primary care: predictors of psychiatric disorders and functional impairment. Arch Fam Med 3:774–779, 1994

LeBlanc LA, Goldsmith T, Patel DR: Behavioral aspects of chronic illness in children and adolescents. Pediatr Clin North Am 50:859–878, 2003

Lewisohn PM, Hops H, Roberst RE, et al: Adolescent psychopathology, I: prevalence and incidence of depression and other DSM-III disorders in high school students. J Abnorm Psychol 102:133–144, 1993

Lustman PJ, Griffith LS, Freedland KE, et al: The course of major depression in diabetes. Gen Hosp Psychiatry 19:138–143, 1997

McDaniel JS, Brown FW, Cole SA: Assessment of depression and grief reactions in the medically ill, in Psychiatric Care of the Medical Patient. Edited by Stoudemire A, Fogel BS, Greenberg DB. Oxford, England, Oxford University Press, 2000, pp 149–164

Ormel J, Von Korff M, Van den Brink WM, et al: Depression, anxiety and social disability show synchrony of change in primary care patients. Am J Public Health 83:385–390, 1993

Rundell JR, Wise MG: Causes of organic mood disorder. J Neuropsychiatry Clin Neurosci 1:398–400, 1989

Schuckit M: Alcoholism and other psychiatric disorders. Hosp Community Psychiatry 34:1022–1027, 1983

Starkstein SE, Pearlson GD, Boston JD, et al: Mania and brain injury: a controlled study of causative factors. Arch Neurol 44:1069–1073, 1987

Sullivan M, LaCroix A, Baum C, et al: Functional status in coronary artery disease: a one-year prospective study of the role of anxiety and depression. Am J Med 103:331–338, 1997

Walker E, Gelfand MD, Gelfand AN, et al: The relationship of current psychiatric disorder to functional disability and distress in patients with inflammatory bowel disease. Gen Hosp Psychiatry 18:220–229, 1996

Waller DA, Rush AJ: Differentiating primary affective disease, organic affective syndromes, and situational depression on a pediatric service. J Am Acad Child Psychiatry 22:52–58, 1983

Wells KB, Kataoka SH, Asarnow JR: Affective disorders in children and adolescents: addressing unmet needs in primary care settings. Biol Psychiatry 49:1111–1120, 2001

Wise MG, Rundell JR: Depression and mania, in Concise Guide to Consultation Psychiatry. Washington, DC, American Psychiatric Press, 1988, pp 55–73

Wolraich ML, Felice ME, Drotar D (eds): The Classification of Child and Adolescent Mental Diagnoses in Primary Care: Child and Adolescent Version. Elk Grove Village, IL, American Academy of Pediatrics, 1996

Yates WR, Wesner RB, Thompson R: Organic mood disorder: a valid psychiatry consultation diagnosis? J Affect Disord 22:37–42, 1991

7

Anxiety Symptoms and Disorders

Anxiety is defined as a state of fear or subjective feeling of apprehension or dread (Colón and Popkin 2002). Symptoms of anxiety are common in patients in the pediatric setting and may significantly impair functioning and recovery. Anxiety may influence aspects of the treatment, including treatment adherence. Anxiety is a risk factor for several general medical conditions (e.g., hypertension) and may exacerbate the symptoms of specific illnesses (e.g., asthma, movement disorders, or irritable bowel syndrome [IBS]). Symptoms of anxiety may be secondary to the direct effects of the illness, be a psychological reaction to the illness, indicate the presence of a comorbid anxiety disorder, or be a combination of all three (Figure 7–1). Physical symptoms, such as tachycardia, shortness of breath, or sweating, are commonly mistaken for anxiety. Anxiety symptoms may be caused or exacerbated by a child's emotional reaction to an acute hospitalization and separation from home. Anxiety symptoms may be present as part of another psychiatric disorder (e.g., depressive or somatoform disorder) or may accompany another disorder as a primary comorbid anxiety disorder. In the pediatric setting, consultants are commonly faced with untangling these diagnostic dilemmas.

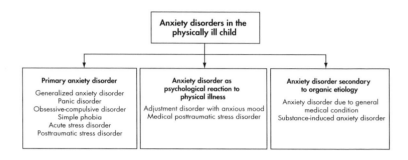

Figure 7–1.   Classification of anxiety disorders in the physically ill child.

Epidemiology

The lifetime prevalence of DSM-IV-TR anxiety disorders is 28.8%, with a median age at onset of 11 years (American Psychiatric Association 2000; Kessler et al. 2005). The age at onset distributions for anxiety disorders are diverse, with specific phobia and separation anxiety disorders having a very early median onset at 7 years, social phobias at 13 years, and other anxiety disorders at ages 19–31 years (Kessler et al. 2005). Girls have a significantly higher risk for anxiety than boys. Patients with chronic physical illnesses have a higher adjusted lifetime prevalence of anxiety disorders (Colón and Popkin 2002). Studies of adult patients suggest that between 4% and 18% of medical patients have a current comorbid anxiety disorder (Colón and Popkin 2002). Frequent users of medical care also display increased rates of anxiety (Barsky et al. 1999). These rates do not differentiate premorbid anxiety disorders from anxiety symptoms that develop in response to the medical illness or its treatment. For instance, Schuckit (1983) reported that 10%–40% of medical patients with anxiety had toxic or medical etiologies for their symptoms. Panic disorder in particular may be more common in physically ill patients, especially those with respiratory disease (Coffman and Levenson 2005).

Etiology

The likelihood of developing anxiety involves a combination of genetic and biological factors, psychological traits, and life experiences. The anxiety symptoms and disorders are so heterogeneous that the relative roles of these factors are likely to differ such that some have a stronger genetic basis whereas others are more rooted in stressful life events.

Psychological Reactions to Stress

Anxiety is a common psychological reaction to the stress of a major physical illness. Patients with genetic and biological vulnerabilities to anxiety symptoms are likely to have more intense reactions to the diagnosis and treatment of a physical illness, although these same conditions can induce disabling anxiety in patients with no prior history of anxiety. Consultants should consider several psychological sources of anxiety during their evaluation (Epstein and Hicks 2005; Goldberg and Posner 2000).

Illness Diagnosis

Patients often experience symptoms of anxiety around the time of diagnosis of a physical illness. Individuals with a family history of a specific medical condition may experience anxiety symptoms due to the excessive fear that they will be similarly affected. This fear can cause elevated symptoms of anxiety related to routine pediatric appointments during the period between the initial evaluation of a symptom and its diagnosis. Anxiety may also occur when a patient has an abnormal laboratory test that does not lead to a diagnosis but does require follow-up or monitoring.

Physical Integrity

Beginning around age 4 or 5, children become more concerned about bodily injury and are more cognitively aware of the physical effects of illness. As a result, they frequently experience anxiety. There may be fears about amputation, loss of vision, or pain. Adolescents in particular may worry about the cosmetic effects of an illness or treatment due to excessive concerns about social stigma.

Hospital Anxiety

Hospitalized children have to adjust to the presence of pediatric staff and to disruptions to their daily routine. These children may experience anxiety about the presence of hospital staff, particularly when the staff becomes associated with stressful medical procedures or the delivery of disturbing medical information. Children younger than ages 4 or 5 years are particularly prone to anxiety when separated from their caretakers. Patients who have not adhered to their medical treatment or who have engaged in risk-taking behaviors may conceal important medical information because of anticipatory anxiety about the potential disapproval of their physicians.

Impact of Illness

Children frequently report symptoms of anxiety related to the impact of the illness on their own lives and on family members. They may be concerned about missing school or falling behind academically. Adolescents may be particularly troubled by their separation from peers as well as by feeling "different" from others. Children may feel guilty about their need for increased parental attention and assistance. Some children report worries about the financial impact of their illness on the family because their parents have to take time off work or because of the costs of treatment.

Prognosis and Death

Patients may experience anxieties about their prognosis and death that can be based on both realistic and unrealistic appraisals of their illness. Children can develop symptoms of anxiety related to fears about the recurrence of an illness such as cancer. Such fears are not necessarily assuaged by a favorable statistical prognosis. A family history of medical illness or knowledge of the death of a family member or peer can influence these fears. Children may also report concerns about the emotional impact of their death on parents or siblings.

Primary Anxiety Disorders

DSM-IV-TR anxiety disorders often present with or are accompanied by physical symptoms. The psychological symptoms of anxiety are routinely associated with physical signs of autonomic activity (e.g., palpitations, shortness of breath, tremulousness, flushing, faintness, dizziness, chest pain, dry mouth, and muscle tension). The physical symptoms of anxiety can present the consultant with particularly complex diagnostic issues in the child with a comorbid general medical condition.

There are several subtypes of primary anxiety disorders seen in the medical setting (Figure 7–1). Separation anxiety disorder involves inappropriate and excessive anxiety concerning separation from caretakers or the home and is particularly common in younger children admitted to the hospital. Generalized anxiety disorder presents with a pattern of excessive anxiety and worry associated with symptoms of restlessness, fatigue, difficulty with concentration, irritability, muscle tension, and sleep disturbance and may also be heightened during the stress of an inpatient admission. Obsessive-compulsive disorder in the physically ill child may include obsessive preoccupation or fears about physical illness. Phobias may be particularly problematic in the pediatric setting in patients with fears about needle sticks and blood. Patients with claustrophobia similarly may have difficulties with procedures such as magnetic resonance imaging or the need for protective isolation due to an infectious disease or immunosuppression. Panic disorders can overlap and blend with the symptoms of the accompanying general medical condition. Studies of adult patients have shown that individuals with panic attacks are high utilizers of medical care (Barsky et al. 1999). This is particularly true for patients who experience chest pain and who repeatedly present at emergency departments or are referred for diagnostic workups. It has been hypothesized that individuals with panic disorder have a heightened sensitivity to normal physiological cardiac symptoms such as palpitations.

Medical Posttraumatic Stress Disorder

There has been increasing recognition of the presence of medically related posttraumatic stress disorder (PTSD) in patients with medical illness (Daviss et al. 2000; Kangas et al. 2002; Tedstone and Tarrier 2003). The PTSD symptom complex of numbness, intrusiveness, and hyperarousal can be remembered using the mnemonic "NIH" as a memory aid. Consultants will commonly come across this symptom complex in the reactions of patients and their families to the "medical trauma" of the physical illness itself or its treatment (Table 7–1). A study of adult cancer survivors revealed a 54% lifetime and a 33% current rate of cancer-related PTSD (Alter et al. 1992). Stuber et al. (1996) examined pediatric cancer survivors and their parents 2 years after treatment and found that 13% of patients, 40% of mothers, and 33% of fathers had severe symptoms of PTSD. PTSD is particularly common in those patients who have traumatic memories of their treatment. Studies reveal that young adult survivors of

Table 7–1. DSM-IV-TR diagnostic criteria for posttraumatic stress disorder

A. The person has been exposed to a traumatic event in which both of the following were present:

  (1) the person experienced, witnessed, or was confronted with an event or events that involved actual or threatened death or serious injury, or a threat to the physical integrity of self or others

  (2) the person's response involved intense fear, helplessness, or horror. **Note:** In children, this may be expressed instead by disorganized or agitated behavior

B. The traumatic event is persistently reexperienced in one (or more) of the following ways:

  (1) recurrent and intrusive distressing recollections of the event, including images, thoughts, or perceptions. **Note:** In young children, repetitive play may occur in which themes or aspects of the trauma are expressed.

  (2) recurrent distressing dreams of the event. **Note:** In children, there may be frightening dreams without recognizable content.

  (3) acting or feeling as if the traumatic event were recurring (includes a sense of reliving the experience, illusions, hallucinations, and dissociative flashback episodes, including those that occur on awakening or when intoxicated). **Note:** In young children, trauma-specific reenactment may occur.

  (4) intense psychological distress at exposure to internal or external cues that symbolize or resemble an aspect of the traumatic event

  (5) physiological reactivity on exposure to internal or external cues that symbolize or resemble an aspect of the traumatic event

C. Persistent avoidance of stimuli associated with the trauma and numbing of general responsiveness (not present before the trauma), as indicated by three (or more) of the following:

  (1) efforts to avoid thoughts, feelings, or conversations associated with the trauma

  (2) efforts to avoid activities, places, or people that arouse recollections of the trauma

  (3) inability to recall an important aspect of the trauma

  (4) markedly diminished interest or participation in significant activities

  (5) feeling of detachment or estrangement from others

  (6) restricted range of affect (e.g., unable to have loving feelings)

Table 7–1. DSM-IV-TR diagnostic criteria for posttraumatic stress disorder *(continued)*

    (7) sense of a foreshortened future (e.g., does not expect to have a career, marriage, children, or a normal life span)

D. Persistent symptoms of increased arousal (not present before the trauma), as indicated by two (or more) of the following:

    (1) difficulty falling or staying asleep

    (2) irritability or outbursts of anger

    (3) difficulty concentrating

    (4) hypervigilance

    (5) exaggerated startle response

E. Duration of the disturbance (symptoms in Criteria B, C, and D) is more than 1 month.

F. The disturbance causes clinically significant distress or impairment in social, occupational, or other important areas of functioning.

Specify if:

  Acute: if duration of symptoms is less than 3 months

  Chronic: if duration of symptoms is 3 months or more

Specify if:

  With delayed onset: if onset of symptoms is at least 6 months after the stressor

Source. Reprinted from *Diagnostic and Statistical Manual of Mental Disorders,* 4th Edition, Text Revision. Washington, DC, American Psychiatric Association, 2000. Used with permission.

childhood cancer have significantly elevated symptoms of PTSD as long as 11 years after completing treatment (Hobbie et al. 2000).

Traumatic reactions that precipitate these PTSD symptoms can occur at the onset of a physical illness, including distressing reactions to the news of its diagnosis. This phenomenon has been labeled an *information stressor* (Green et al. 1997). PTSD can also develop as a reaction to traumatic aspects of the medical treatment, whether acute or chronic. Life-threatening illness differs from other stresses that cause PTSD. In a physical illness, the threat to the individual arises internally and cannot be separated from the patient. There is a qualitative difference between threats to the individual that are externally located (e.g., the threat following an assault or motor vehicle accident) and the threat of a disease that is located within the patient. Intrusive thoughts about physical illnesses tend to be ruminative and future oriented rather than focused on the recollection of a past trauma. This is particularly the case in chronic physical illnesses such as cancer or cystic fibrosis. Similarly, hyperarousal is commonly experienced as increased sensitivity to physical symptoms and may resemble hypochondriasis.

PTSD in children has been classified into two subtypes (Terr 1991). Type I describes single-incident trauma is classically associated with reexperiencing symptoms through flashbacks, intrusive memories, and other mechanisms. Serial exposure to traumatic events causes type II PTSD, characterized by a greater prevalence of numbing, dissociation, and denial. Type I trauma is common after the initial diagnosis of an illness, whereas type II trauma is seen more often in patients with chronic physical illnesses (e.g., long-term survivors of cancer).

Posttraumatic Stress Disorder in Family Members

Stuber et al. (1997) found that 6%–10% of parents of childhood cancer survivors reported high levels of posttraumatic stress symptoms, whereas 20%–40% experienced moderate levels of distress. Parental PTSD has been noted in as much as 50% of parents of pediatric solid organ transplant recipients (Young et al. 2003). Posttraumatic stress symptoms have also been noted in parents of premature infants in a neonatal intensive care unit (Shaw et al. in press). Although a single acute traumatic medical event can trigger posttraumatic stress symptoms, cumulative stress related to a child's illness and subsequent treatment is most commonly involved in symptom development. Parents' appraisal of the potential life threat and intensity of treatment, rather than objective medical measures, are most strongly predictive of posttraumatic stress symptoms. Parents are more at risk for developing PTSD if there is a history of life stress or inadequate levels of social support.

Anxiety Disorder Due to a General Medical Condition

Many medical conditions may result in symptoms of anxiety, and it is important to consider this possibility if the history is not typical for a primary anxiety disorder or if anxiety symptoms are resistant to treatment (Table 7–2). Medical etiologies also are more likely when physical symptoms of anxiety, such as shortness of breath, tachycardia, or tremor, are more marked. It is important to differentiate anxiety that is secondary to a medical condition from comorbid anxiety or anxiety that is a reaction to the underlying medical illness. Table 7–3 lists some of the more common medical conditions that may result in symptoms of anxiety.

Table 7–2.   DSM-IV-TR diagnostic criteria for anxiety disorder due to…[indicate the general medical condition]

A.   Prominent anxiety, panic attacks, or obsessions or compulsions predominate in the clinical picture.

B.   There is evidence from the history, physical examination, or laboratory findings that the disturbance is the direct physiological consequence of a general medical condition.

C.   The disturbance is not better accounted for by another mental disorder (e.g., adjustment disorder with anxiety in which the stressor is a serious general medical condition).

D.   The disturbance does not occur exclusively during the course of a delirium.

E.   The disturbance causes clinically significant distress or impairment in social, occupational, or other important areas of functioning.

Specify if:

With generalized anxiety: if excessive anxiety or worry about a number of events or activities predominates in the clinical presentation

With panic attacks: if panic attacks predominate in the clinical presentation

With obsessive-compulsive symptoms: if obsessions or compulsions predominate in the clinical presentation

Coding note: Include the name of the general medical condition on Axis I, e.g., 293.84 anxiety disorder due to pheochromocytoma, With generalized anxiety; also code the general medical condition on Axis III (see Appendix G for codes).

Source.   Reprinted from *Diagnostic and Statistical Manual of Mental Disorders,* 4th Edition, Text Revision. Washington, DC, American Psychiatric Association, 2000. Used with permission.

Substance-Induced Anxiety Disorder

Anxiety may be induced by a variety of substances or medications, either as a result of the direct effect of a substance or due to a withdrawal reaction (Table 7–4). Corticosteroids, anticholinergic medications, beta-adrenergic agonists, and asthma medications are all potential causes of anxiety, particularly if the medication has recently been started or if there has been a change in dosage (Table 7–5).

Caffeine

Consumption of caffeine may lead to symptoms of insomnia and anxiety, which may occur with surprisingly low doses in sensitive individuals. Patients with generalized anxiety disorder appear to be more sensitive to caffeine in terms of both subjective arousal and physiological effect. Caffeine may also

Table 7–3. Medical conditions etiologically related to anxiety

Neurological disorders
    Encephalopathy
    Mass lesion
    Postconcussive syndrome
    Poststroke
    Seizure
    Vertigo
Endocrine disorders
    Carcinoid syndrome
    Hyperadrenalism
    Hypercalcemia
    Hypocalcemia
    Hypoglycemia
    Hypomagnesemia
    Hyperthyroid
    Hypothyroid
    Pheochromocytoma
Cardiac disorders
    Arrhythmias
    Congestive heart failure
    Hypovolemia
    Valvular disease
Miscellaneous disorders
    Anaphylaxis
    Asthma
    Diabetes mellitus
    Hyperkalemia
    Hyperthermia
    Hypoxia
    Systemic lupus erythematosus
    Pancreatic tumor
    Pneumothorax
    Porphyria
    Pulmonary edema
    Pulmonary embolism

Source. Adapted from Wise and Rundell 1988.

Table 7–4.   DSM-IV-TR diagnostic criteria for substance-induced anxiety disorder

A.   Prominent anxiety, panic attacks, or obsessions or compulsions predominate in the clinical picture.

B.   There is evidence from the history, physical examination, or laboratory findings of either (1) or (2):

  (1)   the symptoms in Criterion A developed during, or within 1 month of, substance intoxication or withdrawal

  (2)   medication use is etiologically related to the disturbance

C.   The disturbance is not better accounted for by an anxiety disorder that is not substance induced. Evidence that the symptoms are better accounted for by an anxiety disorder that is not substance induced might include the following: the symptoms precede the onset of the substance use (or medication use); the symptoms persist for a substantial period of time (e.g., about a month) after the cessation of acute withdrawal or severe intoxication or are substantially in excess of what would be expected given the type or amount of the substance used or the duration of use; or there is other evidence suggesting the existence of an independent non-substance-induced anxiety disorder (e.g., a history of recurrent non-substance-related episodes).

D.   The disturbance does not occur exclusively during the course of a delirium.

E.   The disturbance causes clinically significant distress or impairment in social, occupational, or other important areas of functioning.

Note: This diagnosis should be made instead of a diagnosis of substance intoxication or substance withdrawal only when the anxiety symptoms are in excess of those usually associated with the intoxication or withdrawal syndrome and when the anxiety symptoms are sufficiently severe to warrant independent clinical attention.

  Code [Specific substance]–induced anxiety disorder

    (291.89 alcohol; 292.89 amphetamine (or amphetamine-like substance); 292.89 caffeine; 292.89 cannabis; 292.89 cocaine; 292.89 hallucinogen; 292.89 inhalant; 292.89 phencyclidine (or phencyclidine-like substance); 292.89 sedative, hypnotic, or anxiolytic; 292.89 other [or unknown] substance)

  Specify if:

    With generalized anxiety: if excessive anxiety or worry about a number of events or activities predominates in the clinical presentation

    With panic attacks: if panic attacks predominate in the clinical presentation

    With obsessive-compulsive symptoms: if obsessions or compulsions predominate in the clinical presentation

Table 7–4.   DSM-IV-TR diagnostic criteria for substance-induced anxiety disorder *(continued)*

With phobic symptoms: if phobic symptoms predominate in the clinical presentation

Specify if:

With onset during intoxication: if the criteria are met for Intoxication with the substance and the symptoms develop during the intoxication syndrome

With onset during withdrawal: if criteria are met for withdrawal from the substance and the symptoms develop during, or shortly after, a withdrawal syndrome

Source.   Reprinted from American Psychiatric Association: *Diagnostic and Statistical Manual of Mental Disorders,* 4th Edition, Text Revision. Washington, DC, American Psychiatric Association, 2000. Used with permission.

precipitate panic attacks in patients who have panic disorder. Patients who are chronic users of caffeine may have withdrawal symptoms if their caffeine intake decreases suddenly and may present with symptoms of headache, fatigue, and agitation.

Cocaine

Use of cocaine may be associated with symptoms of anxiety, irritability, tremulousness, and fatigue. There are also reports of cocaine inducing panic attacks in susceptible individuals and potentially precipitating the onset of panic disorder that may continue even after cocaine use ends.

Alcohol

Withdrawal from alcohol, which may be seen in adolescent patients, may be associated with symptoms of anxiety starting approximately 24 hours after cessation of drinking. More serious symptoms include tremulousness, autonomic arousal, and in extreme cases, the onset of an alcohol withdrawal delirium.

Antipsychotic Agents

Antipsychotic agents, in particular risperidone, may be associated with the symptoms of akathisia, which is experienced by the patient as a symptom of internal restlessness, or "restless legs syndrome." Akathisia is best treated with either beta-blockers or benzodiazepines.

Table 7–5. Medications and substances associated with anxiety

Direct effect	Amphetamines
	Androgens
	Anticholinergics
	Antidepressants (including selective serotonin reuptake inhibitors)
	Antiemetics
	Antipsychotics
	Baclofen
	Beta-adrenergic agonists
	Caffeine
	Cocaine
	Corticosteroids
	Dopaminergics
	Estrogens
	Insulin
	Metronidazole
	Progestins
	Sumatriptan
	Sympathomimetics
	Theophylline
	Thyroid preparations
Withdrawal	Alcohol
	Barbiturates
	Benzodiazepines
	Caffeine
	Opiates
	Selective serotonin reuptake inhibitors

Antidepressants

Akathisia can also be caused by some of the selective serotonin reuptake inhibitors, such as fluoxetine. Anxiety or agitation is also a common symptom when treatment is initiated with these medications. Bupropion is also associated with agitation and insomnia.

Opiates

Opiate withdrawal, either from illegal substance abuse or from medically prescribed opiates, is associated with symptoms of anxiety.

Anxiety Symptoms in Specific Physical Conditions

Consultants will observe anxiety symptoms in a wide variety of physical conditions. There will be the noncategorical effects of anxiety that are experienced by all patients facing a physical illness and its treatment. From this perspective, children and their families are seen as experiencing stress in the context of being ill and not as a result of specific factors associated with a particular disease. For example, invasive medical procedures (e.g., venipunctures, intravenous lines) are common across illness types and can cause anxiety. Anxiety symptoms are more dependent on the child's premorbid anxiety vulnerability, developmental stage, family functioning, and degree of psychosocial stress in the environment than on the specific physical illness.

The following section provides brief overviews regarding a number of commonly encountered specific medical conditions associated with symptoms of anxiety.

Cancer

Anxiety is common at various points throughout the diagnosis and treatment of pediatric cancer (Massie and Greenberg 2005). Patients often experience increased anxiety during initial diagnosis, relapse, and even routine follow-up visits to the hospital. Reference has been made to the increased rates of medical PTSD in both patients and family members (Kangas et al. 2002). Anxiety symptoms can interfere with the patient's ability to tolerate important components of their medical treatment, including invasive diagnostic procedures and treatment. Anticipatory nausea and vomiting are also common and frequently have an anxiety component. Several of the medications used in the treatment of cancer include symptoms of anxiety as possible side effects. Antiemetic medications, such as prochlorperazine or metoclopramide, can cause symptoms of akathisia that may be misdiagnosed as anxiety. Anxiety symptoms are also elevated in patients experiencing disease-related pain.

Gastrointestinal Disorders

Studies of patients with inflammatory bowel disease (IBD) suggest that they may be more vulnerable to developing psychiatric disorders, including symptoms of anxiety and depression. As many as 60% of youngsters with IBD have symptoms of anxiety and depression in addition to high rates of phobias, separation anxiety, obsessive-compulsive symptoms, and behavior problems (Bennett 1994). Creed and Olden (2005) found that patients' IBD relapses appeared to occur during times of increased stress. Anxiety symptoms can also occur in the context of any treatment with a corticosteroid.

Patients with IBS also experience higher rates of anxiety disorders. It is unclear if individuals with IBS are more sensitive to stress, more aware of colon spasms, or have an immune system problem that is affected by stress. The onset of the anxiety or mood disorder often coincides with the onset of the gastrointestinal symptoms. There is significant comorbidity between recurrent abdominal pain and anxiety disorders.

Heart Disease

Anxiety symptoms can appear in patients as a direct result of cardiac failure caused by worsening congenital heart disease or an acute myocarditis. Anxiety states can also occur early in the course of a patient with unrecognized subacute bacterial endocarditis. Although the emotional functioning of patients with pediatric heart disease is generally not in the psychopathology range, those children who are at higher risk for anxiety generally have other risk factors (e.g., cognitive or family functioning) that need to be considered (DeMaso 2004).

Hormone-Secreting Tumors

Pheochromocytoma is a rare disorder associated with catecholamine secretion from a tumor in the renal medulla. This secretion results in acute, episodic, or chronic symptoms of anxiety often associated with hypertension. Clinical symptoms include increased heart rate, increased blood pressure, myocardial contractility, and vasoconstriction. Patients may present with headache, sweating, palpitations, apprehension, and a sense of impending doom (Goebel-Fabbri et al. 2005). Other patients may present with classic symptoms of a panic attack. Thyroid adenoma or carcinoma, parathyroid, adrenocorticotropic hormone–producing tumors, and insulinomas are other hormone-secreting tumors associated with anxiety symptoms.

Hyperventilation Syndrome

Hyperventilation syndrome presents with symptoms of anxiety such as faintness, visual disturbances, nausea, vertigo, headaches, palpitations, dyspnea, diaphoresis, and paresthesias. The symptoms may be reproduced by observation of the patient's response to overbreathing. This syndrome is a form of panic disorder in which hyperventilation causes an excessive elimination of carbon dioxide and a reduction in cerebral blood flow.

Poststroke Anxiety

Symptoms of anxiety and generalized anxiety disorder may persist in individuals who have had strokes. Anxiety is associated with right-hemisphere lesions, whereas symptoms of depression are associated with left-hemisphere lesions (Epstein and Hicks 2005). Poststroke anxiety symptoms may include PTSD symptoms of increased somatic preoccupation.

Pulmonary Disease

Hypoxia may provoke anxiety in any individual. The patient experiences symptoms of air hunger. The consultant should be alert to this etiology, particularly in high-risk situations such as occur in the pediatric intensive care unit. After experiencing a lack of oxygen, some patients may develop secondary anxiety symptoms that interfere with efforts to wean them from the ventilator. Posttraumatic stress symptoms have also been reported in patients who experience episodes of acute respiratory distress syndrome (Shaw et al. 2001). Patients may develop posttraumatic stress symptoms without any conscious recollection of the specific traumatic events that occurred during their intensive care unit treatments. Posttraumatic stress symptoms have been reported in pediatric asthma patients who present with symptoms of acute respiratory distress (Shaw et al. 2002).

The strong overlap between symptoms of asthma and anxiety make the differential diagnosis between the two confusing. Asthma and anxiety disorders, particularly panic disorder, often present together in the same individual (Katon et al. 2004). The anxiety may be secondary to the stress of asthma, but it is also possible that hypercapnia and hyperventilation predispose the individual to panic attacks. Episodes of respiratory distress and the side effects of asthma medications may increase anxiety. In addition, anxiety and psychological distress are thought to provoke and increase the severity of asthma attacks.

There is an increased prevalence of anxiety symptoms in pediatric patients with cystic fibrosis, with some studies suggesting rates as high as 50%–60% (Hains et al. 1997). Cystic fibrosis is also associated with increased rates of other psychiatric disorders, such as depression (Coffman and Levenson 2005). Pulmonary embolism is uncommon in children but has been associated with symptoms of anxiety.

Seizure Disorders

Up to one-third of epilepsy patients may experience symptoms of depression and anxiety (Carson et al. 2005). Complex partial seizures can cause symptoms associated with panic disorder including fear, depersonalization, dizziness, and paresthesias. This overlap makes it difficult to differentiate panic attacks from complex partial seizures based purely on the clinical symptoms. There have also been reports of interictal anxiety.

Transplantation

Patients who have undergone solid organ transplantations can develop anxiety symptoms as a direct result of their immunosuppressant medications, particularly corticosteroids. They can experience reactive anxiety symptoms at any point in the treatment course, whether during the waiting period for transplantation, the immediate postoperative time period, rejection episodes, or transitioning to home and school. PTSD in adolescent solid organ transplant recipients is often related to the traumatic aspects of the patient's surgical intensive care treatment and general sequelae of their illness (Shemesh et al. 2000).

Traumatic Brain Injury and Postconcussion Syndrome

Patients who have sustained traumatic brain injury have an increased prevalence of anxiety disorders, including generalized anxiety disorder, panic disorder, obsessive-compulsive disorder, and phobias (Fann et al. 2005). Although these symptoms may be transient, some patients develop more sustained symptoms. Patients with traumatic brain injury also have an increased risk of symptoms of acute stress disorder and subsequent PTSD (Harvey and Bryant 2000). Even when cerebral concussion does not result in any irreversible anatomic lesions, it may be followed with periods of retrograde amnesia. A small proportion of individuals may develop a constellation of symptoms that include anxiety, impairment of sleep and appetite, irritability, lightheadedness, headaches, and poor concentration after receiving a concussion (Goldberg and Posner 2000). Mild head trauma with brief loss of consciousness has been reported to increase the level of catecholamines, which are associated with anxiety.

Thyroid Disease

Patients with thyroid gland disorders often experience anxiety symptoms. Hyperthyroidism is associated with symptoms of anxiety and may be difficult to differentiate from a primary anxiety disorder. Signs indicating thyrotoxicosis include persistent acute anxiety, warm and dry hands, and fatigue accompanied by the desire to be active (Colón and Popkin 2002). Anxiety symptoms usually resolve when the underlying thyroid condition is treated, but anxiety should be treated with beta-blockers during the acute treatment phase. Clinicians should perform routine thyroid function tests in patients presenting with new-onset anxiety, with anxiety disorders that are resistant to treatment, and with anxiety that is accompanied by prominent physical symptoms. Anxiety has also been reported in hypothyroidism.

Assessment

Routine screening laboratory tests that should be performed or reviewed include a complete blood count, glucose, electrolytes, blood urea nitrogen, creatinine, liver enzymes, thyroid function tests, and urinalysis with toxicology screening. Arterial blood gas or oxygen saturation measurements are considerations to rule out respiratory causes of anxiety. If underlying medical conditions are suspected, a chest X ray, electrocardiogram, and 24-hour cardiac monitoring should be considered. Central nervous system scans (e.g., computed tomography, magnetic resonance imaging) and electroencephalography as well as lumbar puncture may be helpful. Table 7–6 outlines evaluative components for the assessment of anxiety in a pediatric setting.

Treatment

Treatment of pediatric anxiety disorders in physically ill children and adolescents follows the same principles as those used in the nonmedical setting. Patients in the acute inpatient setting often require medication at least temporarily while the pediatric team explores other treatment options. Specific details regarding psychopharmacological approaches are described in Chapter 15.

Psychotherapy in the pediatric setting is generally brief, due to the short duration of the patient's hospital stay. Supportive psychotherapy and reassurance play an important role in correcting patients' misconceptions about the

Table 7–6. Evaluative components in assessing anxiety in pediatric setting

Medical-psychiatric history
    Current subjective symptoms
    Sources of anxiety
        Academic and social impact
        Death
        Diagnosis of illness
        Financial burden of illness
        Hospital anxiety
        Impact on family members
        Isolation
        Loss of control
        Loss of privacy
        Pain
        Physical effects of illness
        Uncertainty about prognosis
    Use of prescribed medications (see Table 7–5)
    Use of drugs of abuse
        Alcohol
        Amphetamine
        Barbiturates
        Benzodiazepines
        Caffeine
        Cocaine
    History of psychiatric disorders, especially anxiety disorders
    Family history of psychiatric disorders, especially anxiety disorders
    Vital signs
Mental status examination
    Blood glucose
    Complete blood count
    Electrolytes
    Laboratory evaluation
    Renal/Hepatic function tests
    Serum calcium
    Serum cortisol
    Serum magnesium
    Serum phosphorus

Table 7–6.   Evaluative components in assessing anxiety in pediatric setting *(continued)*

Serum thyroxine
Thyroid function tests
Toxicology screening
Lumbar puncture
Electrocardiogram/24-Hour cardiac monitor
Computed tomography/Magnetic resonance imaging scan
Electroencephalogram

significance of physical symptoms. A meeting with the family and the pediatric team may be necessary to reexplain aspects of the illness and its treatment. Effective treatment of pain is a critical part of the overall approach. Stud'es have shown that cognitive-behavioral therapy is particularly successful in the treatment of anxiety disorders. Its techniques include uncovering and correcting misinterpretations and irrational thoughts associated with symptoms of anxiety. Behavioral tools, such as systematic desensitization, help to treat phobias that interfere with medical treatment. Guided imagery, progressive muscle relaxation, and hypnosis are potentially helpful in the inpatient setting. Principles of individual and family therapy are outlined in Chapters 13 and 14, and treatment of procedural anxiety is addressed in Chapter 16.

References

Alter CL, Pelcovitz D, Axelrod A, et al: The identification of PTSD in cancer survivors. Paper presented at the 39th meeting of the Academy of Psychosomatic Medicine, San Diego, CA, October 1992

American Psychiatric Association: Diagnostic and Statistical Manual of Mental Disorders, 4th Edition, Text Revision. Washington, DC, American Psychiatric Association, 2000

Barsky AJ, Delamater BA, Orav JE: Panic disorder patients and their medical care. Psychosomatics 40:50–56, 1999

Bennett D: Depression among children with chronic medical problems: A meta-analysis. J Pediatr Psychol 19:149–169, 1994

Carson AJ, Zeman A, Myles L, et al: Neurology and neurosurgery, in The American Psychiatric Publishing Textbook of Psychosomatic Medicine. Edited by Levenson JL. Washington, DC, American Psychiatric Publishing, 2005, pp 701–732

Coffman K, Levenson JL: Lung disease, in The American Psychiatric Publishing Textbook of Psychosomatic Medicine. Edited by Levenson JL. Washington, DC, American Psychiatric Publishing, 2005, pp 445–464

Colón EA, Popkin MK: Anxiety and panic, in The American Psychiatric Publishing Textbook of Consultation-Liaison Psychiatry, 2nd Edition. Edited by Wise MG, Rundell JR. Washington, DC, American Psychiatric Publishing, 2002, pp 393–415

Creed F, Olden KW: Gastrointestinal disorders, in The American Psychiatric Publishing Textbook of Psychosomatic Medicine. Edited by Levenson JL. Washington, DC, American Psychiatric Publishing, 2005, pp 465–481

Daviss WB, Mooney D, Racusin R, et al: Predicting posttraumatic stress after hospitalization for pediatric injury. J Am Acad Child Adolesc Psychiatry 39:576–583, 2000

DeMaso DR: Pediatric heart disease, in Handbook of Pediatric Psychology in School Settings. Edited by Brown RT. Hillsdale, NJ, Lawrence Erlbaum Associates, 2004, pp 283–297

Epstein SA, Hicks D: Anxiety disorders, in The American Psychiatric Publishing Textbook of Psychosomatic Medicine. Edited by Levenson JL. Washington, DC, American Psychiatric Publishing, 2005, pp 251–270

Fann JR, Kennedy R, Bombadier CH: Physical medicine and rehabilitation, in The American Psychiatric Publishing Textbook of Psychosomatic Medicine. Edited by Levenson JL. Washington, DC, American Psychiatric Publishing, 2005, pp 787–825

Goebel-Fabbri A, Musen G, Sparks CR, et al: Endocrine and metabolic disorders, in The American Psychiatric Publishing Textbook of Psychosomatic Medicine. Edited by Levenson JL. Washington, DC, American Psychiatric Publishing, 2005, pp 495–515

Goldberg RJ, Posner DA: Anxiety in the medically ill, in Psychiatric Care of the Medical Patient, 2nd Edition. Edited by Stoudemire A, Fogel BS, Greenberg DB. Oxford, England, Oxford University Press, 2000, pp 165–180

Green BL, Epstein SA, Krupnick JL, et al: Trauma and medical illness: assessing trauma-related disorders in medical settings, in Assessing Psychological Trauma and PTSD. Edited by Wilson JP, Keane TM. New York, Guilford, 1997, pp 160–191

Hains AA, Davies WH, Behrens D, et al: Cognitive behavioral interventions for adolescents with cystic fibrosis. J Pediatr Psychol 22:669–687, 1997

Harvey AG, Bryant RA: Two-year prospective evaluation of the relationship between acute stress disorder and posttraumatic stress disorder following mild traumatic brain injury. Am J Psychiatry 157:626–628, 2000

Hobbie WL, Stuber M, Meeske K, et al: Symptoms of posttraumatic stress in young adult survivors of childhood cancer. J Clin Oncol 18:4060–4066, 2000

Kangas M, Henry JL, Bryant RA: Posttraumatic stress disorder following cancer: a conceptual and empirical review. Clin Psychol Rev 22:499–524, 2002

Katon WJ, Richardson L, Lozano P, et al: The relationship of asthma and anxiety disorders. Psychosom Med 66:349–355, 2004

Kessler RC, Berglund P, Demler O, et al: Lifetime prevalence and age-of-onset distributions of DSM-IV disorders in the National Comorbidity Survey Replication. Arch Gen Psychiatry 62:593–602, 2005

Massie MJ, Greenberg DB: Oncology, in The American Psychiatric Publishing Textbook of Psychosomatic Medicine. Edited by Levenson JL. Washington, DC, American Psychiatric Publishing, 2005, pp 517–534

Schuckit M: Anxiety related to medical disease. J Clin Psychiatry 44:31–37, 1983

Shaw RJ, Harvey JE, Nelson K, et al: Linguistic analysis to assess medically related posttraumatic stress symptoms. Psychosomatics 42: 35–40, 2001

Shaw RJ, Robinson TE, Steiner H: Acute stress disorder following ventilation. Psychosomatics 43:74–76, 2002

Shaw RJ, DeBlois T, Ikuta L, et al: Acute stress disorder among parents in the neonatal intensive care nursery. Psychosomatics, in press

Shemesh E, Lurie S, Stuber ML, et al: A pilot study of posttraumatic stress and nonadherence in pediatric liver transplant recipients. Pediatrics 105:E29, 2000

Stuber M, Christakis D, Houskamp B, et al: Posttraumatic symptoms in childhood leukemia survivors and their parents. Psychosomatics 37:254–261, 1996

Stuber ML, Kazak AE, Meeske KM, et al: Predictors of posttraumatic stress symptoms in childhood cancer survivors. Pediatrics 100: 958–964, 1997

Tedstone JE, Tarrier N: Posttraumatic stress disorder following medical illness and treatment. Clin Psychol Rev 23:409–448, 2003

Terr LC: Childhood trauma: an outline and overview. Am J Psychiatry 148:10–20, 1991

Young GS, Mintzer LL, Seacord D, et al: Symptoms of post traumatic stress disorder in parents of transplant recipients: incidence, severity, and related factors. Pediatrics 111:E725–E731, 2003

Wise MG, Rundell JR: Anxiety, panic, and insomnia, in Concise Guide to Consultation Psychiatry. Washington, DC, American Psychiatric Press, 1988, p 77

8

Somatoform Disorders

Medically unexplained physical symptoms are common in children and adolescents. Although frequently chronic and disabling, they do not often result in referrals for psychiatric evaluation or treatment (Campo et al. 1999; Mayou et al. 2003). DSM-IV-TR somatoform disorders are characterized by the presence of one of more physical complaints for which an adequate medical explanation cannot be found (American Psychiatric Association 2000). The symptoms are severe enough to cause significant distress or impairment in functioning and to result in the family seeking medical help. Patients with somatoform disorders are a source of significant health care costs and may undergo unnecessary and potentially harmful medical interventions (Servan-Schreiber et al. 1999).

Somatization can be defined as a pattern of seeking medical help for physical symptoms that cannot be fully explained by pathophysiologic mechanisms but are nevertheless attributed to physical disease by the sufferer (Campo and Fritsch 1994). Somatization has been described as the tendency to experience and express psychological distress through somatic complaints (Abbey 1996). It has been suggested that the somatization occurs universally in young children who have not yet developed the cognitive and linguistic

143

skills needed to comprehend and communicate their feelings (Stoudemire 1991). Somatization is also common in cultures that accept physical illness but not psychological symptoms as an excuse for disability.

Community surveys of children and adolescents suggest that recurrent somatic complaints generally fall into four symptom clusters: cardiovascular, gastrointestinal, pain/weakness, and pseudoneurological (Garber et al. 1991). Large community samples have found that youngsters commonly report recurrent complaints of headache and abdominal pain as well as fatigue and gastrointestinal symptoms (DeMaso and Beasley 1998). The prevalence of somatization is roughly equal among boys and girls in early childhood but appears to rise in adolescence, at which point somatic complaints in girls are five times greater than those in boys. Children and adolescents with a history of somatization are more likely to experience emotional and behavioral difficulties, be absent from school, and perform poorly academically. Pediatric somatization is strongly correlated with the presence of depression and anxiety (Campo et al. 1999).

Risk Factors for Pediatric Somatization

Familial and genetic factors, stressful life events, personality traits and coping styles, learned complaints, family factors, childhood physical illness, and sociocultural background are risk factors that have been associated with somatization in children and adolescents.

Genetic Factors

Somatization clusters in families. This is particularly true for somatization disorder, which occurs in 10%–20% of first-degree relatives of patients with this disorder. Somatization disorders show a concordance rate of 29% in monozygotic twin studies (Kaplan et al. 1994). Rates of anxiety and depression are higher in the family members of somatizing children and adolescents, suggesting a possible genetic etiology (Fritz et al. 1997). Campo and Fritsch (1994) hypothesized that genetic factors contribute to the development of personality traits that may predispose to somatization when combined with environmental factors. Children are believed to be more prone to adopt somatic ways to express emotional distress if they observe their parents using similar strategies, particularly if the emotional expression of distress is considered inappropriate (Stuart and Noyes 1999). Some studies indicate that parental medical illness may be associated with childhood somatization (Kaplan et al. 1994).

Stressful Life Events

Stressful life events, including childhood trauma, have been associated with the development of somatization later in life (Campo and Fritsch 1994). Campo and Fritsch (1994) noted a high correlation of sexual abuse and conversion symptoms. Poikolainen et al. (1995), in a study of Finnish high school students, found significant correlations between somatic symptoms and several psychosocial stressors, including family conflict, physical injury or illness in the family, breakup with a boyfriend or girlfriend, and increased parental absence. In a study of adults with hypochondriasis, Barsky et al. (1994) found that hypochondriacal patients recalled more conflict between parents, more traumatic sexual experiences in childhood, and more victimization by violence than a comparison group.

Personality Traits and Coping Styles

Shapiro (1996) postulated that somatization occurs in individuals who are unable to verbalize emotional distress that instead is expressed in the form of physical symptoms. Physical symptoms have been called a form of body language for children who have difficulty expressing emotions verbally. Examples include individuals who have difficulties with disclosing traumatic events or expressing anger and high-achieving children who cannot admit they are under too much pressure. Personality traits of introspectiveness (the tendency to think about oneself), poor self-concept, and pessimism have been associated with somatization (Abbey 2005). The term *alexithymia* has been used to describe individuals with somatic concerns who do not have a verbal vocabulary to describe their moods (Stoudemire 1991).

Somatic complaints in adults have also been linked to what has been termed *somatosensory amplification*, or the tendency to experience normal somatic sensations as "intense, noxious and disturbing" (Barsky et al. 1988). Patients with this form of somatization tend to be hypervigilant to their own bodily sensations, overreact to these sensations, and interpret them as indicating physical illness (Barsky et al. 1988). Electroencephalographic examinations of evoked potentials suggest that somatizing patients are not able to discriminate between relevant and irrelevant physical stimuli and have an inability to habituate to repetitive stimuli (James et al. 1989).

Learned Complaints

Principles of operant conditioning suggest that behaviors that are rewarded will increase in strength or frequency, whereas behaviors that are inhibited or punished decrease. Attention and sympathy from others or decrease in responsibilities (*secondary gain*) may reinforce somatic complaints. If somatic symptoms are reinforced early in the course of a somatoform disorder, then it is likely that these behaviors will continue. A child or adolescent may learn the benefits of assuming the sick role and may be reluctant to give up their symptoms. Increased parental attention or avoidance of unpleasant school pressures may further reinforce symptoms.

Social learning theory suggests that somatic symptoms may be a result of "modeling" or "observational learning" within the family (Jamison and Walker 1992). Family members with similar physical complaints (*symptom model*) are common in patients with somatoform disorders (DeMaso and Beasley 1998).

Family Factors

Family systems theory postulates that somatization may serve the function of drawing attention away from other areas of tension, as in cases of marital conflict, for example (Stuart and Noyes 1999). The concept of *enmeshment* refers to the blurring of intergenerational boundaries with overinvolved and hyperresponsive family interactions. Minuchin et al. (1978) postulated that family enmeshment, overprotectiveness, rigidity, and lack of conflict resolution predisposed family members to the development of somatization (see Chapter 14). It has been suggested that children in such families with significant degrees of conflict may develop somatic complaints as a mechanism to avoid any emotional expression that may exacerbate familial stress.

Childhood Physical Illness

Although the data are mixed and retrospective, there does appear to be a connection between childhood physical illness and later development of somatization. Hypochondriacal adults have reported being sick more often as children as well as missing school more often for health reasons (Barsky et al.

1994). Persistent abdominal pain in childhood has also been associated with multiple somatic complaints in adulthood (Hotopf et al. 1999). Poikolainen et al. (2000) similarly found that approximately 66% of men and 75% of women who reported frequent somatic symptoms in adulthood had reported frequent somatic symptoms when they were in high school.

Sociocultural Background

Somatoform disorders have been reported to be more common in rural areas and among individuals of lower socioeconomic status (American Psychiatric Association 2000; Gureje et al. 1997). Spells or visions are common aspects of culturally sanctioned religious and healing rituals, and falling down with loss or alteration in consciousness is a feature in a variety of culture-specific syndromes.

The Somatoform Disorders

DSM-IV-TR recognizes five major somatoform disorders, which are summarized in Table 8–1. In the following section, there is a brief review of individual pediatric somatoform disorders followed by discussion of assessment and treatment approaches to these illnesses. Somatoform disorders should be differentiated from malingering, in which the essential feature is the intentional production of false or grossly exaggerated physical or psychological symptoms motivated by external incentives such as avoiding work, obtaining financial compensation, evading criminal prosecution, or obtaining drugs (American Psychiatric Association 2000). Discussion of pain disorders can be found in Chapter 9.

Somatization Disorder

Definition

Somatization disorder is a chronic debilitating illness characterized by the presence of multiple somatic complaints that cannot be adequately explained on the basis of physical or laboratory investigations (Table 8–2). The combination and number of pain, gastrointestinal, sexual/reproductive, and pseudoneurological symptoms required over a several-year time period and the inclusion of criteria that are appropriate only for postpubertal or sexually active

Table 8–1.   Somatoform disorders: a comparison of clinical features

	Somatization disorder	Conversion disorder	Pain disorder	Hypochondriasis	Body dysmorphic disorder
Clinical presentation	Polysymptomatic Recurrent Chronic "Sickly" by history	Monosymptomatic Mostly acute Simulates disease	Pain syndrome simulated or magnified by psychological factors	Disease concern or preoccupation	Subjective feelings of ugliness or concern with body defect
Demographic/ epidemiologic features	Female predominance Familial pattern	Female predominance in adolescence Rural and lower social class Less educated and psychologically unsophisticated	Female predominance (2:1) Familial pattern Up to 40% of pain populations	Equal male:female ratio Previous physical disease	Female predominance Onset during adolescence
Diagnostic features	Review of system profusely positive Multiple physician contacts Polysurgical	Simulation incompatible with known physiologic mechanisms or anatomy	Simulation or intensity incompatible with known physiological mechanisms or anatomy	Disease conviction amplifies symptoms Obsessional	Pervasive bodily concerns
Management strategy	Build therapeutic alliance Schedule regular appointments Requires crisis intervention	Build therapeutic alliance Suggestion and persuasion Multiple techniques	Build therapeutic alliance Redefine goals of treatment Antidepressant medications	Build therapeutic alliance Document symptoms Psychosocial review	Build therapeutic alliance Stress management Psychotherapies Antidepressant medications

Table 8–1. Somatoform disorders: a comparison of clinical features *(continued)*

	Somatization disorder	Conversion disorder	Pain disorder	Hypochondriasis	Body dysmorphic disorder
Prognosis	Poor to fair	Excellent unless chronic	Guarded; variable	Fair to good; waxes and wanes	Fair to good
Associated disturbances	Anxiety and depressive disorder Conduct disorder Substance abuse	Drug/alcohol dependence Somatization disorder Histrionic personality traits	Depression Anxiety Substance use Dependent/Histrionic personality	Depression Panic disorder Obsessive-compulsive disorder	Obsessive-compulsive disorder Anorexia nervosa Psychosocial distress Avoidant/Compulsive personality traits
Primary differential presentation	Physical disease Depression Anxiety	Depression Neurological disease	Depression Psychophysiological Physical disease Malingering	Depression Physical disease Personality disorder Delusional disorder	Delusional psychosis Depression Somatization disorder
Psychological processes contributing to symptoms	Unconscious Cultural Developmental	Unconscious Psychological stress or conflict may be present Secondary gain Symptom model	Unconscious Acute stressor/Developmental Physical trauma may predispose Secondary gain	Unconscious Stress-bereavement Developmental factors	Unconscious Self-esteem factors

Source. Adapted from Folks DG, Ford CV, Houck CA: "Somatoform Disorders, Factitious Disorders, and Malingering," in *Clinical Psychiatry for Medical Students.* Edited by Stoudemire A. Philadelphia, PA, Lippincott Williams & Wilkins, 1998, pp 343–381. Copyright 1998, Lippincott Williams & Wilkins. Used with permission.

Table 8–2.   DSM-IV-TR diagnostic criteria for somatization disorder

A.   A history of many physical complaints beginning before age 30 years that occur over a period of several years and result in treatment being sought or significant impairment in social, occupational, or other important areas of functioning.

B.   Each of the following criteria must have been met, with individual symptoms occurring at any time during the course of the disturbance:

  (1)   *four pain symptoms:*   a history of pain related to at least four different sites or functions (e.g., head, abdomen, back, joints, extremities, chest, rectum, during menstruation, during sexual intercourse, or during urination)

  (2)   *two gastrointestinal symptoms:*   a history of at least two gastrointestinal symptoms other than pain (e.g., nausea, bloating, vomiting other than during pregnancy, diarrhea, or intolerance of several different foods)

  (3)   *one sexual symptom:*   a history of at least one sexual or reproductive symptom other than pain (e.g., sexual indifference, erectile or ejaculatory dysfunction, irregular menses, excessive menstrual bleeding, vomiting throughout pregnancy)

  (4)   *one pseudoneurological symptom:*   a history of at least one symptom or deficit suggesting a neurological condition not limited to pain (conversion symptoms such as impaired coordination or balance, paralysis or localized weakness, difficulty swallowing or lump in throat, aphonia, urinary retention, hallucinations, loss of touch or pain sensation, double vision, blindness, deafness, seizures; dissociative symptoms such as amnesia; or loss of consciousness other than fainting)

C.   Either (1) or (2):

  (1)   after appropriate investigation, each of the symptoms in Criterion B cannot be fully explained by a known general medical condition or the direct effects of a substance (e.g., a drug of abuse, a medication)

  (2)   when there is a related general medical condition, the physical complaints or resulting social or occupational impairment are in excess of what would be expected from the history, physical examination, or laboratory findings

D.   The symptoms are not intentionally produced or feigned (as in factitious disorder or malingering).

Source.   Reprinted from *Diagnostic and Statistical Manual of Mental Disorders,* 4th Edition, Text Revision. Washington, DC, American Psychiatric Association, 2000. Used with permission.

patients mitigate against the diagnosis of somatization disorder in childhood and adolescence (DeMaso and Beasley 1998). As a result, it is likely that this disorder has been underdiagnosed in pediatric patients, leading to suggestions for the development of revised criteria for children and adolescents (Fritz et al. 1997).

Epidemiology

The lifetime prevalence of DSM-IV-TR somatization disorder in adults is estimated to be between 0.2% and 2% for women and less than 0.2% in men (American Psychiatric Association 2000). Women with somatization disorder generally outnumber men by 5–20 times. Somatization disorder is more commonly observed in families where there is a relative with somatization disorder and in children who have been exposed to sexual abuse. Adult patients with this diagnosis often date the onset of their symptoms to their adolescence. Although no data exist regarding the prevalence of somatization disorder in children and adolescents, surveys examining somatic complaints in childhood and adolescence have identified polysymptomatic "somatizers" (Campo and Fritsch 1994). Although the criteria used to define those with frequent unexplained somatic complaints vary, prevalence rates of 4.5%–10% in adolescent boys and 10.7%–15% in adolescent girls have been reported (Campo and Fritsch 1994).

Clinical Features

As noted earlier, children and adolescents rarely present with the full DSM-IV-TR criteria for a somatization disorder. There is commonly a medical history of evolving, recurrent, unexplained physical complaints. Symptoms commonly reported in pediatric patients include headaches, fatigue, muscle aches, abdominal distress, back pain, and blurred vision (Garber et al. 1991). Prepubertal children are more likely to report complaints of headache and abdominal pain, whereas complaints of limb pain, fatigue, and muscle aches appear to increase with age. Specific constellations of symptoms may result in the diagnosis of syndromes such as irritable bowel syndrome, chronic fatigue, or fibromyalgia. There often is history of concurrent treatment from several physicians, which may result in fragmented care and contradictory treatment plans along with multiple workups for the same symptoms. Comorbid anxiety and depressive symptoms are common, as are conduct or substance-related disorders.

Conversion Disorder

Definition

Conversion disorder is defined by the presence of one or more neurological symptoms that cannot be medically explained after thorough investigation (Table 8–3). DSM-IV-TR also specifies that symptoms must be associated

Table 8–3.   DSM-IV-TR diagnostic criteria for conversion disorder

A. One or more symptoms or deficits affecting voluntary motor or sensory function that suggest a neurological or other general medical condition.

B. Psychological factors are judged to be associated with the symptom or deficit because the initiation or exacerbation of the symptom or deficit is preceded by conflicts or other stressors.

C. The symptom or deficit is not intentionally produced or feigned (as in factitious disorder or malingering).

D. The symptom or deficit cannot, after appropriate investigation, be fully explained by a general medical condition, or by the direct effects of a substance, or as a culturally sanctioned behavior or experience.

E. The symptom or deficit causes clinically significant distress or impairment in social, occupational, or other important areas of functioning or warrants medical evaluation.

F. The symptom or deficit is not limited to pain or sexual dysfunction, does not occur exclusively during the course of somatization disorder, and is not better accounted for by another mental disorder.

Specify type of symptom or deficit:

    With motor symptom or deficit
    With sensory symptom or deficit
    With seizures or convulsions
    With mixed presentation

Source.   Reprinted from *Diagnostic and Statistical Manual of Mental Disorders,* 4th Edition, Text Revision. Washington, DC, American Psychiatric Association, 2000. Used with permission.

with psychological factors that include conflicts or other stressors preceding the development or worsening of the conversion symptom. As in other somatoform disorders, the symptom must not be consciously feigned and must produce clinically significant distress or impairment in functioning. The symptoms must also be viewed as abnormal within the individual's own culture.

The term *conversion* derives from the psychoanalytic concept that the somatic symptom is the result of an unconscious resolution of a psychological conflict—commonly a sexual or aggressive impulse—in which the mind "converts" psychological distress into a physical symptom. The resulting reduction in anxiety may explain in part the phenomenon of *la belle indifférence,* or the apparent lack of concern sometimes observed in patients with conversion disorder. *Primary gain* is obtained by keeping the conflict out of consciousness and minimizing anxiety. The symptom allows the partial expression of the forbidden wish, but in a disguised form, so that the patient does not need to consciously confront the unacceptable impulse. *Secondary gain* in the form of increased attention from caregivers or being excused from various pressures or responsibilities may also contribute to the development or continuation of conversion symptoms.

Epidemiology

Conversion disorder is the most common type of somatoform disorder in children and adolescents. In studies of pediatric patients, the incidence varies between 0.5% and 10% (DeMaso and Beasley 1998). Conversion disorder is three times more common in adolescents than preadolescents, and rarely occurs in children younger than age 5 years. Females tend to outnumber males in adolescence, but the ratio is more equal in younger children. Conversion disorder is more common in rural populations, among those from lower socioeconomic status, and in adolescents who are under pressure to perform in academic or athletic settings. The incidence of conversion disorder is also increased following physical or sexual abuse.

Clinical Features

Clinical features of conversion disorder are variable but include motor and sensory symptoms as well as loss of consciousness. Motor symptoms include abnormal movements, disturbances in gait, weakness, paralysis, and tremors. Sensory symptoms include anesthesia and paresthesia, commonly in one of the extremities, as well as deafness, blindness, and tunnel vision. Patients may also present with symptoms of seizures, referred to as *conversion seizures, pseudoseizures, nonelectrical seizures,* or *nonepileptic events.* Symptoms may be modeled after a parent or another important person in the child's life. The presenting symptoms usually do not conform to known physiological pathways or anatomic distribution; for example, sensory deficits may follow a "stocking-glove" distribution and end abruptly at the wrist or ankle. Symptoms may briefly disappear when the patient is distracted.

Table 8–4 lists some of the criteria that may be used to differentiate conversion seizures from epilepsy. The onset of conversion symptoms is generally acute. Individual conversion symptoms are generally short-lived, remitting within 2 weeks in most hospitalized patients (American Psychiatric Association 2000). Good prognostic factors include sudden onset, the presence of an

Table 8–4. Differential diagnosis of conversion seizures and epilepsy

Clinical features	Conversion seizures	Epilepsy
Electroencephalogram: ictal/interictal	Normal	Abnormal/variable
Duration	Often prolonged	Short
Pattern	Variable	Stereotyped
Frequency	Generally higher frequency	Paroxysmal/cluster
Occurring in the presence of others	Yes	Variable
Occurrence during sleep	Rare	Yes
Onset	Gradual	Sudden
Incontinence	Rare	Infrequent
Biting	Tongue	Cheek
Scream	During spell	At onset
Convulsion	Bizarre, thrashing, sexual movements	Tonic/Clonic
Injury	Infrequent, mild	Infrequent and severe
Pupillary reaction	Normal	Slow, nonreactive
Memory of seizure	Variable but sometimes intact	Usually amnestic
Orientation after event	Clear	Confused
Effect of suggestion or hypnosis	Precipitate or terminate	No effect
Effect of antiepileptic medications	Minimal	Decreased seizure frequency

Source.   Adpated from Maldonado and Spiegel 2001.

easily identifiable stressor, good premorbid adjustment, and absence of co-morbid medical or psychiatric disorders. Patients with conversion seizures have a poorer prognosis than those with paralysis or blindness. The recurrence of symptoms is not uncommon, occurring in 20%–25% of cases within 1 year (American Psychiatric Association 2000). Comorbid mood, separation, and other anxiety disorders are common. Stressful family events, such as recent divorce, current marital conflict, or death of a close family member are frequently seen with conversion symptoms (Wyllie et al. 1999). Estimates of the presence of concomitant epilepsy in patients with conversion seizures vary between 10%–58% (Chabolla et al. 1996).

Hypochondriasis

Definition

Hypochondriasis is a preoccupation with the idea that one has or may have a serious disease, despite medical reassurance. This preoccupation is based on the misinterpretation of physical symptoms or signs and is severe enough to cause clinically significant distress or functional impairment but is not of delusional intensity (American Psychiatric Association 2000). The disorder must last at least 6 months to meet DSM-IV-TR criteria (Table 8–5). In contrast to other forms of somatization, it is the significance attached to various symptoms, rather than the physical symptoms themselves, that produces distress.

Epidemiology

Although it is believed that hypochondriasis may have its onset during adolescence, the onset of symptoms is more common in early to middle adulthood, and men and women appear to be equally affected. As such, few data are available regarding the incidence or prevalence of hypochondriasis in children and adolescents. This may be due in part to the fact that children express their concerns via their parents, who are likely to be the main reporters of symptoms to medical providers. In adult patients, prevalence rates of 4%–6% have been reported in a general clinic population (Kaplan et al. 1994).

Clinical Features

Patients with hypochondriasis tend to present with a set of core symptoms that include a fear of disease, the conviction of having a disease, and bodily preoccupation or absorption associated with multiple somatic complaints

Table 8–5. DSM-IV-TR diagnostic criteria for hypochondriasis

A. Preoccupation with fears of having, or the idea that one has, a serious disease based on the person's misinterpretation of bodily symptoms.
B. The preoccupation persists despite appropriate medical evaluation and reassurance.
C. The belief in Criterion A is not of delusional intensity (as in delusional disorder, somatic type) and is not restricted to a circumscribed concern about appearance (as in body dysmorphic disorder).
D. The preoccupation causes clinically significant distress or impairment in social, occupational, or other important areas of functioning.
E. The duration of the disturbance is at least 6 months.
F. The preoccupation is not better accounted for by generalized anxiety disorder, obsessive-compulsive disorder, panic disorder, a major depressive episode, separation anxiety, or another somatoform disorder.

Specify if:

With poor insight: if, for most of the time during the current episode, the person does not recognize that the concern about having a serious illness is excessive or unreasonable

Source. Reprinted from *Diagnostic and Statistical Manual of Mental Disorders,* 4th Edition, Text Revision. Washington, DC, American Psychiatric Association, 2000. Used with permission.

(Folks et al. 2000). Patients often complain of poor relationship with their physicians and feelings of frustration and anger, and they are prone to "doctor shopping." Patients with hypochondriasis are particularly prone to somatosensory amplification and may experience significant secondary gain as a result of their ability to adopt the sick role. Complications may arise as the result of exposure to unnecessary treatments and procedures. Adolescents may manifest subclinical forms of the disorder—for example, they may have unrealistic concerns about having AIDS or cancer (Fritz et al. 1997). Hypochondriasis is commonly associated with both mood and anxiety disorders and has features in common with obsessive-compulsive disorder.

Body Dysmorphic Disorder

Definition

Body dysmorphic disorder, formerly known as dysmorphophobia, is characterized by an excessive preoccupation with a defect in appearance. This defect is either imagined or is too minor to warrant the degree of concern and dis-

Table 8–6. DSM-IV-TR diagnostic criteria for body dysmorphic disorder

A.   Preoccupation with an imagined defect in appearance. If a slight physical anomaly is present, the person's concern is markedly excessive.
B.   The preoccupation causes clinically significant distress or impairment in social, occupational, or other important areas of functioning.
C.   The preoccupation is not better accounted for by another mental disorder (e.g., dissatisfaction with body shape and size in anorexia nervosa).

Source.   Reprinted from *Diagnostic and Statistical Manual of Mental Disorders,* 4th Edition, Text Revision. Washington, DC, American Psychiatric Association, 2000. Used with permission.

tress felt by the individual. Symptoms cannot be better accounted for by another mental illness—for example, the concern with being overweight in a patient with anorexia nervosa (Table 8–6).

Epidemiology

Although there are no epidemiological data on pediatric patients, estimates of the prevalence of this disorder in adults range from 1.9% in a nonclinical sample to 12% in a sample of psychiatric outpatients (Allen and Hollander 2000). The onset of the disease is believed to most often occur during adolescence or early adulthood, although childhood cases have been reported. Patients may wait a mean of 6 years before seeking treatment (Phillips 1991). Unlike many other somatoform disorders, the ratio of men to women is nearly equal. Many people with the disorder do not seek psychiatric help, but rather seek treatment from dermatologists and plastic surgeons, which may influence efforts to study the psychological aspects of this disorder.

Clinical Features

Although any body part or aspect of physical appearance may be a source of concern and several body parts may be involved simultaneously, concerns generally focus on the patient's face or head (e.g., size or shape of the nose, eyes, lips, teeth, or other facial features; thinning hair or excessive facial hair; acne, wrinkles, or scars). The onset of the disorder is usually gradual because individuals with body dysmorphic disorder are intensely ashamed of their imagined defect and are often reluctant to discuss it, let alone seek psychiatric treatment. They may spend hours each day checking the defect, engage in excessive grooming or exercising to minimize or erase the defect, or even become housebound. This disorder shares much in common with obsessive-compulsive disorder. Both disorders are characterized by the presence of intrusive thoughts and repetitive behaviors as well as the need to seek reassurance. DSM-IV-TR, however, differentiates obsessive-compulsive disorder based on obsessions and compulsions that are not restricted to concerns about physical appearance. Those individuals with body dysmorphic disorder who are successful in obtaining surgery may continue to be concerned about the perceived defect or may shift the focus of attention to other aspects of their appearance (Phillips 1991). Substantial comorbidity exists between body dysmorphic disorder and depression, obsessive-compulsive disorder, social phobia, delusional disorder, anorexia nervosa, gender identity disorder, and narcissistic personality disorder. As many 20% of affected patients have been reported to have attempted suicide (Kaplan et al. 1994).

Assessment

The biological, psychiatric, and social dimensions need to be evaluated both separately and in relation to each other in all somatoform disorders (Richtesmeier and Aschkenasy 1988). Patients should have a complete and comprehensive medical workup to rule out serious medical illness, combined with an effort to avoid unnecessary and potentially harmful tests and procedures. Ideally, if somatization is suspected, psychiatric consultation should be included early in this workup process. Campo and Fritz (2001) noted that when somatization was presumed, the likelihood of subsequently discovering a previously undiagnosed physical disease is less than 10%. Nevertheless, certain physical illnesses are notoriously overlooked and should be carefully considered as part of the diagnostic workup (Table 8–7). It is also important to note that the presence of physical illness does not definitively exclude the possibility of pediatric somatization.

The psychiatric differential diagnosis includes mood, generalized anxiety, panic, separation anxiety, and obsessive-compulsive disorders. In addition, the presence of intentionally produced symptoms is not uncommon in somatization disorder; however, most symptoms are not consciously produced, as in either malingering or factitious disorders.

Referral by the medical team for psychiatric consultation is a difficult step for many families. These patients and families present with the belief that there is a medical cause for their problem. The most common response is for

Table 8–7. Selected medical differential diagnosis for somatoform disorders

AIDS	Lyme disease
Acquired myopathies	Migraine headaches
Acute intermittent porphyria	Multiple sclerosis
Angina	Myasthenia gravis
Basal ganglia disease	Narcolepsy
Brain tumors	Optic neuritis
Cardiac arrhythmias	Periodic paralysis
Chronic systemic infections	Polymyositis
Creutzfeldt-Jakob disease	Seizure disorders
Guillain-Barré syndrome	Superior mesenteric artery
Hyperparathyroidism	syndrome
Hyperthyroidism	Systemic lupus erythematosus

the family to react adversely and think that their child's symptoms are not being taken seriously. It is helpful for the primary care physician to frame the consultation as a routine part of a comprehensive work-up as well an opportunity to assess the level of stress connected with the current physical symptoms. The primary managing physician or medical team should not send the family away after consultation but rather communicate to the family that the psychiatric results will be integrated into their findings to obtain a more complete understanding of the child's symptoms. The psychiatric consultant must be prepared to address the same family concerns and to reassure the family that this does not mean that the medical workup has been abandoned.

Somatoform disorders are not diagnoses of exclusion. Table 8–8 provides a detailed outline for the psychiatric assessment of these disorders. Although no single element is conclusive, psychiatric and social factors may increase the likelihood of somatization (Fritz and Campo 2002). Particular factors to consider in the assessment include the presence of psychosocial stressors, comorbid depression or anxiety disorders, a history of somatization in the child or the parents, the presence of a model of illness behavior, and evidence of secondary gain resulting from the symptoms. Symptoms may not follow known physiological principles or anatomical patterns and may respond to suggestion or placebo. The possibility of sexual or physical abuse must be carefully investigated. Any comorbid psychiatric disorders must also be diagnosed and treated.

Table 8–8.   Key elements in the psychiatric assessment of pediatric somatoform disorder

Medical findings suggesting somatoform disorder

1. Absence of findings despite thorough medical workup
2. Inconsistent findings on examination
    Sensory changes inconsistent with anatomical distribution (e.g., splitting at the midline; loss of sensation of entire face but not scalp; discrepancy between pain and temperature sensation; absence of Romberg sign)
    Absence of functional impairment despite claims of profound weakness (e.g., impairment of fine motor function on testing, yet able to dress and undress)
    Face-hand test (deflecting falling arm from face)
    Hoover's sign (patient pushes down with "paretic" leg when attempting to raise unaffected leg and fails to press down with unaffected leg when raising "paretic" leg)
    Astasia-abasia (staggering gait, momentarily balancing, but never actually falling)
    Dragging a "weak" leg as though it were a totally lifeless object instead of circumduction of the leg
    Patients with psychogenic deafness responding to unexpected words or noises
    Tunnel vision
    Movement disorder with normal concurrent electroencephalogram
    Symptoms suggestive of conversion seizures (see Table 8–4).
    Increased symptoms in the presence of family or medical staff
    Periods of normal function when distracted
3. Relationship between onset of symptom and psychosocial stressor

Family beliefs regarding somatoform symptoms

1. Belief in a single undiagnosed primary medical cause
    Investment in further medical workup
    Fear about serious medical illness
2. Belief in the role of environmental triggers
3. Belief in the role of psychological factors
4. Beliefs regarding symptom management
    Awareness of nonpharmacological approaches
    Belief that the child should rest and be excused from usual responsibilities

History of childhood trauma

Family medical history

1. Family history of unexplained somatic symptoms
2. Pattern of reinforcement of illness behavior in the family

Table 8–8. Key elements in the psychiatric assessment of pediatric somatoform disorder *(continued)*

Impact of somatoform symptoms

1. Emotional (e.g., depression or anxiety vs. *la belle indifférence*)
2. Family (e.g., disruption of work schedule, impact on marital relationship, impact on distraction from family conflict)
3. Social and peer relationships
4. Academic (e.g., absenteeism, placement in home teaching)

Reinforcement of somatoform symptoms

1. Reinforcement by parents
      Medical journals and diaries of symptoms kept by parents
      Parent home from work
2. Increased attention from family/friends
3. Increased attention from medical providers
4. Avoidance of school, social, or athletic stressor

Video-electroencephalographic monitoring has been increasingly used to investigate seizure disorders. The lack of electrical evidence in the face of a seizure makes pseudoseizure or conversion disorder a likely diagnosis. Drug-assisted interviews (e.g., amobarbital, thiopental, or methohexital) have been found to be useful in some children and adolescents (Weller et al. 1985). Somatic symptoms may disappear transiently or even permanently after a drug-assisted interview.

Treatment

Table 8–9 outlines guidelines for a stepwise approach to developing an integrated medical and psychiatric treatment approach to somatoform disorders. The formulation of the problem is the crucial first step in treatment. Patients and their families present to their physicians with the belief that their symptoms are caused by a general medical condition. This view of the problem needs to be reframed from a narrow model view to a comprehensive biopsychosocial understanding. With completion of the psychiatric assessment, the consultant should begin by communicating the formulation to the medical team. In doing so, the consultant should be alert to the frustration engendered in physicians by these patients, whom they may feel are not "deserving"

Table 8–9.   Guidelines to a stepwise approach to developing an integrated medical and psychiatric treatment approach to somatoform disorders

1. Complete a psychiatric assessment
     Review histories, examinations, and studies by pediatrician and pediatric specialists
     Perform patient and family interviews
     Elicit diagnostic criteria
     Develop a developmental biopsychosocial formulation of the patient and family

2. Convey the biopsychosocial formulation to the pediatrician and medical team
     Remember that somatoform illness is not a diagnosis by exclusion
     Remember that symptoms can be in significant excess of what would be expected from the physical findings that are present
     Remember that physical findings may have accounted for early symptoms but may no longer be the etiology for the current symptoms

3. Convene an informing conference between the pediatrician and the family
     Convey integrated medical and psychiatric findings to family
     Because the family has a medical model as their frame of reference, help reframe this understanding of symptoms into a developmental biopsychosocial formulation

4. Implement treatment interventions in *both* medical and psychiatric domains
     Consider the following medical interventions:
     Set up ongoing pediatric follow-up appointments
     Physical therapy or other face-saving remedies may be added depending on symptoms

5. Consider the following psychiatric interventions:
     Implement cognitive-behavioral intervention
     Implement psychotherapy
     Implement family therapy
     Assess for the presence of target symptoms for psychotropic medications

Source.   Adapted from DeMaso DR, Beasley PJ: "The Somatoform Disorders," in *Clinical Child Psychiatry*, 2nd Edition. Edited by Klykylo WM, Kay JL. Indianapolis, IN, Wiley, 2005, pp 471–486. Used with permission.

of the sick role (DeMaso and Beasley 1998). Other reactions have included dismissing the patient as being "hysterical" or pursuing the "million dollar workup" (Stinnett 1987).

  After the formulation is accepted by the medical team, the next step is an "informing conference" that includes both the primary managing physician

Table 8–10.   Presenting the diagnosis of a conversion disorder

1.   Present objective evidence of absence of seizure activity associated with episodes.
2.   Explain the common reasons for seizure episodes (e.g., epilepsy, cardiac, and/ or emotional).
3.   Give the good news that the patient does not have epilepsy.
4.   Cite common examples of physical phenomena, such as fainting or hand sweating, that may be related to emotional arousal.
5.   Acknowledge the patient's suffering.
6.   Acknowledge the family's concern.
7.   Emphasize that the events are not under voluntary control.
8.   Explain that remote and recent events may contribute to the episodes, even if the patient is not feeling stressed.
9.   Emphasize the physically disabling nature of the events and the importance of prompt, intensive, and appropriate treatment.

Source.   Adapted from Chabolla et al. 1996.

and family (DeMaso and Beasley 1998). It is important in this meeting that the managing physician present the medical and psychosocial findings to the patient and the family in a supportive and nonjudgmental manner. If patients and their families believe that the primary physician understands and empathizes with the degree of distress the somatic symptoms have produced, then they are more likely to be active participants in treatment. Table 8–10 provides guidelines on how to present the diagnosis of a conversion disorder to the family, which may be modified for other types of somatoform disorders. The psychiatric consultant may or may not attend this meeting, depending on the comfort and expertise of the pediatrician.

Unfortunately, it is not uncommon for some families to remain resistant to mental health intervention. In these situations, the consultant can be helpful to the medical team by advising alternative ways in which they can decrease reinforcement for the sick role and lessen psychosocial stressors. The psychiatrist can also help advise regarding the needs for social service intervention in cases of parental or medical neglect, such as seeking multiple unnecessary medical procedures or failing to pursue necessary mental health treatment (DeMaso and Beasley 1998).

Once the family has accepted a new formulation of the problem, an integrated medical and psychiatric treatment approach should be developed (De-

Maso and Beasley 1998). In the treatment of somatization disorders, it is helpful to establish realistic goals that emphasize improvements in functioning rather than the illusion that the symptoms can be completely removed. This approach includes ongoing monitoring and treatment for possible physical illness by the pediatrician as well as the interventions by the mental health professional.

Role of the Primary Care Physician

Primary care physicians can schedule frequent, brief, and ongoing medical visits while avoiding unnecessary medical investigations and procedures. This arrangement allows the patient to receive attention from his or her doctor without having to develop somatic symptoms. This practice has been shown to reduce overall health care utilization and to improve patient satisfaction. Over time, the physician may learn more about the connections between psychosocial stressors and the patient's somatic complaints. It may be helpful for attention to be paid to the anxiety the patient experiences in relation to the physical symptoms rather than the symptoms themselves. Reassurance that a serious or life-threatening illness is not present is necessary but generally insufficient to alleviate the anxiety of the patient (Campo and Fritz 2001).

The Rehabilitation Model

A rehabilitative approach may be useful in the treatment of these patients. This perspective shifts the focus away from finding a cure for symptoms and instead emphasizes a return to normal functioning (Campo and Fritz 2001). The patient becomes an active participant in his recovery, which means that the sick role must be relinquished. Parents must be encouraged to view their child as capable, strong, and competent rather than passive, helpless, and fragile. Success is measured by the ability to return to school and the resumption of normal social and recreational activities.

Treatment approaches include the use of intensive physical and occupational therapy that emphasizes the recovery of function and offers face-saving remedies for the patient. Physical therapy may be particularly helpful in restoring function in cases of conversion disorder (Abbey 2005). This approach can be combined with a behavioral modification program, with incentives for improvements in functioning, while removing secondary gain for illness behavior. In severely disabled patients, it may be preferable to recommend admission to an inpatient treatment program that specializes in the treatment of somatoform disorders. Another useful option to consider is that of partial hospitalization. These approaches have the benefit of temporarily removing the child from the home environment, where the family may be playing an unwitting role in reinforcing the child's symptoms.

Cognitive-Behavioral Therapy

Treatment approaches that have included cognitive-behavioral interventions aimed at correcting distorted beliefs about the meaning of somatic symptoms have been shown to be effective. For example, cognitive-behavioral therapy has been used successfully in the treatment of both body dysmorphic disorder and recurrent abdominal pain (Allen and Hollander 2000). In cognitive therapy, attention is drawn to the factors that increase worries about health, including excessive focus on physical symptoms or the misinterpretation of these symptoms. Cognitive-behavioral therapy is generally more effective when combined with a package of multimodal treatment interventions. A variety of self-management strategies have been employed in treatment of somatoform disorders in children and adolescents, including relaxation training, self-hypnosis, and biofeedback (Campo and Fritz 2001). Hypnosis, which may be used as a diagnostic technique in conversion disorder, may be used as a treatment technique by providing the patient with a face-saving method of obtaining control over their symptoms (Maldonado and Spiegel 2000).

Psychotherapy

Both individual and family therapies have been found useful in the treatment of patients with somatization disorder and have resulted in reduced health care expenditures (Kaplan et al. 1994). Insight-oriented psychotherapy may have a role in the treatment of children with conversion disorder. Patients are encouraged to express their underlying emotions and to develop alternative ways with which to express their feelings of distress. Family therapy may be helpful in changing family members' views of the patient's physical impairment and helplessness. As they cease to see the somatizing patient as permanently or severely ill, parents and siblings may stop reinforcing illness behavior. Family therapy may reveal important family stresses or dysfunctional family dynamics that are relevant in terms of the etiology of the child's symptoms.

Psychopharmacology

There is little literature pertaining to pharmacological treatment of somatoform disorders in the pediatric population. Clinical experience suggests that mood and anxiety disorders will respond to medications even when somatization complicates the picture (Fritz et al. 1997). Although data are not available for pediatric patients, some adult studies suggest that antidepressants may be helpful with certain somatic symptoms, such as functional gastrointestinal disorders. Benzodiazepines may ameliorate distress and anxiety in anxious somatizing patients (Campo and Fritz 2001).

References

Abbey SE: Somatization and somatoform disorders, in Textbook of Consultation-Liaison Psychiatry. Edited by Rundell JR, Wise MG. Washington, DC, American Psychiatric Press, 1996, pp 369–401

Abbey SE: Somatization and somatoform disorders, in The American Psychiatric Publishing Textbook of Psychosomatic Medicine. Edited by Levenson JL. American Psychiatric Publishing, 2005, pp 271–296

Allen A, Hollander E: Body dysmorphic disorder. Psychiatr Clin North Am 23:617–628, 2000

American Psychiatric Association: Diagnostic and Statistical Manual of Mental Disorders, 4th Edition, Text Revision. Washington, DC, American Psychiatric Association, 2000

Barsky AJ, Goodson JD, Lane RS, et al: The amplification of somatic symptoms. Psychosom Med 50:510–519, 1988

Barsky AJ, Wool C, Barnett MC, et al: Histories of childhood trauma in adult hypochondriacal patients. Am J Psychiatry 151:397–401, 1994

Campo J, Fritsch S: Somatization in children and adolescents. J Am Acad Child Adolesc Psychiatry 33:1223–1235, 1994

Campo JV, Fritz G: A management model for pediatric somatization. Psychosomatics 42:467–476, 2001

Campo JV, Jansen-McWilliams L, Comer DM, et al: Somatization in pediatric primary care: association with psychopathology, functional impairment, and use of services. J Am Acad Child Adolesc Psychiatry 38:1093–101, 1999

Chabolla DR, Krahn LE, So El, et al: Psychogenic nonepileptic seizures. Mayo Clin Proc 71:493–500, 1996

DeMaso DR, Beasley PJ: The somatoform disorders, in Clinical Child Psychiatry. Edited by Klykylo WM, Kay JL, Rube DM. Philadelphia, PA, WB Saunders, 1998, pp 429–444

Folks DG, Feldman MD, Ford CV: Somatoform disorders, factitious disorders, and malingering, in Psychiatric Care of the Medical Patient, 2nd Edition. Edited by Stoudemire A, Fogel BS, Greenberg DB. Oxford, England, Oxford University Press, 2000, pp 459–476

Fritz GK, Campo JV: Somatoform disorders, in Child and Adolescent Psychiatry: A Comprehensive Textbook, 3rd Edition. Edited by Lewis M. Philadelphia, PA, Lippincott Williams & Wilkins, 2002, pp 847–857

Fritz GK, Fritsch S, Hagino O: Somatoform disorders in children and adolescents: a review of the past ten years. J Am Acad Child Adolesc Psychiatry 36:1329–1338, 1997

Garber J, Walker LS, Zeman J: Somatization symptoms in a community sample of children and adolescents: further validation of the children's somatization inventory. Psychol Assess 3:588–595, 1991

Gureje O, Simon GE, Ustun TB, et al: Somatization in cross-cultural perspective: a World Health Organization study in primary care. Am J Psychiatry 154:989–995, 1997

Hotopf M, Mayou R, Wadsworth M, et al: Childhood risk factors for adults with medically unexplained symptoms: results from a national birth cohort study. Am J Psychiatry 156:1796–1800, 1999

James L, Gordon E, Kraiuhin C, et al: Selective attention and auditory event-related potentials in somatization disorder. Compr Psychiatry 30:84–89, 1989

Jamison RN, Walker LS: Illness behavior in children of chronic pain patients. Int J Psychiatry Med 22:329–342, 1992

Kaplan HI, Sadock BJ, Grebb JA: Somatoform disorders, in Kaplan and Sadock's Synopsis of Psychiatry: Behavioral Sciences/Clinical Psychiatry, 7th Edition. Baltimore, MD, Williams & Wilkins, 1994, pp 617–631

Maldonado JR, Spiegel D: Medical hypnosis, in Psychiatric Care of the Medical Patient, 2nd Edition. Edited by Stoudemire A, Fogel BS, Greenberg DB. Oxford, England, Oxford University Press, 2000, pp 73–90

Maldonado JR, Spiegel D: Conversion disorder, in Review of Psychiatry, Vol 20. Edited by Phillips K. Washington, DC, American Psychiatric Publishing, 2001, pp 95–128

Mayou R, Levenson J, Sharpe M: Somatoform disorders in DSM-V. Psychosomatics 44:449–451, 2003

Minuchin S, Rosman BL, Baker L: Psychosomatic families: anorexia nervosa in context. Cambridge, MA, Harvard University Press, 1978

Phillips KA: Body dysmorphic disorder: the distress of imagined ugliness. Am J Psychiatry 148:1138–1149, 1991

Poikolainen K, Kanerva R, Loonqvist J: Life events and other risk factors for somatic symptoms in adolescence. Pediatrics 96:59–63, 1995

Poikolainen K, Aalto-Setala T, Tuulio-Henriksson A, et al: Predictors of somatic symptoms: a five year follow up of adolescents. Arch Dis Child 83:388–392, 2000

Richtesmeier AJ, Aschkenasy JR: Psychological consultation and psychosomatic diagnosis. Psychosomatics 29:338–341, 1988

Servan-Schreiber D, Kolb R, Tabas G: The somatizing patient. Prim Care 26:225–242, 1999

Shapiro CM: Alexithymia: a useful concept for all psychiatrists? J Psychosom Res 41:503–504, 1996

Stinnett JL: The functional somatic symptom. Psychiatr Clin North Am 10:19–33, 1987

Stoudemire A: Somatothymia. Psychosomatics 32:365–381, 1991

Stuart S, Noyes R: Attachment and interpersonal communication in somatization. Psychosomatics 40:3–43, 1999

Weller EB, Weller RA, Fristad MA: Use of sodium amytal interviews in pre-pubertal children: indications, procedure, and clinical utility. J Am Acad Child Psychiatry 24:747–749, 1985

Wyllie E, Glazer JP, Benbadis S, et al: Psychiatric features of children and adolescents with pseudoseizures. Arch Pediatr Adolesc Med 153:244–248, 1999

9

Pediatric Pain

The International Association for the Study of Pain defines *pain* as "an unpleasant sensory and emotional experience associated with actual or potential tissue damage, or described in terms of such damage" (Merskey and Bogduk 1994, p. 209). Although the experience of pain is universal, each person's experience is subjective and may be shaped by past experiences. For the psychiatric consultant, pain behavior generally represents an important clinical dilemma in which psychosocial factors and physical illness interact to varying degrees to determine a patient's individual pain experience. It is the consultant's goal to understand this interaction so that the pediatric team can develop and implement focused treatments designed to relieve, remove, or reduce a patient's suffering.

Classification

There are several ways to classify pain, including systems based on quality, duration, or etiology. Pain may be described as being nociceptive, neuropathic, or related to sympathetic overactivity (Table 9–1). Pain occurs when partial de-

Table 9–1. Classification of pain

Pain	Location of injury	Character of pain
Nociceptive pain		
Visceral	Hollow organs (bowel, bladder)	Dull, crampy, heavy, crushing, and poorly localized
Somatic	Skin, connective tissue, bone, muscle	Dull, heavy, crushing, sometimes worse with movement (bone pain)
Neuropathic pain/ Neuralgia	Primary lesion or disturbance to peripheral or central nervous system	Burning, electrical tingling, pricking, shooting, stabbing, itching, cold
		Allodynia (pain resulting from mild stimulation of normal tissue)
		Hyperalgesia (greater than expected pain from noxious stimulation)
		Hyperalgia (persistence of pain at primary or remote site)
Pain exacerbated by sympathetic activity (complex regional pain syndrome)	Autonomic dysfunction Association with nerve injury	Burning, allodynia, paresthesia, hyperalgesia to cold
		Signs of autonomic dysfunction (cyanosis, mottling, hyperhidrosis, edema, cooling of extremity)

struction or injury to the tissues adjacent to nerve fibers results in the release of chemicals such as neuropeptides. The quality of the pain experienced is related to the type of nociceptor activated. Activation of the cutaneous Aδ receptors that are myelinated and of large diameter leads to a pricking pain sensation. Activation of the cutaneous C receptors, which are thin and unmyelinated, results in pain with a dull or burning sensation. Activation of muscle nociceptors results in pain that has an aching quality. Acute pain signals injury and promotes action to prevent further damage and enhance healing. Repeated injury to nerve fibers may lead to a surge in nerve growth factor and sprouting of nerves in inappropriate locations leading to aberrant innervation and potentially lower pain thresholds.

Pain may be described as acute, recurrent, or chronic in nature. *Acute* pain generally refers to a discrete episode of pain with complete resolution. *Recurrent* pain refers to discrete episodes of pain that are generally of brief duration with complete recovery between episodes. For example, recurrent abdominal pain is defined as three or more episodes of abdominal pain severe enough to affect a child's activities over a period longer than 3 months, generally with complete recovery between episodes (Fritz et al. 1997). *Chronic* pain persists on a daily basis for longer that what would generally be expected for healing of the underlying physical pathology. It may or may not be associated with tissue damage. Chronic pain is often associated with depressed mood and the restriction of functional and physical activities. Both emotional and physical factors generally play an important role in chronic pain.

In DSM-IV-TR, psychological factors can play an important role in the onset, severity, exacerbation, or maintenance of pain as well as cause significant distress or functional impairment (American Psychiatric Association 2000). DSM-IV-TR divides pain disorders into 1) disorders associated with psychological factors in which emotional factors alone are judged to play a major role; 2) disorders associated with psychological factors and a general medical condition in which both together are deemed to have important roles; and 3) disorders entirely related to a general medical condition. The first two are coded as mental disorders on Axis I and the latter is coded on Axis III (Table 9–2).

Epidemiology

Between 25% and 44% of children and adolescents report somatic complaints such as pain and headaches that are generally transient in nature. Headaches and limb pains are more frequently seen in the 11- to 13-year age group, whereas older adolescents are most likely to report headaches, chest pain, and abdominal pain. Approximately 10%–20% of children younger than 10 years report recurrent headaches, and the frequency of migraine increases significantly after puberty, particularly in adolescent girls (Hämäläinen and Masek 2003). Complaints of recurrent abdominal pain complaints have been reported in 10%–25% of school-age children and adolescents and account for 2%–4% of pediatric office visits. The gender ratio is equal in early childhood, but girls are more symptomatic in later childhood and adolescence (Fritz and Campo 2002). Symptoms of pain also increase significantly in patients with underlying physical conditions. Approximately 25% of pediatric cancer patients report daily pain episodes, and pain is a common symptom in 60% of children with HIV (Galloway and Yaster 2000).

Table 9–2. DSM-IV-TR diagnostic criteria for pain disorder

A. Pain in one or more anatomical sites is the predominant focus of the clinical presentation and is of sufficient severity to warrant clinical attention.

B. The pain causes clinically significant distress or impairment in social, occupational, or other important areas of functioning.

C. Psychological factors are judged to have an important role in the onset, severity, exacerbation, or maintenance of the pain.

D. The symptom or deficit is not intentionally produced or feigned (as in factitious disorder or malingering).

E. The pain is not better accounted for by a mood, anxiety, or psychotic disorder and does not meet criteria for dyspareunia.

Code as follows:

307.80 Pain disorder associated with psychological factors: psychological factors are judged to have the major role in the onset, severity, exacerbation, or maintenance of the pain. (If a general medical condition is present, it does not have a major role in the onset, severity, exacerbation, or maintenance of the pain.) This type of pain disorder is not diagnosed if criteria are also met for somatization disorder.

Specify if:

Acute: duration of less than 6 months

Chronic: duration of 6 months or longer

307.89 Pain disorder associated with both psychological factors and a general medical condition: both psychological factors and a general medical condition are judged to have important roles in the onset, severity, exacerbation, or maintenance of the pain. The associated general medical condition or anatomical site of the pain (see below) is coded on Axis III.

Specify if:

Acute: duration of less than 6 months

Chronic: duration of 6 months or longer

Note: The following is not considered to be a mental disorder and is included here to facilitate differential diagnosis.

Table 9–2. DSM-IV-TR diagnostic criteria for pain disorder *(continued)*

Pain disorder associated with a general medical condition: a general medical condition has a major role in the onset, severity, exacerbation, or maintenance of the pain. (If psychological factors are present, they are not judged to have a major role in the onset, severity, exacerbation, or maintenance of the pain.) The diagnostic code for the pain is selected based on the associated general medical condition if one has been established (see Appendix G) or on the anatomical location of the pain if the underlying general medical condition is not yet clearly established—for example, low back (724.2), sciatic (724.3), pelvic (625.9), headache (784.0), facial (784.0), chest (786.50), joint (719.40), bone (733.90), abdominal (789.0), breast (611.71), renal (788.0), ear (388.70), eye (379.91), throat (784.1), tooth (525.9), and urinary (788.0).

Source.   Reprinted from *Diagnostic and Statistical Manual of Mental Disorders,* 4th Edition, Text Revision. Washington, DC, American Psychiatric Association, 2000. Used with permission.

Developmental Factors

There have been historic fears and misperceptions regarding the treatment of pain. These fears have included concern about causing drug addiction, doing harm (e.g., respiratory depression), giving the impression of giving up, and hastening the demise of a physically ill child as well as worry about diversion of medication to family members. Although young children may lack the vocabulary and sophistication to articulate their experiences of pain, they may demonstrate pain by social withdrawal or changes in their patterns of sleep and eating and in their level of activity. Infants as young as age 18 months will make efforts to localize pain and seek reassurance from adult figures, whereas 2-year-old children are able to use specific words to indicate the presence of pain. As the understanding of pediatric pain has grown, there is now recognition of the need to proactively address pain across the entire age spectrum.

Cognitive Theories Related to Pain

Piagetian stages of cognitive development are helpful in understanding the developmental issues related to a child or adolescent's experience of pain (Gaffney et al. 2003).

Preoperational

In the preoperational phase of development children are generally confused about the causes of pain and may view pain as a punishment for the real or imagined transgression of rules. They have a tendency toward magical thinking and may develop idiosyncratic explanations for their pain. Assessment of pain in this stage is complicated because young children do not have the ability for measurement of continuous qualities and tend to choose the end points of scales. Requests to imagine the "worst pain imaginable" are complicated because children in the preoperational phase cannot yet understand the abstract concept of possibility. In addition, they are generally not able to separate the physical and affective components of pain and differentiate pain from anxiety or fear until the age of 10–12 years. During this stage, children are not able to use self-generated coping strategies and tend to rely on their environment (i.e., the support of adults).

Concrete Operations

By age 7–8 years, children have more developed abilities for measurement, assessment, and seriation (the ability to accurately place items in ascending or descending order). The ability to seriate physical qualities of pain develops before children are able to differentiate the associated emotional components of pain. Children's understanding broadens during this phase to include awareness of associated negative affects. The capacity for increasingly logical thought processes leads to a greater understanding of pain, although children may still attribute pain to punishment. The ability to localize pain becomes more differentiated, and the ability to use self-initiated coping strategies such as distraction or guided imagery increases. Pain that limits school and physical activities may have particularly adverse effects at this stage because self-esteem is dependent on the child's ability to obtain mastery.

Formal Operations

Children enter the phase of formal operations around ages 11–14 years. Adolescents develop an increased capacity for abstract thought and introspection and become more aware of the psychological aspects of pain and its protective function. They may be increasingly able to differentiate the emotional aspects of pain and make use of behavioral interventions to reduce pain symptoms. However, the adolescent's greater ability to focus on future events may lead to greater worries and concerns about the recurrence of pain and disease and potential disabilities.

Measurement of Pain

Pain is measured by self-report, observation, or physiological measures. It is critical to use measures that are developmentally appropriate for assessment. Because direct report is not feasible with infants and younger children, it is often necessary to rely on observational reports from family members or the pediatric team.

Self-Report Measures

Self-report measures are generally valid for children as young as 4–5 years. These measures are usually combined with parent observations. Self-report measures are limited by difficulties in discriminating between intensity and duration and between the physical and emotional components of pain. It is important to also ask about physical sensations (i.e., heat, burning, or skin sensitivity that occur in neuropathic pain) that may accompany pain complaints. The following self-report measures have been used (Leo 2003; Figure 9–1).

Verbal Descriptor Scale

The verbal descriptor scale requires the child to rate the pain experienced according to one of five to seven verbal descriptors, with a limited range of options offered. The child must have adequate verbal skills and ability to use this scale, and its use may not be appropriate in younger children.

Numeric Rating Scale

With the widely used numeric rating scale, the child is asked to rate their pain on an 11-point scale anchored at one end by *no pain* (or 0) and at the other by *worst pain possible* (or 10). These ratings are reliable and correlate well with other simple assessment measures. The child must have intact language and cognitive skills.

Visual Analog Scale

Similar to the numeric rating scale, the visual analog scale consists of a line with descriptive or numerical anchors on a continuum of pain intensity, sim-

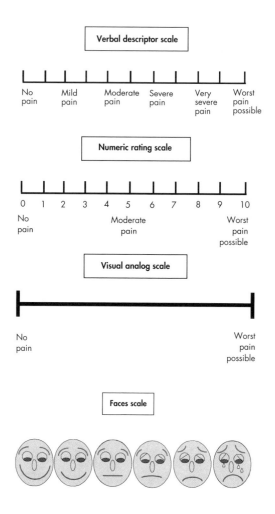

Figure 9–1.   Pain assessment instruments.

Source.   Reprinted from Leo RJ: "Evaluation of the Pain Patient," in *Concise Guide to Pain Management for Psychiatrists.* Washington, DC, American Psychiatric Publishing, 2003, p 52. Used with permission.

ilar to a Likert scale (Gaffney et al. 2003). The scale, anchored at one end by *no pain* (or 0) and at the other by *worst pain possible* (or 10), is presented to patients who are asked to describe their current pain by making a mark across the line. This scale is valid and reliable for children ages 8 years or older.

Faces Scale

The faces scale consists of six faces depicting different intensities of pain (Wong et al. 2001). It is a useful measure for children older than ages 6–8 years and is thought to be more direct and less complex than visual analog scales.

Pain Diary

Pain diaries may be used by older children and adolescents to report their pain experience at the time it occurs in order to avoid errors associated with retrospective recall. Pain diaries provide good baseline data prior to intervention and may include comments about functional ability, pain triggers, coping strategies, and medications used and their efficacy. Pain diaries may also be contrasted with parent reports of their child's pain.

Psychiatric Assessment

Psychiatric assessment may be requested when there is suspicion that the patient's symptoms or response to treatment have an emotional component. In approaching such referrals, it is important to avoid the dichotomy between a medical versus psychiatric etiology for the pain. Explanations of how emotional factors may exacerbate the child's experience of underlying physical pain are more successful in engaging the patient and family. It is important to validate the child's experience of pain and to explore the impact the pain has had on all members of the family. Sociodemographic, medical, treatment, situational, and psychological variables are key to understanding a child or adolescent's response to pain (Table 9–3).

Sociodemographic Variables

Pain responses have been noted to be associated with several sociodemographic variables, including the patient's age, gender, and ethnic background. Young children, for example, are more likely to experience distress during pain episodes or painful procedures partly due to their less mature coping skills (Schechter 2002). Firstborn children appear to have lower pain thresh-

Table 9–3.   Key elements in the psychiatric assessment of pediatric pain

Characteristics of pain

1. Location/radiation
2. Quality
3. Intensity
4. Duration and frequency (e.g., acute, recurrent, chronic, during procedures)
5. Level of distress and assessment of its relationship with severity of underlying etiology

Precipitating or exacerbating factors

1. Eating
2. Motion
3. Menstrual cycle
4. Stress
5. Bright lights
6. Lack of sleep/Fatigue

Alleviating factors

1. Distraction
2. Vomiting
3. Touch
4. Bathing
5. Heat
6. Cold

Use and efficacy of past and current treatment interventions

1. Pharmacological
   Types of medication used
   Schedule of medications (e.g., scheduled vs. as-needed dosing)
   Frequency of missed treatments (i.e., treatment adherence)
   Reasons for missed treatments
   Efficacy of previous treatment
   Side effects of treatment

Table 9–3.   Key elements in the psychiatric assessment of pediatric pain *(continued)*

2. Nonpharmacological
      Physical therapy
      Biofeedback
      Guided imagery
      Hypnosis
      Distraction

Impact of pain

1. Emotional (e.g., depression, anxiety, posttraumatic stress disorder)

2. Family (e.g., disruption of work schedule, impact on marital relationship, impact on siblings, distraction from family conflict)

3. Social and peer relationships

4. Academic (e.g., absenteeism, placement in home teaching)

Family beliefs regarding pain

1. Belief in single, undiagnosed primary medical cause for the pain
      Investment in further medical workup
      Unjustified concerns about potential medical illness

2. Belief in role of environmental triggers

3. Belief in role of psychological factors

4. Beliefs regarding pain control
      Awareness of pharmacological strategies
      Awareness of nonpharmacological approaches
      Belief that child should rest and be excused from responsibilities during pain episodes

Family medical history

1. Family history of unexplained somatic symptoms

2. Pattern of reinforcement of illness behavior in the family

Reinforcement of pain behaviors

1. Reinforcement by parents
      Medical journals and diaries of symptoms kept by parents
      Parent home from work

2. Increased attention or sympathy from family/friends

3. Increased attention from medical providers

4. Avoidance of school, social, or athletic stressor

olds, which may in part be due to greater reinforcement of pain complaints that may occur with first-time parents. Girls, especially as adolescents, generally report lower pain tolerance and a higher frequency of pain complaints compared with boys, a finding hypothesized to be related to cultural and societal variables (Dahlquist and Switkin 2003). Culture and ethnicity play an important role in determining how much expression of pain is acceptable.

Medical Variables

Pain duration and predictability as well as disease severity influence the experience of pain. Prior negative experiences with painful procedures are associated with more patient distress. It appears to be the adverse nature of the prior experience rather than the number of pain episodes that is of greater significance. Sleep deprivation affects pain perception and may interfere with efforts to divert attention from pain sensations. Similarly, increased muscle tension or protective posturing secondary to pain may increase the child's experience of pain.

Treatment Variables

The choice and dosage of pain medications prescribed can influence the pain experience. Suboptimal dosing or the use of "as-needed" medication for breakthrough pain rather than scheduled dosing can contribute adversely to the pain experience. Forgetfulness, lack of supervision, or nonadherence due to the patient's or the family's reluctance to take medications may play significant roles. The consultant should inquire about current or past use of nonpharmacological interventions.

Situational Variables

Children who lack age-appropriate information about their illness and its treatment are more likely to experience distress. This is particularly so when children have little perceived control over the treatment. Children need adequate preparation for procedures whenever possible and should receive instruction in effective coping methods (e.g., distraction techniques). Pain tolerance is negatively affected when there are inconsistencies in the procedure expected or in the response by pediatric staff or parents. It is important to ensure that the children have parental support during pain episodes and procedures.

Psychological Variables

Meaning of Pain

Children's knowledge, attitudes, and beliefs about their illness may influence their perception of pain and their response to treatment. Pain may be viewed as a punishment, a challenge, or in some cases as a character-building experience. Pain that is perceived as having little benefit or that is associated with potential disfigurement or disability is likely to be less well tolerated (Schechter 2002). Similarly, a child with a diagnosis of cancer may interpret pain as an indication of disease progression or relapse and experience increased anxiety or depression.

Personality Characteristics

Personality characteristics affecting the child's response to pain include the tendency to withdraw from others in response to pain, the ability to seek support, and coping style. For example, children with low adaptability tend to report more distress during painful procedures, and those with negative thinking or a tendency to catastrophize tend to report more psychological distress and need for medication. Patients may be classified based on their habitual tendency to approach or avoid new situations. Although there is no definitive coping style associated with adaptation to pain, the critical dimension appears to be whether the child has the freedom to use his or her own specific approach.

Stress

Pain is frequently correlated with stressful life events. School-related stressors (e.g., performance anxiety related to tests or sports), family stressors (e.g., deaths, abuse, divorce, or new siblings), and stressors related to the illness (e.g., immobilization or disfigurement) might all play important roles in the development or exacerbation of pain.

Psychiatric Comorbidity

Psychiatric comorbidity is common and often overlooked in children with pain, partly because of the difficulties making a psychiatric diagnosis in the physically ill child. Although depression may be secondary to the physical illness or its treatment, the presence of a depressive disorder increases the risk of developing chronic pain conditions. There is a strong relationship between pain and anxiety. Pain often results in symptoms of anxiety, and anxiety may decrease the pain threshold and increase the sensation of pain (Green and Kowalik 1994). The possibility of substance abuse is an important consideration in the adolescent age group. Patients with chronic recurrent pain (e.g., sickle cell crises) may be at risk of developing a dependence on narcotic medication that begins with benign use but evolves into a pattern of drug-seeking behavior.

Family Influences

Parents play an important role in both mediating and promoting the child's experience of pain, and there is a tendency for pain to aggregate in families. Parents with a history of multiple chronic pain symptoms are more likely to have children with impairment and disability. Parents who are more somatically focused are more likely to take medications for physical symptoms and may encourage their child's own pain complaints. The consultant should be alert to ways that parents wittingly or unwittingly might reinforce their child's pain behavior.

Secondary Gain

Pain symptoms may be promoted by secondary gain, which is the avoidance of a stressful or unpleasant situation. Pain behaviors may allow the child to remain home from school and avoid a stressful academic or social activity. Pain may provide the child with a legitimate excuse for dropping out of competitive sports. In families with high levels of dysfunction, pain may serve the function of diverting family attention away from a problematic conflict (e.g., marital problems) or provide a way for a parent to meet his or her own unresolved needs for attention through interactions with pediatric care providers or through sympathy and attention from friends and family members.

Principles of Pain Management

Principles of pain management are similar to those outlined for the treatment of the somatoform disorders (see Chapter 8). The first step is for the consultant to arrive at developmental biopsychosocial formulation of the problem (see Chapter 3). In particular, the consultant needs to determine the roles that psychological factors and the pediatric illness itself play in the pain experience. This formulation should be communicated to the patient, family, and pediatric team. The consultant can use the steps outlined in Table 9–4 for implementing an integrated medical and psychiatric treatment program. Depending

Table 9–4. Guidelines to developing an integrated medical and psychiatric treatment approach to pediatric pain

1. Complete a psychiatric assessment

   Use guidelines for the psychiatric assessment of pediatric pain (see Table 9–3)

   Develop a developmental biopsychosocial formulation of pain experience

   Determine contributing roles of emotional factors and the physical illness

2. Convey the biopsychosocial formulation to the pediatric team

   Remember symptoms can be in significant excess of what would be expected from the physical findings that are present

   Remember that physical findings may have accounted for early symptoms, but may no longer be the etiology for the current symptoms

3. Convene an informing conference between the pediatrician and the family

   Convey integrated medical and psychiatric findings to the family

   Because the family has a medical model as their frame of reference, help reframe this understanding of symptoms into a developmental biopsychosocial formulation

4. Implement treatment interventions

   Consider the following pharmacological interventions:

   Nonsteroidal anti-inflammatory drug

   Opioid

   Antidepressant

   Anticonvulsant

   Antiarrhythmic

   Clonidine

   Psychostimulants

   Antipsychotic

   Anxiolytic

   Topical anesthetic

5. Consider the following nonpharmacological interventions:

   Physical therapy

   Biofeedback

   Relaxation

   Guided imagery and hypnosis

   Transcutaneous electrical nerve stimulation

Table 9–4. Guidelines to developing an integrated medical and psychiatric treatment approach to pediatric pain *(continued)*

Operant interventions

Family therapy

Individual psychotherapy

Rehabilitation model

Source. Adapted from DeMaso DR, Beasley PJ: "The Somatoform Disorders," in *Clinical Child Psychiatry*, 2nd Edition. Edited by Klykylo WM, Kay JL. Indianapolis, IN, John Wiley and Sons, Inc., 2005, pp 471–486. Used with permission.

on the formulation of the pain experience, specific treatment recommendations fall into nonpharmacological and pharmacological categories.

The Rehabilitation Model

A subset of patients may develop symptoms of chronic pain with severe impairment in their level of functioning. The ongoing experience of pain can result in a sensitization of the nervous system that produces physiological and neuroanatomical changes. Disuse may lead to further pain and disability. The term *pain-associated disability syndrome* has been used to describe this presentation (Bursch et al. 2003). Patients may experience a downward spiral of increasing disability and pain in which acute symptom-focused treatment is not found to be helpful. A chronic illness model is required in which pain is accepted as a symptom that may not go away. This implies the decision to stop any further medical workup and instead focus on efforts to improve independent functioning and skill building to improve coping.

Adoption of a rehabilitation model frequently requires a large paradigm shift on the part of the patient and family. Explanation of the fact that the pain is "real" may seem in conflict with a decision to stop making inquiry about the symptoms. It is important to explain how biological and psychological factors interact with the child's social environment to influence pain and disability. Families may interpret the proposal to use nonpharmacological interventions as a statement that the child's pain complaints are only psychologically based. Specific goals of treatment are introduced that do not include the absence of pain. By contrast, progress is measured by changes in the child's level of adaptive functioning, including the ability to return to school and to resume normal social and recreational activities.

Nonpharmacological Management

Several principles are useful when developing a treatment intervention for pediatric pain that incorporates nonpharmacological approaches.

- Pain is a subjective sensation, and it is important to believe the child's experience of pain.
- Developmentally appropriate measures should be used to assess pain and the child's response to treatment.
- It is important to try to avoid the dichotomy between organic and nonorganic pain by assuming that both factors may be relevant.
- Treatment should be multimodal and multidisciplinary in nature and incorporate both pharmacological and nonpharmacological approaches.
- Nonpharmacological interventions can be helpful even with pain for which emotional factors make little contribution to the pain experience.

Education

Parents and family members often require education about treatment approaches for chronic pain. It is important to help the family differentiate the appropriate response of sympathy and attention during an episode of acute pain from responses that reinforce chronic pain behaviors. Parents may mistakenly believe that the child should be allowed to rest during pain episodes. Excessive attention to the child's pain symptoms may inadvertently encourage the child to scan his or her body for somatic cues and reinforce somatic vigilance. Parents need to learn how to acknowledge their child's pain but at the same time encourage the use of distraction and other active coping strategies. Other common misconceptions include the belief in a single, as yet undiagnosed, cause of pain as well as an inaccurate understanding of the interplay with stress or other psychological factors. Parents require education about the appropriate use of analgesia and possible misconceptions about addiction. Education about the secondary effects of inactivity and muscle tension may be helpful.

Physical Therapy

Physical therapy is used to increase flexibility and mobility as well as endurance and stamina. Stretching and massage may reduce muscle tension that is often a secondary cause of pain in patients with chronic pain. Physical therapy introduced in association with changes to the medication regimen, or following a nerve block, may allow the resumption of physical activities that have not been possible for many months, with the hope that these activities will be sustained after the block is discontinued (McCarthy et al. 2003).

Biofeedback

Biofeedback refers to the procedure in which physical parameters such as muscle tension or temperature are continuously monitored and fed back to the patient, who then attempts to alter the parameter. Although the measurement and control of physiological responses are usually not thought to be under voluntary control, biofeedback is based on the principle that it is possible to amplify and transform the response in such a way that it can be monitored and understood by the patient. Muscle tension and finger temperature are the most common physical functions measured in the treatment of pain. Biofeedback uses electrical equipment that allows the use of auditory and visual feedback from a physiological function (e.g., muscle contraction or relaxation). The patient's increased ability to monitor and control the muscle tension is then applied to controlling or altering the physiological process thought to cause the pain sensations (McGrath et al. 2003). For example, in the treatment of tension headaches associated with increased tension in the frontalis muscle, the patient is taught to reduce muscle tension in this muscle. Biofeedback results in an increased sense of mastery and control for patients (ages 6 years and older), who are generally enthusiastic and receptive to this intervention.

Transcutaneous Electrical Nerve Stimulation

Transcutaneous electrical nerve stimulation (TENS) units are used for localized pain, complex regional pain syndromes, and postoperative pain (McCarthy et al. 2003). Electrodes are placed around the painful region, along peripheral nerve routes, or at spinal segments. Electrical stimulation of large afferent A nerve fibers by the TENS unit is believed to inhibit pain transmission to the spinal cord that ordinarily occurs via the smaller-diameter nerve fibers, with the result that the child feels tingling and vibrating sensations rather than aching pain. It is also believed that TENS units may activate the release of endogenous opioids. Patients are trained on the use of TENS units during physical therapy sessions and then wear the unit at home and during normal activities, including school.

Cognitive-Behavioral Therapy

Progressive Muscle Relaxation

Several methods of progressive muscle relaxation are used to distract patients from their pain and to reduce subjective pain intensity. In the tension-relaxation method, the child is taught to constrict the muscles for 5–10 seconds and then relax specific muscle groups. This technique can be combined with suggestions of relaxation, heaviness, and warmth and images of relaxing situations. In the suggestion method, the patient is given repeated suggestions of calmness, relaxation, heaviness, and warmth combined with pleasant imagery, but without instructions to tense the muscles. With differential relaxation, the child learns to relax one part of the body while maintaining tension in other part. For example, in the treatment of a migraine the patient learns to relax the jaw and shoulders but keeps tension in arms and trunks in order to be able to continue school activities.

Guided Imagery and Hypnosis

Guided imagery and hypnosis, described in Chapter 16, are commonly used as part of a pain management intervention.

Behavior Modification

Behavior modification interventions are introduced when the target is not specifically the pain complaints but rather the associated pain behaviors, including the pain disability. Programs include incentives for improvements in functional ability and decreased attention to complaints of pain.

Psychotherapy

Individual psychotherapy can play an important role in helping change a child's erroneous cognitions about his or her ability to resume functioning. Encouragement of more adaptive coping strategies can become a focus of the therapy. It is helpful to explore potential sources of stress and gain understanding of the emotional factors that may perpetuate pain behaviors.

Family therapy is designed to help the family support healthy, functional behaviors and reduce support for pain behaviors. Treatment should also address family conflicts that may be causing stress for the child or interfering with efforts to cope with pain. Children with chronic pain may unconsciously use their symptoms to avoid stressful school or social situations or as a response to competitive athletic pressures. Parents similarly may receive secondary gain from their child's pain behavior—for example, by avoiding work or gaining increased closeness with their child. Illness behavior in general tends to promote or maintain maladaptive patterns of family interaction that need to be explored in family therapy. In addition, family members may experience feelings of frustration related to the disruption to family life caused by their child's pain. Families may harbor feelings of pessimism that no treatment will help, or they may fear the possibility of increased pain and disability. There may be strong feelings of anger directed toward health care providers. Therapy should be directed toward reducing feelings of anxiety and hopelessness and toward promoting active coping.

Pharmacological Management

Pharmacological measures include the use of nerve block procedures and epidurals to allow the child to begin physical therapy. Adjunctive pain medications and medications for anxiety or depression may also be required. By contrast, the decision may be made to wean patients from chronic, ineffective opioid regimens by using blinded pain cocktails. This section summarizes the common pharmacological agents used in the treatment of pediatric pain (Table 9–5).

When using analgesic medications it is important to adopt a preventative approach to pain management by treating pain early and aggressively and by adhering to the following principles:

- Use scheduled rather than as-needed medications.
- Adopt an effective system for the assessment of pain and treatment response.
- Titrate one medication at a time.
- Initiate new medications at the lowest possible dosage.
- Slowly titrate every 3–7 days depending on medication and patient characteristics (e.g., age, prior experience with medications, other medications).
- Titrate to end point of maximal significant pain relief (>50%) or intolerable side effects, or toxic serum level for tricyclic antidepressants or mexiletine.

Table 9–5. Pharmacological agents used to treat pediatric pain

Drug		Route	Pediatric dosing	Important side effects
Nonsteroidal anti-inflammatory drugs	Aspirin	po	10–15 mg/kg every 4–6 hours	Antiplatelet effect, gastrointestinal upset, tinnitus, association with Reye's syndrome
	Ibuprofen	po	5–10 mg/kg tid–qid	
	Indomethacin	po/iv/pr	1–3 mg/kg bid–tid	
Acetaminophen		po/pr	20–30 mg/kg every 6 hours po	Hepatotoxic (massive overdosage)
			40–60 mg/kg every 6 hours pr	
Opiates	Morphine	iv	0.1 mg/kg every 2–3 hours	Nausea, vomiting, constipation, itching, sedation, respiratory depression/arrest, urinary retention
			0.02–0.03 mg/kg/hour for PCA	
	Meperidine	iv	1.0–3.0 mg/kg every 3–4 hours	Meperidine may cause tachycardia
	Fentanyl	iv	1.0–3.0 μg/kg every 1–2 hours	Fentanyl may cause bradycardia
	Codeine	po	0.5–1.0 every 4 hours	
	Hydromorphone	iv	0.05–1.0 mg/kg every 3 hours	
	Oxycodone	po	0.05–0.1 mg/kg every 4 hours	
Antidepressants	Amitriptyline	po	0.05–2 mg/kg/day	Anticholinergic side effects, autonomic side effects (orthostatic hypotension, sweating), electrocardiographic changes
	Nortriptyline	po	0.05–2 mg/kg/day	
	Venlafaxine	po	1–2 per day divided bid or tid	Headache, initial anxiety, sustained hypertension

Table 9–5. Pharmacological agents used to treat pediatric pain *(continued)*

Drug		Route	Pediatric dosing	Important side effects
Anticonvulsants	Carbamazepine	po	15–30 mg/kg divided bid–tid	Sedation, ataxia, dizziness, blood dyscrasias including aplastic anemia, hepatotoxicity
	Sodium valproate	po	10–60 mg/kg divided bid–tid	Sedation, blood dyscrasias, hepatotoxicity, weight gain, polycystic ovarian syndrome
	Gabapentin	po	5–30 mg/kg divided tid–qid	Somnolence, dizziness, ataxia, aggressive behavior
Membrane stabilizers	Lidocaine	iv	150 µg/kg/hour	Sedation, nausea
	Mexiletine	po	10–15 mg/kg divided tid	Sedation, fatigue, confusion, nausea, hypotension
Antihypertensive	Clonidine	po/td/ epidural infusion	0.05–0.2 µg/kg/hour	Sedation, hypotension, bradycardia, potential for rebound hypertension

Note. iv=intravenously; po=orally; pr=rectally; td=transdermally.
Source. Krane et al. 2003; Maunuksela and Olkkola 2003; Yaster et al. 2003.

- Continue chronic use only if significant pain relief, tolerable side effects, and increased activity and functioning of patient occur.
- Introduce polypharmacy only if the first medication produces only partial pain relief and higher dosage produces side effects.
- Supplement medication treatment with nonpharmacological interventions.

Nonsteroidal Anti-Inflammatory Drugs

The nonsteroidal anti-inflammatory drugs (NSAIDs), also referred to as *antipyretic analgesics,* include a large group of medications that are often first-line choices for all classes of pain. They are used in the treatment of rheumatoid arthritis, dental pain, bone pain, muscle pain, and menstrual cramps. They are particularly useful in trauma where swelling and inflammation play a role in producing pain. The mechanism of action involves inhibition of the cyclooxygenase and lipoxygenase enzyme pathways resulting in decreased production of the prostaglandins (specifically thromboxanes and leukotrienes) that result in inflammation and pain. Effects on platelet aggregation, gastric mucosa, and renal parenchyma bleeding may limit their use. NSAIDS have the benefit of not causing dependence or respiratory depression.

Acetaminophen

Acetaminophen, which is one of the most commonly prescribed analgesics for mild to moderate pain, appears to inhibit the cyclooxygenase enzyme pathway in the central nervous system. Given that it does not inhibit tissue prostaglandin synthesis or platelet aggregation, acetaminophen has no significant anti-inflammatory effect. There are no gastrointestinal or renal side effects analogous to the NSAIDs. Taken in excess, acetaminophen does have the potential to cause hepatotoxicity. Unlike the NSAIDS, the use of acetaminophen is not associated with Reye's syndrome.

Opioids (or Narcotics)

Opioid medications act centrally by binding with the central nervous system's opioid μ receptors. These receptors are subdivided into the μ_1 receptors, which cause supraspinal analgesia, and the μ_2 receptors, which cause respiratory depression, inhibition of gastrointestinal motility, and spinal analgesia.

Opioids mimic the action of endogenous opioids to inhibit the release of pain neurotransmitters. Opioids produce analgesia, respiratory depression, euphoria, and physical dependence. Data support the safety and effectiveness of opioids in the treatment of infants, children, and adolescents with moderate to severe pain (Yaster et al. 2003).

Opioids are classified based on their strength and their duration of action. Short-acting opioids include fentanyl, morphine, and meperidine and long-acting opioids include methadone, codeine, and oxycodone. Codeine and oxycodone are commonly used for moderate pain in association with NSAIDs. Morphine, meperidine, and fentanyl are more effective for severe pain. Because of its relatively brief duration of action, fentanyl is useful for short, painful procedures.

Patient-controlled analgesia (PCA) is a pain-control system that uses a computerized pump to deliver pain medication at predetermined dosages when the patient pushes a button (Ferrante et al. 1990). PCA has been found to be effective in children as young as 1 year of age (Yaster et al. 2003). PCA results in immediate pain relief and provides the child with a greater sense of control over their pain. It has been used for postsurgical recovery, cancer pain, flares of inflammatory diseases, sickle cell crises, and burn pain in children as young as age 6 or 7 years.

Side effects common to all opioids include decreased gastrointestinal motility with constipation and nausea, itching, sedation, respiratory slowing, and at high dosages respiratory arrest (Table 9–6). Because the immature blood-brain barrier is permeable to morphine, children younger than age 3 months require 25% of the traditional dosage. Physical dependence occurs with all opioids within 7 days and may result in patients having to be weaned, with a reduction in dosage by 10%–20% per day.

Antidepressants

As noted previously, there is a clear relationship between pain and depression. Tricyclic antidepressants (TCAs) and serotonin-norepinephrine reuptake inhibitors (SNRIs) have been used as adjuncts in the pharmacological treatment of pain, with most of the data derived from studies of adult patients (Ansari 2000; Carter and Sullivan 2002; Krane et al. 2003). Although there has been interest in the use of the selective serotonin reuptake inhibitors, they have generally not been found to be as effective in pain treatment, with the excep-

Table 9–6. Management of side effects of opiates

Side effect	Treatment intervention	Route	Dosage	Side effects
Nausea Vomiting	Metoclopramide	iv	1–2 mg/kg	Sedation, fatigue, confusion, headache, extrapyramidal symptoms
	Promethazine	iv, im	0.25–0.5 mg/kg qid	Blurred vision, confusion, urinary difficulties, dry mouth, nervousness
	Dolasetron	po, iv	1.8 mg/kg (100 mg max)	Diarrhea, headache
	Lorazepam	po, iv	2–6 mg/day bid/tid	Ataxia, dizziness, drowsiness, slurred speech
Constipation	Docusate sodium	po	>12 years, 50–360 mg/day <12 years, 50–150 mg/day	Stomach/intestinal cramps, allergic reactions
	Milk of magnesia	po	80 meq single dose	Diarrhea, polydipsia, stomach cramps
	Lactulose	po	10 g in 120 mL of water	Diarrhea, stomach cramps, gas
	Senna	po	>12 years, 15 mg/day <12 years, 5–10 mg/day	Electrolyte and fluid imbalance, nausea/vomiting, stomach cramps
	Bisacodyl	po	>12 years, 10–15 mg single dose 6–12 years, 5 mg single dose	Diarrhea, cramps
	Magnesium citrate	po	80 meq single dose	Diarrhea, stomach cramps
Pruritus	Diphenhydramine	po, iv	12.5–25 mg qid	Drowsiness, delirium, thickening of bronchial secretions
	Hydroxyzine	po, iv	>6 years, 50–100 mg/day <6 years, 50 mg/day	Drowsiness, thickening of bronchial secretions

Table 9–6. Management of side effects of opiates *(continued)*

Side effect	Treatment intervention	Route	Dosage	Side effects
Pruritus *(continued)*	Fexofenadine	po	>12 years, 60 mg bid <12 years, 30 mg bid	Headache, coughing
Sedation	Adjust dose Change opioid Adjust schedule to normalize sleep-wake cycle Avoid other sedating medications Change route of administration			

Note.   bid = twice a day; iv = intravenously; po = orally; qid = four times a day; tid = three times a day.

tion of one recent trial of citalopram to treat recurrent abdominal pain in pediatric patients (Campo et al. 2004).

Tricyclic Antidepressants

In most studies, TCAs have been found to be superior to placebo in the treatment of pain (Carter and Sullivan 2002). Evidence suggests that TCAs have a direct analgesic effect that is separate from their efficacy in treating depression or insomnia. Different mechanisms have been suggested, including increased availability of serotonin, endogenous opioid peptide release, and a direct action on opioid receptors (Gray et al. 1998). TCAs may also potentiate the action of opioids, allowing a reduction in chronic opioid requirements. The effect of TCAs on pain reduction and improved sleep is more rapid (3–7 days) at lower dosages (0.1–0.2 mg/kg/day) than is expected in the treatment of depression.

Amitriptyline is one of the most widely studied TCAs and has been found to be effective in a wide range of pediatric pain syndromes, including migraine, peripheral neuropathies, phantom limb pain, fibromyalgia, and pain related to the invasion of nerves by tumors. Studies have emphasized the helpfulness of even low dosages as well as benefit from the drug's sedation. Nevertheless, there is no theoretical or empirical basis to suggest that amitriptyline has any unique efficacy in pain management compared with other TCAs. Where sedation is problematic or the patient is particularly susceptible to anticholinergic side effects, imipramine and nortriptyline are alternate considerations.

TCAs may have anticholinergic side effects including dry mouth, constipation, blurred vision, urinary retention, confusion, and delirium. Autonomic side effects include orthostatic hypotension, profuse sweating, palpitations, tachycardia, and high blood pressure. Electrocardiographic changes include flattened T-waves; prolonged QT, QRS, and PR intervals; and depressed ST segments. Electrocardiographic monitoring is recommended at baseline and after the patient has been stabilized at a therapeutic dosage (see Chapter 15).

Serotonin-Norepinephrine Reuptake Inhibitors

There has been increasing interest in the SNRIs, including venlafaxine and duloxetine, which some authors have suggested are at least as effective as the TCAs and with fewer side effects (Goldstein et al. 2004). Venlafaxine has been used effectively in the treatment of adults with headache, neuropathic

196 Clinical Manual of Pediatric Psychosomatic Medicine

pain, fibromyalgia, diabetic peripheral neuropathy, and reflex sympathetic dystrophy (Kiayias et al. 2000).

Anticonvulsants

Carbamazepine, clonazepam, and phenytoin have been widely used in the treatment of migraine and neuropathic pain, and divalproex sodium has been used for migraine prophylaxis. Newer agents such as topiramate and lamotrigine have been used for diabetic neuropathy and trigeminal neuralgia. Anticonvulsants have certain drawbacks, including the potential to cause behavioral changes and the requirement for serum level monitoring because of their narrow therapeutic window (see Chapter 15). Table 9–7 lists the anitconvulsants used for pain management.

Gabapentin is one of the most promising agents used to treat neuropathic pain associated with postherpetic neuralgia, post-poliomyelitis neuropathy, complex regional pain syndrome, phantom limb pain, and diabetic/HIV neuropathy (Krane et al. 2003). Gabapentin has fewer side effects and fewer drug interactions than other anticonvulsants and does not require serum level monitoring. Gabapentin appears to be helpful in reducing spontaneous paroxysmal pain with burning and lancinating quality as well as allodynia to cold and tactile stimuli.

Membrane Stabilizers

Membrane-stabilizing agents have been used to enhance the efficacy of opioids, antidepressants, and anticonvulsants. Lidocaine and mexiletine are thought to act through a sodium channel binding mechanism. Lidocaine is used as an adjunct medication for mucositis pain related to chemotherapy agents, refractory cancer pain, and neuropathies and to predict the potential efficacy of mexiletine. In a lidocaine test for tolerance, lidocaine is administered over 30 minutes by continuous infusion with close electrocardiographic and blood pressure monitoring. The infusion is stopped if the patient develops drowsiness or dysarthria or intolerable side effects such as tinnitus, dysphoria, dysrhythmias, or seizures. A reduction in pain during the lidocaine test suggests that mexiletine, the oral analogue of lidocaine, may be useful in longer-term treatment of the patient's pain symptoms (Krane et al. 2003). Mexiletine's most common side effects include nausea, vomiting, sedation, confusion, diplopia, and ataxia. Verapamil has been used to treat migraines and cluster headaches.

Table 9–7. Use of anticonvulsants for pain management

Drug	Mechanism of action	Pharmacology	Adverse effects	Clinical applications
Carbamazepine	Inhibits norepinephrine uptake Prevents repeated discharges in neurons Blocks sodium channels	Slow absorption Protein bound Hepatic metabolism Urinary excretion t½ = 10–20 hours	Sedation, nausea, diplopia, vertigo, hematological abnormalities, jaundice, oliguria, hypertension, acute left ventricular heart failure Monitor complete blood count and liver function tests	Diabetic neuropathy Trigeminal neuralgia
Oxcarbamazepine	Prevents repeated discharges in neurons Binds to sodium channels Increases potassium conductance	Metabolized to 10-monohydroxy metabolite with t½ = 9 hours	Dizziness, somnolence, diplopia, fatigue, ataxia, nausea, abnormal vision, hyponatremia	Trigeminal neuralgia Neuropathic pain syndromes
Topiramate	Blocks sodium channels Inhibits calcium channels Potentiates GABA-ergic inhibition	Rapid oral absorption t½ = 21 hours 70% eliminated unchanged in urine	Kidney stones, somnolence, dizziness, ataxia, paresthesias, nervousness, abnormal vision, weight loss, cognitive slowing	Migraine headaches Neuropathic pain Diabetic neuropathy

Table 9–7. Use of anticonvulsants for pain management *(continued)*

Drug	Mechanism of action	Pharmacology	Adverse effects	Clinical applications
Gabapentin	Possible increase in total brain concentration of GABA	Not metabolized Not protein bound Renal excretion t½=5–7 hours	Somnolence, dizziness, ataxia, fatigue, concentration difficulties, gastrointestinal disturbance, nystagmus, pedal edema	First-line drug for pain management Complex regional pain syndrome Postherpetic neuralgia Diabetic neuropathy Phantom limb pain Multiple sclerosis Possible use for inflammatory pain
Lamotrigine	Blocks sodium channels Inhibits glutamate release Modulates calcium and potassium currents	Complete oral absorption 98% bioavailability t½=24 hours Hepatic metabolism Drug–drug reactions with other anticonvulsants	Dizziness, nausea, headache, ataxia, diplopia, blurred vision, somnolence, Stevens-Johnson syndrome	Complex regional pain syndrome Trigeminal neuralgia Spinal core injury Multiple sclerosis Central poststroke pain
Levetiracetam	Reduces high-voltage calcium currents Opposes inhibition of GABA Affects potassium conductance	Rapid oral absorption t½=7–11 hours Renal excretion No hepatic metabolism	Somnolence, asthenia, dizziness, depression, nervousness	Migraine prophylaxis Postherpetic neuralgia Neuropathic pain

Table 9–7. Use of anticonvulsants for pain management *(continued)*

Drug	Mechanism of action	Pharmacology	Adverse effects	Clinical applications
Pregabalin	GABA analogue Increases neuronal GABA concentration	90% oral bioavailability t½=6 hours 99% excreted unchanged in urine	Dizziness, somnolence, headache	Diabetic neuropathy Postherpetic neuralgia
Zonisamide	Blocks sodium and calcium channels, facilitates serotonin and dopamine transmission Increases GABA release	100% oral bioavailability t½=60 hours Renal excretion	Somnolence, ataxia, anorexia, difficulty with concentration, agitation, headache, Stevens-Johnson syndrome	Neuropathic pain Migraine headaches

Note. GABA=γ-aminobutyric acid; t½=drug half-life.
Source. Adapted from Hayes K: "Adjuvant Treatments," in *The Massachusetts General Hospital Handbook of Pain Management,* 3rd Edition. Edited by Ballantyne JC. Philadelphia, PA, Lippincott, Williams & Wilkins, 2006, pp 127–140. Copyright 2006, Lippincott, Williams and Wilkins. Adapted with permission.

Clonidine

Clonidine, an α_2-adrenergic agonist, has been used in the treatment of diabetic neuropathy and postherpetic neuralgia. Intrathecal clonidine has also been used to reduce muscle spasms in patients with spinal cord injuries. Clonidine may work both peripherally and centrally by increasing conduction of potassium. Clonidine is generally considered a second-line drug after antidepressants and anticonvulsants, but it does have some unique advantages, such as its transdermal route of administration. Its sedative effect may also be advantageous. Side effects include hypotension and sedation. Abrupt cessation may result in rebound hypertension and nervousness.

Psychostimulants

Psychostimulant medications are believed to have antinociceptive properties that may be mediated by norepinephrine, serotonin, dopamine, or endogenous opioid mechanisms. Indications for psychostimulants include reduction of drowsiness caused by narcotic medications as well as the potential to reduce the dosage of narcotics without diminution of the analgesic effect. Methylphenidate and dextroamphetamine have been found to be safe and effective adjuncts to opiate analgesia and have also been used in the treatment of spasmodic torticollis, spastic colon, and headaches.

Antipsychotic Agents

Antipsychotic agents have been used in the treatment of many chronic pain syndromes, including cancer, arthritis, migraine, neuropathy, and phantom limb pain. The mechanism of action is unknown, but these medications may have a local anesthetic action in spinal nerves. Chlorpromazine and haloperidol have been used to treat nausea associated with the use of opiates or pain. However, ondansetron, a $5\text{-}HT_3$ receptor antagonist, is still the first-line treatment for opioid-induced nausea and vomiting.

Anxiolytic Agents

Benzodiazepines do not have any direct analgesic action but may be useful in treatment of pain by reducing comorbid symptoms of anxiety and insomnia. Benzodiazepines may also decrease pain by reducing muscle spasm. Anxiolytics may be useful as a premedication to alleviate anticipatory anxiety and to cause anterograde amnesia when prescribed at adequate dosages. Short-term use of benzodiazepines can be effective in postoperative pain and sickle cell crises. Hydroxyzine similarly may have an application in the augmentation of opioids in sickle cell crises.

Topical Anesthetics

EMLA, a formulation of lidocaine and prilocaine under an occlusive dressing, has been used to provide anesthesia to a skin depth of 2–4 mm to reduce pain from needle procedures. EMLA needs to be applied 1 hour prior to the procedure to provide anesthesia. Tetracaine applied as gel or cream has a more rapid onset of action than EMLA and causes vasodilatation, which may be an advantage during blood draws. Vapocoolant spray has also been used to reduce the pain from injections. Capsaicin, derived from chili peppers, depletes substance P in small afferent neurons, and it has been used for diabetic neuropathy and postherpetic neuralgia. Capsaicin requires regular and multiple daily applications for a 3- to 4-week period. Its application may be limited by a burning sensation necessitating pretreatment with lidocaine cream.

References

American Psychiatric Association: Diagnostic and Statistical Manual of Mental Disorders, 4th Edition, Text Revision. Washington, DC, American Psychiatric Association, 2000

Ansari A: The efficacy of newer antidepressants in the treatment of chronic pain: a review of the current literature. Harv Rev Psychiatry 7:257–277, 2000

Bursch B, Joseph MH, Zeltzer LK: Pain-associated disability syndrome, in Pain in Infants, Children and Adolescents, 2nd Edition. Edited by Schechter NL, Berde CB, Yaster M. Philadelphia, PA, Lippincott Williams & Wilkins, 2003, pp 841–848

Campo JV, Perel J, Lucas A, et al: Citalopram treatment of pediatric recurrent abdominal pain and comorbid internalizing disorders: an exploratory study. J Am Acad Child Adolesc Psychiatry 43:1234–1242, 2004

Carter GT, Sullivan MD: Antidepressants in pain management. Curr Opin Invest Drugs 3:454–458, 2002

Dahlquist LM, Switkin MC: Chronic and recurrent pain, in Handbook of Pediatric Psychology, 3rd Edition. Edited by Roberts MC. New York, Guilford, 2003, pp 198–215

Ferrante FM, Ostheimer GW, Covino BG: Patient-Controlled Analgesia. Boston, MA, Blackwell Scientific, 1990

Fritz GK, Campo JV: Somatoform disorders, in Child and Adolescent Psychiatry: A Comprehensive Textbook, 3rd Edition. Edited by Lewis M. Philadelphia, PA, Lippincott Williams & Wilkins, 2002, pp 847–858

Fritz GK, Fritsch S, Hagino O: Somatoform disorders in children and adolescents: a review of the past 10 years. J Am Acad Child Adolesc Psychiatry 36:1329–1338, 1997

Gaffney A, McGrath PJ, Dick B: Measuring pain in children: developmental and instrument issues, in Pain in Infants, Children and Adolescents, 2nd Edition. Edited by Schechter NL, Berde CB, Yaster M. Philadelphia, PA, Lippincott Williams & Wilkins, 2003, pp 128–141

Galloway KS, Yaster M: Pain and symptom control in terminally ill children. Pediatr Clin North Am 47:711–746, 2000

Goldstein DJ, Lu Y, Detke MJ, et al: Effects of duloxetine on painful physical symptoms associated with depression. Psychosomatics 45:17–28, 2004

Gray AM, Spencer PS, Sewell RD: The involvement of the opioidergic system in the antinociceptive mechanism of action of antidepressant compounds. Br J Pharmacol 124:669–674, 1998

Green WH, Kowalik SC: Psychopharmacologic treatment of pain and anxiety in the pediatric patient. Child Adolesc Psychiatr Clin N Am 3:465–483, 1994

Hämäläinen M, Masek BJ: Diagnosis, classification, and medical management of headache in children and adolescents, in Pain in Infants, Children and Adolescents, 2nd Edition. Edited by Schechter NL, Berde CB, Yaster M. Philadelphia, PA, Lippincott Williams & Wilkins, 2003, pp 707–718

Kiayias JA, Vlachou ED, Lakka-Papadodima E: Venlafaxine HCl in the treatment of painful peripheral diabetic neuropathy. Diabetes Care 23:699, 2000

Krane EJ, Leong MS, Golianu B, et al: Treatment of pediatric pain with nonconventional analgesics, in Pain in Infants, Children and Adolescents, 2nd Edition. Edited by Schechter NL, Berde CB, Yaster M. Philadelphia, PA, Lippincott Williams & Wilkins, 2003, pp 225–240

Leo RJ: Evaluation of the pain patient, in Concise Guide to Pain Management for Psychiatrists. Washington, DC, American Psychiatric Publishing, 2003, pp 35–62

Maunuksela E-L, Olkkola KT: Nonsteroidal anti-inflammatory drugs in pediatric pain management, in Pain in Infants, Children and Adolescents, 2nd Edition. Edited by Schechter NL, Berde CB, Yaster M. Philadelphia, PA, Lippincott Williams & Wilkins, 2003, pp 171–180

McCarthy CF, Shea AM, Sullivan P: Physical therapy management of pain in children, in Pain in Infants, Children and Adolescents, 2nd Edition. Edited by Schechter NL, Berde CB, Yaster M. Philadelphia, PA, Lippincott Williams & Wilkins, 2003, pp 434–448

McGrath PJ, Dick B, Unruh AM: Psychologic and behavioral treatment of pain in children and adolescents, in Pain in Infants, Children and Adolescents, 2nd Edition. Edited by Schechter NL, Berde CB, Yaster M. Philadelphia, PA, Lippincott Williams & Wilkins, 2003, pp 303–316

Merskey H, Bogduk N (eds): Classification of Chronic Pain: Descriptions of Chronic Pain Syndromes and Definitions of Pain Terms, 2nd Edition. Seattle, WA, IASP Press, 1994, pp 209–214

Schechter NL: The development of pain perception and principles of pain control, in Child and Adolescent Psychiatry: A Comprehensive Textbook, 3rd Edition. Edited by Lewis M. Philadelphia, PA, Lippincott Williams & Wilkins, 2002, pp 404–413

Wong DL, Hockenberry-Eaton M, Wilson D, et al: Wong's Essentials of Pediatric Nursing, 6th Edition. St. Louis, MO, Mosby, 2001

Yaster M, Kost-Byerly S, Maxwell LG: Opioid agonists and antagonists, in Pain in Infants, Children and Adolescents, 2nd Edition. Edited by Schechter NL, Berde CB, Yaster M. Philadelphia, PA, Lippincott Williams & Wilkins, 2003, pp 181–224

10

Solid Organ Transplantation

Solid organ transplantation has evolved from an experimental surgical procedure to what is now an established part of pediatric medical care. Improved surgical techniques and the development of effective immunosuppressant medications, particularly the introduction of cyclosporine in 1983, have led to enhanced survival rates and improved medical outcomes. More sophisticated immunological subtyping has also led to decreased rates of organ rejection due to improved matches between donors and recipients.

The United Network for Organ Sharing (UNOS) was established in 1984 under the directorship of the U.S. Department of Health and Human Services to set the standards regarding transplant procedures and accreditation of transplant centers (United Network for Organ Sharing 2004). UNOS also directs the national Organ Procurement and Transplantation Network (OPTN) and the U.S. Scientific Registry on Organ Transplantation. It is responsible for the fair and equitable allocation and distribution of organs based on specific criteria that include organ type, tissue match, blood type, length of time on the waiting list, geographic location, and immune status (Slater 2002). UNOS collects data about all transplant procedures in the United States and maintains information regarding waiting lists and survival rates, which can be accessed through its Web site, http://www.optn.org.

Enhanced survival has led to an increased need to understand the psychological issues involved in organ transplantation for both recipients and their families. The initial focus of psychiatric consultation in organ transplantation was on screening potential recipients to determine whether they were eligible for transplant. Prediction of posttransplant adherence was of great interest, because failure to take immunosuppressant medications results in organ rejection and potential loss of life. A lack of a sufficient number of donors to meet the national demand for organs as well as increased attention to the medical economics associated with these costly and high-risk procedures have led to more scrutiny of the suitability of candidates identified as having a medical need for transplantation (Mai 1993). In addition to this focus on recipient suitability, psychiatric consultation has focused on posttransplant adjustment and health-related quality of life. Other questions posed to the consultant include those regarding informed consent, ethical dilemmas, developmental considerations, and management of pain and procedural anxiety.

Epidemiology

The greatest limiting factor in organ transplantation is the significant shortage of donated organs. The number of patients on the waiting lists for kidney and liver transplants in the United States has increased steadily over the past 5–10 years. An estimated 10%–15% of liver, heart, and lung transplant candidates die while on a transplant waiting list (OPTN 2006).

Patient and Graft Survival

Regardless of age, the 1-year patient survival rates for the recipients of transplanted organs are intestinal, 97%; kidney, 95%; heart, 87%; liver, 86%; and lung, 77% (OPTN 2006). In general, the survival rates for children are comparable with those of adult patients. Table 10–1 outlines survival rates for children and adolescents. Currently, heart, kidney, and liver transplants have better 5-year survival rates associated with them (63%–81% depending on recipient age and organ) than do intestinal and lung transplants (36%–54%).

Length of Waiting List and Time on the Waiting List

The number of patients on organ transplant waiting lists has more than doubled in the past 12 years, from 35,751 in 1994 to 95,070 in 2006 (OPTN

Table 10-1. Survival rates for pediatric organ transplantation, 2006

Organ	Child age (years)	1-Year survival	3-Year survival	5-Year survival
Heart	1–5	86.6	77.7	66.6
	6–10	89.4	82.9	70.6
	11–17	87.2	78.0	66.4
Liver	1–5	75.2	77.8	66.2
	6–10	81.7	76.5	73.8
	11–17	84.7	70.9	63.8
Intestine	1–5	62.1	41.1	41.4
	6–10	77.3	73.1	53.6
	11–17	73.7	50.0	—*
Kidney	1–5	91.6	86.89	81.1
	6–10	95.0	88.89	81.0
	11–17	93.8	79.9	66.9
Lung	1–5	100.0	46.2	41.9
	6–10	87.5	55.4	31.6
	11–17	71.2	47.7	36.0

*Graft survival not computed because $N < 10$.
Source. From OTPN 2006.

2006). This continued growth in waiting list sizes, as well as the long wait times for listed transplant candidates, highlights the critical shortage of donor organs. Time spent on the waiting list is affected by several factors, including organ type, recipient blood type, and severity of the recipient's illness at the time of listing. The national shortage of cadaveric donors has led to the use of living related donors for kidney and liver transplantation and, in rare cases, for lung transplantation.

Pretransplant Psychiatric Assessment

Most of the literature on psychosocial assessments of patients prior to transplant has focused on adults. These evaluations are used to help determine a candidate's psychosocial eligibility for transplant as well as to identify psychiatric issues that need to be addressed before and after transplantation. These assessments have been particularly emphasized in candidates with histories of alcohol or substance abuse, obesity, poor adherence, or other problematic health care behaviors.

In contrast to work with adult patients, there has generally not been the same emphasis on routine use of pretransplant psychosocial evaluations in the pediatric literature (Shaw and Taussig 1999). This is surprising given that several pediatric transplant studies have documented psychological difficulties and family dysfunction among transplant candidates (DeMaso et al. 1995, 2004). A variety of reasons likely underlie this lack of emphasis, including the shortage of trained child mental health professionals with the necessary skills to conduct these assessments and difficulties in obtaining adequate reimbursement for these services. In a pretransplant evaluation (Table 10–2) the psychiatric consultant evaluates both the child and the family with the goal of identifying psychosocial risk factors and psychopathology that are likely to be associated with poor posttransplant adjustment or treatment nonadherence.

Problems that may be anticipated in pediatric transplantation include those related to isolation from peers, the need for frequent medical follow-up, adherence to treatment, enforcing limitations on physical activity, and sibling reactions (House 2000). In light of this, it is helpful to identify factors that have the potential to interfere with the parents' ability to provide adequate emotional and medical support. This is particularly relevant in younger transplant recipients for whom the burden of the medical care falls most heavily on parents.

Beginning the Pretransplant Assessment

Clarify Evaluation Expectations

It is important for the consultant and the transplant program to have a mutual understanding of the purpose of the pretransplant evaluation. A clinician from the transplant team should clearly explain to the child and family the purpose of the assessment. It is important to state explicitly whether the evaluation will be used to determine the patient's suitability for transplant as well as to clarify with the family who has ultimate decision-making responsibility regarding transplantation.

Anticipate Family Reactions

When the consultant is viewed as a member of the transplant team, families are generally very accepting of the assessment. The consultant is in a position to frame his or her role as a source of patient support throughout the transplant process and as someone who can assist the family with developmental

Table 10–2. The pediatric pretransplant psychiatric assessment

Understanding of illness and expectations of transplant

1. Understanding of illness
2. Understanding of surgery process
3. Understanding of posttransplant treatment expectations
4. Cognitive issues affecting comprehension of illness and treatment (cognitive impairment, mental retardation, stage of cognitive development)
5. Motivation for transplant
6. Anxieties about transplant surgery
7. Attitude toward transplant donor
8. Attitude toward having a transplanted organ (e.g., gender, ethnicity)
9. Anxieties about posttransplant treatment
10. Posttransplant goals

Past psychiatric history

1. Psychiatric comorbidity
2. History of outpatient psychiatric treatment
3. History of psychiatric medications
4. History of psychiatric hospitalizations
5. History of risk-taking behaviors

Substance abuse history

1. History of alcohol, substance, and nicotine use
2. Previous history of substance abuse treatment
3. Legal problems related to substance abuse

Family issues

1. Family psychiatric illness
2. Family history of alcohol or substance abuse
3. Marital conflict
4. History of domestic violence
5. Involvement with Child Protective Service agencies
6. Presence of social support
7. Work issues (e.g., work schedule, work flexibility)
8. Financial issues (e.g., financial resources, insurance coverage)

Table 10–2. The pediatric pretransplant psychiatric assessment *(continued)*

Treatment adherence

1. Past history of treatment adherence
   Medications
   Appointments
   Laboratory tests
   Diet
   Exercise
2. Family support for treatment
   Family availability to provide supervision of treatment
   Presence of family conflict or disagreement affecting treatment

Relationship with medical providers

1. Relationship of family with medical providers (e.g., trust, confidence, anger, feelings of entitlement)
2. Previous experiences with medical providers

Previous hospital experiences

1. Prior history of traumatic medical experiences
2. Prior history of procedural anxiety
3. Prior history of difficulties with pain management
4. Coping styles utilized during stressful procedures

issues, management of pain and anxiety, and general adjustment. The consultant can also play an important role in facilitating communication between the family and the medical team. The consultant should be alert to helping the family process their reactions to the child's diagnosis of a serious and potentially life-threatening illness. It is important for the consultant to keep in mind that anxiety may influence the way family members respond during the pretransplant assessment. It is common for both patients and parents to have difficulties integrating the large amount of information that is given to them during this time period.

Provide Feedback to the Family

It is important for the consultant to provide feedback to the transplant team. This should include not only a written report but also a face-to-face meeting to allow for discussion of issues and recommendations raised. The consultant's formulation and recommendations should be communicated directly to the patient and family. In some cases, the consultant and transplant team together may develop a written family contract to help minimize any potential confusion or misinterpretation on the part of the patient and the family. This contract may include techniques to assist the child in preparation for painful and stressful procedures, recommendations for mobilizing family supports and resources, or interventions to address factors that may prejudice the transplant outcome.

Be Alert to Developmental Issues

It is important to assess the patient's level of cognitive and emotional development and to anticipate the relevant developmental vulnerabilities that may affect the transplant process. For example, preschool-age children with immature cognitive abilities may interpret invasive procedures as a punishment for perceived past misbehavior and may be unable to comprehend abstract concepts such as the finality and irreversibility of death. Developmental issues in adolescence include possible concerns about medication side effects, including growth retardation, hirsutism, breast enlargement, weight gain, and delayed development of secondary sex characteristics. Children and adolescents may need advice on ways to explain their transplant when they return to school so that they are prepared to respond to possible queries and misconceptions from peers.

Consider Cognitive and Developmental Assessments

Assessment of cognitive functioning is important for several reasons. Many patients with end-stage renal, liver, and cardiac diseases have cognitive and academic delays resulting from their illnesses (DeMaso 2004). For example, patients with hepatic encephalopathy may present with a constellation of symptoms that includes cognitive impairment, confusion, disorientation, and affective dysregulation (DiMartini et al. 2005). Complex cyanotic cardiac lesions are associated with significant cognitive, developmental, and neurological abnormalities (DeMaso 2004). Such cognitive and developmental difficulties may affect the patient's ability to understand the transplant process or follow the lifelong treatment requirements.

Understanding and Expectations of Transplantation

The consultant should assess the child's and the family's understanding and expectations of the transplant. It is important to determine whether the patient and family are competent to give assent and consent for the transplant process. Both cognitive and emotional issues can interfere with family members' abilities to assimilate information and fully understand the implications of the proposed transplant. Prior to the psychiatric evaluation, the family should have met with the transplant team and received a thorough explanation of the transplant process. The consultant should assess the patient and family's response to and understanding of this information as well as their motivation to undergo transplantation and participate in the long-term care that will be required.

Psychiatric Comorbidity

The finding of DeMaso et al. (2004) that pretransplant emotional functioning is correlated with posttransplant emotional functioning emphasizes the importance of identifying comorbid psychosocial problems prior to transplantation. Body image and self-esteem concerns are common in children with chronic physical illnesses and take on particular relevance in adolescents, for whom peer issues and social acceptance are of special importance (Wallander and Thompson 1995). It is important to recognize that emotional and behavioral problems have been related to poor treatment adherence. Given the apparent high prevalence of emotional problems in transplant recipients, identification of psychiatric disorders before transplant can afford the consultant an opportunity to be helpful in treating, mitigating, or even preventing problems after transplantation (DeMaso et al. 2004).

Substance Abuse

Although less prevalent than among adult transplant candidates, substance abuse is a risk factor to consider for adolescent transplant candidates. Pretransplant histories of alcohol, tobacco, or other substance abuse, as well as a family history of substance misuse, are associated with a greater risk of posttransplant substance abuse. These same factors have been shown to be associated with greater postoperative complications, more hospital admissions, and lower quality of life after transplantation (Shapiro et al. 1995). In the presence of substance abuse, the consultant should attempt to estimate the patient's potential for rehabilitation as well as his or her risk for relapse. Transplant programs commonly require a defined period of abstinence that may range from 6 to 24 months prior to listing for transplant (House 2000).

Family Issues

The pretransplant psychiatric assessment should include a family psychiatric history, history of substance abuse in the family, and assessment of general sibling adjustment. The consultant should assess the family's available social support network. Transplantation generally results in frequent medical appointments, unexpected complications, lengthy hospitalizations, and invasive procedures that are disruptive to family functioning. Families with poor social support, lack of adequate parental supervision, or poor patterns of communication are particularly at risk for poor treatment adherence after the transplant surgery (Schweitzer and Hobbs 1995). Inquiring about the potential impact of the hospitalization on the parent's employment may help to identify potential issues prior to surgery.

Treatment Adherence

Adherence to prescribed treatment regimens, including cooperation with necessary procedural interventions, remains one of the most frustrating and problematic areas of transplant medicine (see Chapter 11). The consultant must estimate the patient's prior history of treatment adherence because past behavior appears to be the single best predictor of future adherence. For example, among those children who lose one kidney because of poor treatment adherence, 50% are likely to lose their second kidney for the same reason, even with psychosocial interventions (Fine et al. 1987).

Relationship With Care Providers

The likelihood of a successful transplant outcome is increased if there is trust and respect between the family and the transplant team. If the family perceives that their concerns are not being considered, there may be feelings of anxiety or anger that undermine the family's confidence in the transplant team and result in the family acting out through critical aspects of the treatment, including adherence. It is important to be aware of potential countertransference reactions on the part of the transplant clinicians (e.g., negative reactions toward adolescents who become candidates for liver transplantation after acetaminophen overdoses).

Prior Hospital Experiences

Knowledge of a family's previous experiences with inpatient hospitalizations can help identify potential areas of difficulty for the upcoming surgery. For example, children who have had to deal with multiple invasive and painful procedures or who have experienced excessive pain or anxiety during an earlier hospitalization may be at particular risk for having these difficulties during the transplant process. Conversely, the pretransplant evaluation may identify particularly successful coping strategies used during previous hospitalizations that may be helpful during the transplant process.

Living Donor Assessment

The number of living related organ donors has increased significantly in recent years because of the shortage of cadaveric donors. Survival rates of patients receiving living donor transplants are comparable with, if not in some instances superior to, survival rates of those receiving cadaveric transplants. Living organ donation does involve significant donor risks, including adverse medical events, financial expense, inconvenience, and negative psychological consequences (DiMartini et al. 2005). Although mortality rates among kidney and liver donors are less than 1%, up to 33% of these donors have significant medical complications (Brown et al. 2003). Possible psychological problems in living donor transplants include frustration with the shift in attention from the donor to the recipient postoperatively, feelings of hostility between the donor and the recipient, and a sense of indebtedness on the part of the recipient (House 2000). Psychiatric evaluation of the donor is often overlooked in pediatric transplant cases, unless there is severe donor psychopathology or doubt about the competency of the donor to give informed consent. Although it is rare to refuse a donor on psychological grounds, careful psychological assessment of the donor is recommended given the significant risks just delineated. This assessment should establish whether the donor is fully informed and able to provide consent and whether there is any evidence of family coercion (Table 10–3).

Transplant Process

The transplant process can be conceptualized as an interconnected series of phases of varying durations consisting of decision and preparation, listing and waiting, surgery and hospitalization, and posttransplant adjustment. Each phase has characteristic psychological challenges that must be faced by the patient, family, and transplant team.

Table 10–3.   Psychiatric assessment of the organ donor

1. Relationship of donor to potential recipient
2. Quality of relationship between donor and potential recipient
3. Donor understanding of transplant process and its effects (e.g., loss of a kidney)
4. Motivation of donor
   Ambivalence
   Feelings of guilt
   Family pressure
5. Presence of social support
6. Financial resources
7. Psychiatric comorbidity
8. Likely reactions in the event of organ rejection
9. Risks of communicable disease (e.g., sexual activity, drug use)

Decision and Preparation

The pretransplant assessment allows the consultant to assist the family in adjusting to the need and decision to go forward with an organ transplant. Parents commonly request assistance with ways to inform and prepare their child or adolescent for the transplant. Most transplant programs have preparation protocols that may include manuals, videotapes, or photographs that explain the transplant process. Many families find it helpful to hear the stories of successful transplant recipients, and some hospitals have programs in which new potential organ recipients have the opportunity to meet with patients and parents who have successfully gone through the transplant process. The transplant programs at Children's Hospital Boston and the Neuropsychiatric Institute at University of California–Los Angeles have collaborated on a Web site for parents facing organ transplantation. It contains both factual information and stories from patients and their parents. The site can be viewed at http://www.experiencejournal.com/transplant (DeMaso et al. 2006).

The consultant can use his or her knowledge of child development and the transplant process to help prepare the patient. In contrast to many parents' expectations, children generally do well with frank and open discussion of the need and reasons for transplant surgery. In younger patients, preparation begins with the parents being educated about the importance of being open, honest, and age-appropriate about the child's illness and treatment.

Parents can elect to speak with their child alone but more often choose to have a transplant team physician join them for the informing and preparation discussion.

Listing and Waiting

Listing for a transplant occurs after parents have given consent for the surgery. Listing generally heralds a period of enormous anxiety on the part of the patient and the family while they anticipate a donor organ becoming available. The wait between listing and surgery can extend from weeks to months or even years. During this period, the patient is at risk for acute medical decompensation as a result of events that include infection, stroke, and progressive organ dysfunction. Rates of delirium are elevated in patients waiting for transplant and may be overlooked unless the patient is carefully monitored. There is always the potential that a donor will not be identified in time to save the child's life.

In addition to these medical uncertainties, the waiting period is often characterized by a variety of psychosocial stressors for families. Parents may have strong feelings of guilt related to the knowledge that another child needs to die in order for their child to have a chance to live. There may be concerns regarding competition for organs as well as anger about the process of organ allocation. Children and adolescents are often hospitalized at transplant centers that are located far away from their home community. It is not unusual for families to be temporarily separated during the waiting period. These events can lead to significant emotional distress and potential conflict between parents as well as creating a situation in which the healthy siblings' emotional needs become neglected. Siblings can develop feelings of anxiety and resentment toward the ill child. Finally, there are generally unwelcome financial costs and burdens.

Surgery and Hospitalization

When families receive the call telling them that a donor has been found, the news is often greeted with both relief and anxiety. Families are relieved that the child's life may be saved but also acutely anxious about the transplant operation. After a common "honeymoon period of elation" following the transplant, the patient and his or her family members slowly begin to face the realities of living with a new chronic medical illness. Patients and families may be disappointed to find the need for continued isolation from school or a slow recovery after the surgery. The consultant can provide the patient and family with the opportunity to discuss and understand this process. The time immediately following the transplant surgery is when patients and families have the most interest in the child's donor and may make requests to find out more about the donor's identity. Feelings of sadness or guilt commonly arise in parents as their own child becomes more stable. Many recipients have found it helpful to write an anonymous letter of thanks to the donor's family (Strouse et al. 1996).

In the immediate postoperative period, the consultant must be alert to acute disabling mental status changes. The postsurgical recovery may be quite variable, with the potential for a number of acute serious medical events (Strouse et al. 1996). Delirium, with its fluctuating consciousness, confusion, and sleep disruptions, may be the result of sepsis, electrolyte imbalances, residual effects of general anesthesia, hypoxic episodes, immunosuppressants, or analgesic medications. Studies have found delirium of varying levels of severity in as many as 25%–50% of patients (House 2000). The consultant should be familiar with the side effects of the various immunosuppressant medications (Table 10–4). Neurotoxicity due to immunosuppressants can occur at any time after the transplant. Corticosteroids are well known for inducing mood lability, hypomania, and psychosis. These symptoms are more common with prednisone dosages greater than 40 mg/day. Headaches resembling classic migraines are increased in patients receiving cyclosporine. In addition, many of the immunosuppressant medications are associated with symptoms of depression and anxiety. Neurological symptoms include tremor, cerebral dysfunction, cortical blindness, dysarthria, and hemiplegia.

Posttransplant Adjustment

To understand and assess the impact of chronic physical illness on children and adolescents, researchers have increasingly broadened their focus from purely physiological concepts such as morbidity and mortality to include dimensions such as psychological and social functioning (Spieth and Harris 1996). There are four commonly accepted "core" health-related quality-of-life domains that are considered: disease state, functional status, emotional adjustment, and social functioning.

Table 10–4. Side effects of immunosuppressant medications

Immunosuppressant medication	Potential side effects
corticosteroids	*Central nervous system:* Increased intracranial pressure with papilledema (pseudotumor cerebri), seizures, vertigo, headache, psychosis, hypomania, mood lability, depression, cognitive impairment *Gastrointestinal:* Peptic ulcer, pancreatitis, abdominal distention, ulcerative esophagitis *Endocrine:* Menstrual irregularities, Cushingoid state, growth suppression, diabetes mellitus *Dermatological:* Impaired wound healing, thin fragile skin, petechiae, facial erythema, increased sweating *Ophthalmic:* Posterior subcapsular cataracts, increased intraocular pressure, glaucoma, exophthalmos *Electrolyte disturbances:* Sodium retention, fluid retention, congestive heart failure, hypertension *Musculoskeletal:* Muscle weakness, steroid myopathy, loss of muscle mass, osteoporosis, vertebral compression fractures, aseptic necrosis of femoral and humeral heads, pathologic fracture
cyclosporine (Gengraf, Neoral, Sandimmune)	*Central nervous system:* Tremor, restlessness, headache, acute confusional state, psychosis, speech apraxia, cortical blindness, seizures, coma *Gastrointestinal:* Diarrhea, nausea, vomiting, abdominal discomfort *Renal:* Renal dysfunction *Cardiovascular:* Hypertension *Hematological:* Lymphoma, leukopenia *Endocrine:* Gynecomastia *Dermatological:* Hirsutism, gum hyperplasia, acne
azathioprine (Azasan, Imuran)	*Gastrointestinal:* Nausea, vomiting, diarrhea, abdominal discomfort, hepatotoxicity, veno-occlusive disease *Hematological:* Leukopenia, thrombocytopenia, lymphoma *Dermatological:* Rash, alopecia

Table 10–4. Side effects of immunosuppressant medications *(continued)*

Immunosuppressant medication	Potential side effects
muromonab-CD3 (OKT3)	*Central nervous system:* Agitation, aphasia, cerebral edema, cerebral herniation, cerebrovascular accident, central nervous system infection or malignancy, cranial nerve VI palsy, encephalitis, hyperreflexia, involuntary movements, intracranial hemorrhage, impaired cognition, myoclonus, status epilepticus, stupor, transient ischemic attack, vertigo *Gastrointestinal:* Bowel infarction *Cardiovascular:* Cardiovascular collapse, hemodynamic instability *Renal:* Delayed graft function, renal insufficiency/renal failure occasionally in association with cytokine release syndrome *Hematological:* Aplastic anemia, disseminated intravascular coagulation, neutropenia, pancytopenia *Dermatological:* Erythema, flushing, Stevens-Johnson syndrome, urticaria *Special senses:* Blindness, blurred vision, deafness, diplopia, otitis media, nasal and ear stuffiness, papilledema
mycophenolate mofetil (CellCept)	*Central nervous system:* Agitation, convulsion, delirium, depression, emotional lability, hallucinations, neuropathy, paresthesia, psychosis, somnolence, vertigo *Gastrointestinal:* Anorexia, dysphagia, gastrointestinal hemorrhage, gingivitis, gum hyperplasia, jaundice, liver damage, mouth ulceration, nausea, vomiting *Cardiovascular:* Angina pectoris, arrhythmias, congestive heart failure, palpitation, postural hypotension, pulmonary hypertension, syncope *Renal:* Acute kidney failure, hematuria, urinary frequency, urinary incontinence, urinary retention *Endocrine:* Cushing's syndrome, diabetes mellitus, hypothyroidism, parathyroid disorder *Hematological:* Coagulation disorder, ecchymosis, pancytopenia *Dermatological:* Acne, alopecia, hirsutism, pruritus, rash, skin carcinoma, sweating, rash *Respiratory:* Apnea, asthma, epistaxis, hemoptysis, hiccup *Special senses:* Abnormal vision, deafness, tinnitus

Table 10–4. Side effects of immunosuppressant medications *(continued)*

Immunosuppressant medication	Potential side effects
tacrolimus (FK-506, Prograft)	*Central nervous system:* Tremor, restlessness, headache, insomnia, vivid dreams, hyperesthesias, agitation, cognitive impairment, dysarthria, delirium, focal neurological abnormalities, speech disturbances, hemiplegia, cortical blindness, seizures, coma, leukoencephalopathy (demyelination in parieto-occipital region) *Gastrointestinal:* Diarrhea, nausea, vomiting, abdominal pain *Cardiovascular:* Chest pain, hypertension *Hematological:* Anemia, leukopenia *Endocrine:* Cushing's syndrome, diabetes mellitus *Dermatological:* Acne, alopecia, exfoliative dermatitis, hirsutism, skin discoloration
sirolimus (Rapamune)	*Central nervous system:* Anxiety, confusion, depression, dizziness, emotional lability, hypesthesia, hypotonia, insomnia, neuropathy, paresthesia, somnolence *Gastrointestinal:* Anorexia, dysphagia, flatulence, gastritis, gum hyperplasia, ileus, liver function tests abnormal, mouth ulceration *Renal:* Bladder pain, dysuria, hematuria, nocturia, urinary incontinence, urinary retention *Cardiovascular:* Atrial fibrillation, congestive heart failure, hemorrhage, syncope, tachycardia, venous thromboembolism *Hematological:* Ecchymosis, leukocytosis, lymphadenopathy, thrombotic thrombocytopenic purpura (hemolytic-uremic syndrome) *Endocrine:* Cushing's syndrome, diabetes mellitus *Dermatological:* Hirsutism, pruritus, skin hypertrophy, skin ulcer, sweating *Musculoskeletal system:* Arthrosis, bone necrosis, leg cramps, myalgia *Special senses:* Abnormal vision, cataract, conjunctivitis, deafness, ear pain, otitis media, tinnitus

Medical Issues

Improvements in disease state and functional status are easily demonstrated following pediatric solid organ transplantation. Children who are no longer on dialysis have more time for age-appropriate academic and social activities. Similarly, heart transplant recipients are able to be home rather than in the hospital receiving continuous intravenous medications or cardiac support. Improvements in physical health after organ transplantation are associated with reduced hospitalizations, shorter lengths of stay, and decreased reliance on medications, all of which can facilitate improvements in emotional, family, and academic functioning

Despite clear medical benefits, the first year after transplantation is characterized by the need for close medical follow-up to monitor for potential organ rejection. It is a period of frequent appointments, regular biopsies and procedures, and multiple medication changes. It is generally a time of heightened anxiety as the patient is gradually reintroduced into peer and academic settings and the parents relinquish their heightened supervisory roles. Entrance into the second year generally heralds a reduction in the intensity and frequency of medical monitoring as well as a lessening of special attention and treatment for the patient.

Emotional Adjustment

Although solid organ transplant survivors are generally reported to have good physical and functional quality of life domains, the results regarding emotional adjustment are mixed. This variability in psychological functioning is likely reflective of limited research, particularly the paucity of longer-term or longitudinal follow-up studies. The incidence of psychological difficulties may also vary with the type of transplant. Pediatric kidney transplantation has been associated with improved overall emotional health, although there may be persistent difficulties with peer relationships and treatment adherence (Bursch and Stuber 2005). Although a majority of youngsters have healthy emotional functioning following heart transplantation, more than 25% present with significant emotional difficulties (DeMaso et al. 2004; Wray et al. 2001). Children with liver and lung transplants have been found to have psychosocial functioning similar to that of a normal population despite significant differences in physical functioning (Alonso et al. 2003; Hirshfeld et al. 2004). Pretransplant psychopathology and a lack of social support appear to increase the risk for psychopathology in transplant survivors (Dew et al. 2001). Pretransplant psychological dysfunction in either the child or the family has been correlated with poor posttransplant adjustment in heart transplant recipients (DeMaso et al. 1995; 2004). Conversely, patients with higher levels of perceived support, adaptive functioning, and quality of life prior to transplantation have improved rates of posttransplant survival (Trzepacz and DiMartini 1992). Children whose sense of self has been based on having a chronic physical illness may have significant difficulties leaving the "sick role" behind and adjusting to the new expected "healthy role" after transplantation (DiMartini et al. 2005). By contrast, patients who experienced acute medical decompensation prior to their transplant may have heightened denial and strong wish to resume normal functioning that may be associated with vulnerabilities to treatment nonadherence.

Academic Adjustment

Patients with chronic renal and liver disease, particularly those whose disease had an early onset, have been found to have delays in cognitive and motor functioning. Studies have shown that transplantation may lead to a recovery of some of these losses, although the degree of recovery may depend on the age at onset and duration of illness prior to transplant. Liver transplant recipients continue to have impairments in intellectual and academic functioning, learning, memory, abstraction, concept formation, visuospatial functioning, and motor skills following transplant (Stewart et al. 1991). Longer-term studies of pediatric liver transplant recipients have shown that patients may fail to make significant gains and tend to have lower levels of academic achievement in general (Kennard et al. 1999). Todaro et al. (2000) reported that following heart transplantation children functioned within the normal range on most measures of cognitive functioning, although a complicated transplant course may place the child at increased risk for cognitive difficulties. O'Brien et al. (1987) found that 80% of heart transplant patients required special school services for some period of time following transplant.

Together these findings outline the importance of the consultant investigating the academic functioning of all transplant recipients, particularly those with known or suspected central nervous system vulnerabilities. Early intervention and close liaison with schools is indicated to reduce psychological morbidity and enhance adaptation within the school environment (Wray et al. 2001).

Treatment Adherence

Nonadherence is estimated to occur in 20%–40% of transplant patients. Nonadherence is associated with acute and chronic rejection, graft loss, and death. It is also one of the most common reasons for late rejection in transplant recipients, suggesting that even the potential for a fatal outcome may not protect patients from failing to take their medications as directed. Further details regarding the issue of treatment adherence are given in Chapter 11.

References

Alonso EM, Neighbors K, Mattson C, et al: Functional outcomes of pediatric liver transplantation. J Pediatr Gastroenterol Nutr 37:155–160, 2003

Brown RS Jr, Russo MW, Lai M, et al: A survey of liver transplantation from living adult donors in the United States. N Engl J Med 348:818–825, 2003

Bursch B, Stuber M: Pediatrics, in The American Psychiatric Publishing Textbook of Psychosomatic Medicine. Edited by Levenson JL. Washington, DC, American Psychiatric Publishing, 2005, pp 761–786

DeMaso DR: Pediatric heart disease, in Handbook of Pediatric Psychology in School Settings. Edited by Brown RT. Hillsdale, NJ, Lawrence Erlbaum Associates, 2004, pp 283–297

DeMaso DR, Twente AW, Spratt EG, et al: Impact of psychologic functioning, medical severity, and family functioning in pediatric heart transplantation. J Heart Lung Transplant 14:1102–1108, 1995

DeMaso DR, Kelley SD, Bastardi H, et al: The longitudinal impact of psychological functioning, medical severity, and family functioning in pediatric heart transplantation. J Heart Lung Transplant 23:473–480, 2004

DeMaso DR, Marcus N, Kinnamon C, et al: Transplant Experience Journal: A Computer-Based Intervention for Families Facing Pediatric Organ Transplantation. July 2004. Available online at http://www.experiencejournal.com/transplant/. Accessed April 23, 2006.

Dew MA, Kormos RL, DiMartini AF, et al: Prevalence and risk of depression and anxiety-related disorders during the first three years after heart transplantation. Psychosomatics 42:300–313, 2001

DiMartini AF, Mew MA, Trzepacz PT: Organ transplantation, in The American Psychiatric Publishing Textbook of Psychosomatic Medicine. Edited by Levenson JL. Washington, DC, American Psychiatric Publishing, 2005, pp 675–700

Fine RN, Salusky IB, Ettinger RB: The therapeutic approach to the infant, child, and adolescent with end-stage renal disease. Pediatr Clin North Am 34:789–801, 1987

Hirshfeld AB, Kahle AL, Clark BJ, et al: Parent-reported health status after pediatric thoracic organ transplant. J Heart Lung Transplant 23:1111–1118, 2004

House RM: Transplantation surgery, in Psychiatric Care of the Medical Patient, 2nd Edition. Edited by Stoudemire A, Fogel BS, Greenberg DB. Oxford, England, Oxford University Press, 2000, pp 1051–1067

Kennard BD, Stewart SM, Phelan-McAuliffe D, et al: Academic outcome in long-term survivors of paediatric liver transplantation. J Dev Behav Pediatr 20:17–23, 1999

Mai FM: Psychiatric aspects of heart transplantation. Br J Psychiatry 163:285–292, 1993

O'Brien BJ, Buxton MJ, Ferguson BA: Measuring the effectiveness of heart transplant programmes: quality of life data and their relationship to survival analysis. J Chronic Dis 40:137S–158S, 1987

Organ Procurement and Transplantation Network (OPTN): Available at http://www.OPTN.org. Accessed April 23, 20056.

Schweitzer JB, Hobbs SA: Renal and liver disease: end-stage and transplantation issues, in Handbook of Pediatric Psychology, 2nd Edition. Edited by Roberts MC. New York, Guilford, 1995, pp 424–445

Shapiro PA, Williams DL, Foray AT, et al: Psychosocial evaluation and prediction of compliance problems and morbidity after heart transplantation. Transplantation 60:1462–1466, 1995

Shaw RJ, Taussig HN: The pediatric psychiatric pre-transplant evaluation. Clin Child Psychol Psychiatry 4:353–365, 1999

Slater JA: Psychiatric issues in pediatric bone marrow, stem cell, and solid organ transplantation, in Child and Adolescent Psychiatry: A Comprehensive Textbook, 3rd Edition. Edited by Lewis M. Philadelphia, PA, Lippincott Williams & Wilkins, 2002, pp 1147–1175

Spieth LE, Harris CV: Assessment of health-related quality of life in children and adolescents: an integrative review. J Pediatr Psychol 21:175–193, 1996

Stewart SM, Silver CH, Nici J, et al: Neuropsychological function in young children who have undergone liver transplantation. J Pediatr Psychol 16:569–583, 1991

Strouse TB, Wolcott DL, Skotzo CE: Transplantation, in Textbook of Consultation-Liaison Psychiatry. Edited by Rundell JR, Wise MG. Washington, DC, American Psychiatric Press, 1996, pp 641–670

Todaro JF, Fennell EB, Sears SF, et al: Review: cognitive and psychological outcome in pediatric heart transplantation. J Pediatr Psychol 25:567–576, 2000

Trzepacz PT, DiMartini A: Survival of 247 liver transplant candidates: relationship to pretransplant psychiatric variables and presence of delirium. Gen Hosp Psychiatry 14:380–386, 1992

Wallander JL, Thompson RJ: Psychosocial adjustment of children with chronic physical conditions, in Handbook of Pediatric Psychology, 2nd Edition. Edited by Roberts MC. New York, Guilford, 1995, pp 124–141

Wray J, Long T, Radley-Smith R, et al: Returning to school after heart or heart-lung transplantation: how well do children adjust? Transplantation 72:100–106, 2001

11

Treatment Adherence

Treatment adherence, or *treatment compliance,* has been defined as the "extent to which a person's behavior…coincides with medical or health advice" (Haynes 1979, p. 1–2). Nonadherence frequently results in increased rates of medical morbidity and mortality. The failure to follow through on prescribed medical treatments such as medications, diet, and laboratory monitoring is a common reason for psychiatric consultation in the pediatric setting. Problems with treatment adherence frequently arise in adolescents who have chronic illnesses such as diabetes mellitus or in organ transplant recipients who may have complex medication regimens or stringent requirements for medical monitoring or dietary restrictions (Smith and Shuchman 2005).

Epidemiology

Rates of treatment adherence vary widely depending on the nature of the medical condition, the type of treatment prescribed, and the criteria used to define adherence (La Greca 1990). Reviews of relevant studies suggest that 33% of patients with acute medical conditions and 50%–55% of those with chronic illnesses fail to adhere to their treatment regimens (Shaw et al. 2003).

Rates of adherence to medication are frequently higher than adherence to other treatment measures such as dietary restrictions for diabetes or physical therapy for cystic fibrosis. The complexities of treatment regimens appear to result in higher rates of nonadherence. Estimates of nonadherence are often based on patient report or provider estimates that likely underestimate the true rate of nonadherence.

Consequences of Nonadherence

Nonadherence with medical treatment may result in adverse consequences that include medical, financial, and quality-of-life outcomes.

Medical Outcomes

Studies have shown a direct relationship between nonadherence and morbidity and mortality in several chronic illnesses, including asthma and diabetes. Ettenger et al. (1991) found that two-thirds of adolescent renal transplant recipients failed to adhere to their immunosuppressant medications. Within this group, 15% experienced graft rejection and 26% had graft dysfunction. In adult patients, nonadherence has been cited as the third leading cause of graft loss after rejection and systemic infection (Didlake et al. 1988). In a study of heart transplant recipients, Cooper et al. (1984) reported that nonadherence accounted for up to 26% of deaths. Nonadherence in patients with infectious diseases such as tuberculosis or HIV is related to increased morbidity and to the emergence of drug-resistant infectious organisms. Finally, nonadherence can interfere with medical treatment decisions by leading physicians to misattribute treatment failures to ineffective treatment agents or by exposing patients to unnecessary diagnostic procedures.

Financial Outcomes

The increased morbidity associated with nonadherence has also been related to higher health care costs due to unnecessary or extended hospital admissions. A patient who loses a renal transplant may require hemodialysis, which imposes enormous costs on the health care system. Nonadherence can also burden family members who must miss work or incur childcare and transportation expenses. Berg et al. (1993) estimated that nonadherence costs the U. S. health care system as much as $100 billion a year.

Quality-of-Life Outcomes

Nonadherence affects the quality of life of both the child and other family members. The medical consequences of nonadherence can lead to decreased physical ability to participate in recreational and social activities. Children hospitalized for medical complications of nonadherence experience other negative consequences such as missing school, which frequently leads to lower academic performance.

Risk Factors

There has been fairly extensive research on the correlates of treatment adherence (see Table 11–1). The results of these studies have been used to identify subjects at particular risk and to develop treatment interventions (Rapoff 1999).

Patient Correlates

Several studies have established a relationship between treatment adherence and the presence of individual psychopathology. Behavioral and emotional problems, feelings of pessimism, and denial of the illness have all been correlated with poor adherence in patients with renal disease and diabetes (Brownbridge and Fielding 1994; Kovacs et al. 1992). Patients who are less knowledgeable about their disease also have lower rates of adherence (La Greca et al. 1990). Adolescent patients, especially those with comorbid psychiatric illness, are at particular risk. A patient's past record of adherence is one of the strongest predictors of current and subsequent adherence.

Family Correlates

Many studies have shown that adaptation to chronic illness is closely related to family functioning (Lorenz and Wysocki 1991). Greater family support, expressiveness, harmony, cohesion, empathy, organization, and good conflict resolution skills are all positive aspects associated with successful adaptation. By contrast, parental depression and anxiety have been correlated with poor adherence in children and adolescents with renal disease and seizure disorders (Brownbridge and Fielding 1994). Additional family variables associated with nonadherence include the presence of family conflict, lack of parental supervision and support, and problematic communication styles.

Table 11–1.   Risk factors associated with pediatric treatment nonadherence

Correlates	Risk factors
Individual	Past history of poor adherence
	Adolescence
	History of behavioral difficulties
	Past emotional difficulties
	Presence of denial regarding illness
	Lack of knowledge about disease
	Feelings of pessimism regarding illness
	Low self-esteem
	Internal locus of control
Family	Lack of parental supervision
	Parental conflict
	Parental psychopathology
	Poor family support
	Low socioeconomic status
	Lack of family cohesion
	Poor pattern of family communication
Disease	Long duration of illness
	Few or no symptoms
Treatment	Complexity of the treatment regimen
	Unpleasant medication side effects
	Low level of perceived efficacy of treatment
	High financial costs

Disease Correlates

Nonadherence is associated with diseases of long duration, and adherence has been found to decline over time in patients with diabetes and arthritis and following renal transplantation. Adherence may decline more frequently in patients who are asymptomatic, such as organ transplant recipients. Perceptions of disease severity may also influence adherence. Parental perceptions of higher disease severity are associated with higher rates of adherence, whereas patient perceptions of severity are negatively associated with adherence, possibly because of feelings of pessimism and hopelessness.

Treatment Correlates

Rates of adherence tend to be lower for illnesses with complex or difficult treatment regimens. Nonadherence is more likely when the treatments have unpleasant or cosmetic side effects, a particular issue for adolescent patients. Rates of adherence are higher for treatments that have a high level of perceived efficacy and for those that benefit the patient immediately and measurably. In lower-income families, treatment cost can negatively affect adherence.

Developmental Influences

Data from studies on treatment adherence suggest that specific developmental factors play an important role. Numerous studies have shown that difficulties with treatment adherence increase markedly during adolescence (La Greca et al. 1990). These findings may be understood by considering the developmental issues in adolescence that may directly interfere with an adolescent's ability to adapt to the diagnosis of a chronic illness. These issues include separation-individuation conflicts, difficulties with risk assessment, and peer group affiliations (Shaw 2001).

Separation-Individuation

The developmental task of separation-individuation is a core issue for adolescents that can result in parent–child conflict. There has been little empirical study of this issue in children with chronic illness, but clinical observations suggest that adolescents act out conflicts with their parents by overt or covert refusal to adhere to medications or treatment. Stein et al. (1999) suggested that some adolescents decide to limit or avoid treatment in an effort to reduce feelings of dependency on their parents.

Separation-Individuation and Treatment Adherence

Chronic illness can interfere with the adolescent's separation from his or her parents if it creates physical limitations or the need for increased levels of parental involvement due to the demands of treatment. A struggle around the medical treatment may result in overt nonadherence and treatment refusal. Other adolescents persistently maintain that they are fully adherent with their treatment despite clear medical evidence to the contrary. Lask (1994) classified these groups as either "refusers" or "deniers."

Response by Caretakers

Parental reactions to the diagnosis of a serious medical illness in their child can enhance the potential for conflict around adherence. Parents who experience guilt related to their child's illness may compensate for these feelings by failing to set limits on their child's behavior. This type of parenting can indirectly encourage acting-out behaviors such as nonadherence. Some parents of children with potentially life-threatening diseases such as leukemia or asthma respond with increased anxiety and hypervigilance. This anxiety often fosters overprotectiveness that clashes with the adolescent's need for autonomy.

Difficulties With Risk Assessment

Patients usually cannot accurately assess the risks of nonadherence. Child and parent perceptions of the seriousness of the child's health condition as well as maternal perceptions of risks related to nonadherence are related to treatment adherence (Riekert and Drotar 2000). Adolescents may be particularly prone to misjudging the consequences of medical nonadherence due to cognitive difficulties in assessing personal risk, lack of experience with the consequences of risk, ignorance, and denial (Brooks-Gunn 1993).

Cognitive Immaturity

Piaget's theory of cognitive development provides a model to understand the developmental issues that contribute to poor treatment adherence (Inhelder and Piaget 1958). Young adolescents are likely to employ concrete operations in making treatment decisions and to perceive only a narrow range of solutions to difficulties related to their treatment. Adolescents tend to ignore long-term consequences and make premature decisions when faced with the need to conform to family or peer pressures.

Adolescent Omnipotence

Adolescents often feel invulnerable, and this feeling can contribute to a sense that they are immune to the potential negative consequences of high-risk behavior (Elkind 1967). This observation has led to speculation that poor adherence to medical treatment may be based on the patient's belief that he or she can get away with failing to adhere to the prescribed treatment.

Cognitive Limitations

Cognitive limitations related to the illness or treatment can interfere with the adolescent's ability to assess risk. Many chronic illnesses, such as renal and liver failure, directly affect cognitive and academic functioning. In addition, medications such as anticonvulsants and immunosuppressants used to treat many chronic medical conditions may impair cognitive functioning.

Affiliation With the Peer Group

The adolescent's desire for acceptance and conformity with his or her peers often conflicts with treatment adherence (Brooks-Gunn 1993). Chronic illness carries a stigma, and the pressures for conformity may result in resistance to treatment recommendations, particularly those that have cosmetic side effects (Friedman and Litt 1987). For example, corticosteroid medications used in asthma and juvenile rheumatoid arthritis as well as organ transplantation may result in significant changes in physical appearance (e.g., weight gain) that are troubling to adolescents. To reduce the stigma of their illness, some individuals avoid taking their medications in front of their peers or stop taking them altogether (Conrad 1985).

Psychiatric Factors Affecting Adherence

Nonadherence is common among adolescents, but there is a smaller subset of physically ill adolescents who engage in severe risk-taking behaviors, including nonadherence, that indicate the presence of psychiatric comorbidity.

Mood Disorders

Depressed patients may forget or ignore their medical treatment or, in severe cases, intentionally miss medications as an expression of their hopelessness or suicidality. Studies of patients on renal dialysis have demonstrated an association between poor treatment adherence and depression and suicidal behavior (Brownbridge and Fielding 1994). Patients with terminal illnesses may also consciously refuse treatment when they judge that the costs of treatment outweigh the benefits.

Posttraumatic Stress Disorder

There are a number of studies that have found symptoms of medical posttraumatic stress disorder as a consequence of physical trauma and medical illness (Green et al. 1997). Shemesh et al. (2000) have shown that there may be a direct relationship between symptoms of posttraumatic stress and nonadherence in pediatric liver transplant recipients. Patients who desire to avoid stimuli that remind them of their medical illness may avoid their medications or medical appointments.

Parent–Child Conflict

Family function plays a crucial role in the adaptation of children and adolescents to chronic illness (Lorenz and Wysocki 1991). Numerous studies have shown a direct relationship between family conflict and treatment adherence (Christiaanse et al. 1989). Other family correlates of adherence include parental coping, family support, family cohesion, efficacy of family communication, and parental supervision of the medical treatment (Beck et al. 1980; Hauser et al. 1990). Parental support is critical to ensure adequate treatment adherence, and families with excessive levels of conflict are at particular risk for nonadherence.

Assessment of Treatment Adherence

To assess adherence, clinicians must evaluate the different components of the treatment regimen. Common components include medications, diet, exercise, and monitoring, such as blood glucose or drug assays. Assessment of adherence in pediatric patients is more complicated because of the parental supervisory role. When children are younger and their parents are exclusively responsible for the treatment, the evaluation should focus on parental behavior. With adolescents, the situation is more complex because responsibility is shared between the patient and the parents (Smith and Shuchman 2005). Table 11–2 presents guidelines for the clinical assessment of treatment adherence.

Treatment Interventions

Studies on the efficacy of treatment interventions for adherence in children with chronic illnesses have been limited by several factors. It is difficult to obtain adequately sized samples and to standardize the definitions and measurement of adherence. Many studies have been single-sample studies that help to delineate intervention models but cannot be easily generalized to patients with different illness types or demographics (Shaw et al. 2001). There are few data on long-term outcome secondary to difficulties in recruitment and retention of study subjects.

Table 11–2. Clinical assessment of pediatric treatment adherence

Treatment regimen

Describe the frequency and timing of each component of the prescribed treatment regimen:

1. Medications
2. Outpatient appointments
3. Laboratory tests
4. Monitoring (e.g., blood glucose)
5. Diet (e.g., diabetes diet, fluid restrictions)
6. Exercise

Patient's understanding of illness and treatment

Describe the patient's understanding of the illness and treatment regimen, including:

1. Understanding of illness
2. Understanding of treatment regimen
3. Understanding of consequences of nonadherence

Treatment protocol

Describe the system used by the patient and family for taking the prescribed treatment:

1. Where are medications kept?
2. Who is responsible for remembering the treatment?
3. What is the degree of family supervision of the treatment?
   Direct observation of treatment
   Parent dispenses or administers treatment
   Calls to remind patient
   Absence of supervision
4. What aids are used to facilitate treatment?
   Medication dispensers/Pillboxes
   Pagers/Alarm clocks
   Telephone calls
   Signs posted around house
5. What are patient's responses to missed treatment?
   No response
   Additional make-up treatment
   Checks blood sugar and adjusts next insulin dose

Pattern of adherence

Describe the pattern of missed treatments, including:

1. Frequency of missed treatment (e.g., once a day, once a week, etc.)

Table 11–2.   Clinical assessment of pediatric treatment adherence *(continued)*

2. Days, times, and places of most frequently missed treatments (e.g., school days, weekends, mornings, evenings, home, school)
3. Circumstances associated with missed treatments (e.g., with one parent and not the other, in separated families; while one parent is away or out of town; when one parent is working longer hours; school vacations; sleepovers)
4. Patient's level of distress associated with missed treatments

Major reasons for nonadherence

1. Forgetfulness
2. Reluctance to take treatment
    Taste
    Difficulty swallowing
    Side effects (e.g., cosmetic, nausea, low energy)
    Embarrassment/Teasing/Social stigma
    Lack of confidence in efficacy/Lack of trust in doctor
    Hopelessness about disease
3. Treatment too complicated or difficult
4. Lack of resources
    Cost of medications
    Transportation difficulties
5. Anger and acting out in relationship to the medical team
6. Lack of awareness or belief in possibility of negative medical consequences
7. Lack of supervision
    Working parents
    Parental resistance to providing supervision
8. Family psychopathology
    Parental conflict
    Parental disorganization
    Poor communication
    Parental psychiatric illness (e.g., depression, substance abuse)
9. Psychiatric illness
    Depression
    Attention-deficit/hyperactivity disorder
    Posttraumatic stress symptoms
    Oppositional defiant disorder
    Cognitive deficits

To develop effective treatment interventions it is critical to establish conceptual models of treatment adherence (Shaw and Palmer 2004). Research on the correlates of nonadherence is a useful first step that helps identify certain high-risk groups (e.g., adolescents). This research also suggests specific interventions, such as treatment aimed at reducing family conflict or improving family cohesion and communication. Conceptual models help to identify factors such as psychiatric comorbidity that may reduce the efficacy of treatment interventions. Rapoff (1999) emphasized that the family should be the primary focus of interventions designed to improve adherence to therapeutic regimens in pediatric populations. This conclusion is particularly important when parents have the primary responsibility for ensuring treatment adherence because of the child's age (La Greca et al. 1990). Treatment approaches based on the major etiologic factors related to nonadherence are given in Table 11–3.

Educational Interventions

Written and verbal educational interventions should be part of the routine care provided when patients are first diagnosed or when there is a simple goal, such as helping adolescents take on increased responsibility. The consultant must assess the knowledge of the patient and family regarding the illness and its treatment before initiating any adherence-enhancing program. It is important to review with the family the common principles of adolescent development and how they relate to treatment adherence. This assessment should emphasize the family's role in supporting their child's treatment by providing adequate supervision and should help the family anticipate difficulties that may interfere with adherence. The family should also receive guidance on how to respond to nonadherence. Families often react in an overly strong and punitive manner and withdraw privileges rather than increasing levels of supervision until such time that the adolescent demonstrates greater ability to take responsibility for the treatment.

Organizational Interventions

Simplification of the Medical Regimen

It is always important to simplify the treatment regimen wherever possible. Patients with chronic illnesses may be seen by several subspecialties, each of which may be prescribing medications without awareness of the total burden of the treatment on the individual.

Table 11–3. Treatment approaches for pediatric treatment adherence

Primary reason for nonadherence	Treatment modality
Forgetfulness	Increased parental supervision Memory aids (e.g., pillboxes, pagers, telephone reminders)
Inadequate awareness of consequences of nonadherence	Reeducation of patient and family regarding medical issues

Lack of appropriate parental supervision of treatment
    Lack of awareness of need for parental supervision
    Logistical issues (e.g., working parents)
	Education of the family regarding adolescent developmental need for supervision
	Establishment of effective system for supervision of treatment

Adolescent developmental issues
    Cognitive immaturity
    Acting out of separation conflicts
    Adolescent omnipotence/denial
    Peer group issues
	Education of the family
	Increased parental supervision
	Behavioral interventions (i.e., incentives, behavior modification programs)
	Possible referral for individual and/or family therapy in refractory cases

Family psychopathology
    Parental conflict
    Parental disorganization
    Poor communication
    Parental psychiatric illness (e.g., depression, substance abuse)
	Family therapy
	Possible referral of parent for individual psychiatric treatment

Psychiatric illness
    Depression
    Attention-deficit/Hyperactivity disorder
    Posttraumatic stress symptoms
    Oppositional defiant disorder
	Individual psychotherapy
	Family therapy
	Possible use of psychiatric medications

Memory Aids

Helpful strategies to remind patients about their treatments include the use of pagers, alarm clocks, and telephone calls from parents or medical clinics. Other strategies include using pillboxes, storing medications in highly visible places, and posting reminders around the house.

Enhanced Supervision

The first step in treating a nonadherent patient is to increase the level of supervision. This increase may involve parental observation or administration of treatments, more frequent clinic visits, or laboratory monitoring.

Behavioral Interventions

Data support the conclusion that interventions that integrate behavioral approaches including the use of incentives are more effective than programs based on educational and organizational approaches alone. To implement these strategies families need to understand the importance of reinforcing desired behaviors by providing incentives rather than focusing on negative behaviors. Specific behavioral plans with appropriate incentives and an effective system of monitoring and rewards should be tailored for each patient. For younger children, the program may involve a sticker chart tied to age-appropriate incentives. For adolescents adherence may be tracked using signatures on a chart with a similar system of short- and longer-term incentives.

Psychotherapy Interventions

In situations in which psychiatric comorbidity has been identified, the patient and family may be referred for psychotherapy. Treatment may involve both individual and family therapy, with the goals of helping the family develop insight into the issues affecting adherence behaviors and promoting a sense of greater personal responsibility. Referrals for family therapy are specifically indicated for families who are unable to provide adequate supervision despite clear education about its importance. Family therapy may also be indicated when significant family conflict leaves the parents unable to coordinate their treatment efforts and motivates the child to act out family conflicts in the form of nonadherent behavior. Treatment intervention studies have targeted family variables, such as parent–adolescent conflict, in an effort to improve treatment adherence (Wysocki et al. 2000).

References

Beck DE, Fennell RS, Yost RL, et al: Evaluation of an educational program on compliance with medication regimens in pediatric patients with renal transplants. J Pediatrics 96:1094–1097, 1980

Berg JS, Dischler J, Wagner DJ, et al: Medication compliance: a healthcare problem. Ann Pharmacother 27:2–21, 1993

Brooks-Gunn J: Why do adolescents have difficulties adhering to health regimes? Hillsdale, NJ, Lawrence Erlbaum Associates, 1993

Brownbridge G, Fielding DM: Psychosocial adjustment and adherence to dialysis treatment regimens. Pediatr Nephrol 8:744–749, 1994

Christiaanse ME, Lavigne JV, Lerner CV: Psychosocial aspects of compliance in children and adolescents with asthma. J Dev Behav Pediatr 10:75–80, 1989

Conrad PC: The meanings of medication: another look at compliance. Soc Sci Med 20:29–37, 1985

Cooper DKC, Lanza RP, Barnard CN: Noncompliance in heart transplant recipients: the Cape Town experience. Heart Transplant 3:248–253, 1984

Didlake RH, Dreyfus K, Kerman RH, et al: Patient noncompliance: a major cause of late graft failure in cyclosporine-treated renal transplants. Transplant Proc 20:63–69, 1988

Elkind D: Egocentrism in adolescence. Child Dev 38:1025–1034, 1967

Ettenger RB, Rosenthal JT, Marik JL, et al: Improved cadaveric renal transplant outcome in children. Pediatr Nephrol 5:137–142, 1991

Friedman IM, Litt IF: Adolescents' compliance with therapeutic regimens: psychological and social aspects and intervention. J Adolesc Health Care 8:52–67, 1987

Green BL, Epstein SA, Krupnick JL, et al: Trauma and medical illness: assessing trauma-related disorders in the medical settings, in Assessing Psychological Trauma and PTSD. Edited by Wilson JP, Keane TM. New York, Guilford, 1997

Hauser ST, Jacobson AM, Lavori P, et al: Adherence among children and adolescents with insulin-dependent diabetes mellitus over a four-year longitudinal follow-up, II: immediate and long term linkages with the family milieu. J Pediatr Psychol 15:527–542, 1990

Haynes RB: Introduction, in Compliance in Health Care. Edited by Haynes RB, Taylor DW, Sackett DL. Baltimore, MD, Johns Hopkins University Press, 1979, pp 1–18

Inhelder B, Piaget J: The Growth of Logical Thinking From Childhood to Adolescence. New York, Basic Books, 1958

Kovacs M, Goldston D, Obrosky DS, et al: Prevalence and predictors of pervasive noncompliance with medical treatment among youths with insulin-dependent diabetes mellitus. J Am Acad Child Adolesc Psychiatry 31:1112–1119, 1992

La Greca AM: Issues in adherence with pediatric regimens. J Pediatr Psychol 15:423–436, 1990

La Greca AM, Follansbee D, Skyler JS: Developmental and behavioral aspects of diabetes management in youngsters. Child Health Care 19:132–137, 1990

Lask B: Non-adherence to treatment in cystic fibrosis. J R Soc Med 87:25–27, 1994

Lorenz RA, Wysocki T: From research to practice: the family and childhood diabetes. Diabetes Spectrum 4:261–292, 1991

Rapoff MA: Adherence to Pediatric Medical Regimens. New York, Kluwer Academic/ Plenum, 1999

Riekert KA, Drotar D: Adherence to medical treatment in pediatric chronic illness: critical issues and answered questions, in Promoting Adherence to Medical Treatment in Chronic Childhood Illness: Concepts, Methods, and Interventions. Edited by Drotar D. Mahwah, NJ, Lawrence Erlbaum Associates, 2000, pp 1–32

Shaw RJ: Treatment adherence in adolescents: development and psychopathology. Clin Child Psychol Psychiatry 6:137–150, 2001

Shaw RJ, Palmer L: Consultation in the medical setting: a model to enhance treatment adherence, in The Stanford University School of Medicine Handbook of Psychiatric Treatment of Children and Adolescents: Treatment from a Developmental Perspective. Edited by Steiner H, Chang K, Lock J, et al. San Francisco, CA, Jossey-Bass, 2004, pp 917–941

Shaw RJ, Palmer L, Hyte H, et al: Case study: treatment adherence in a 13-year-old deaf adolescent male. Clin Child Psychol Psychiatry 6:551–562, 2001

Shaw RJ, Palmer L, Blasey C, et al: A typology of nonadherence in pediatric renal transplant recipients. Pediatr Transplant 7:489–493, 2003

Shemesh E, Lurie S, Stuber ML, et al: A pilot study of posttraumatic stress and non-adherence in pediatric liver transplant recipients. Pediatrics 105:e29, 2000

Smith BA, Shuchman M: Problem of nonadherence in chronically ill adolescents: strategies for assessment and intervention. Curr Opin Pediatr 17:613–618, 2005

Stein MT, Shafer MA, Elliott GR, et al: An adolescent who abruptly stops his medication for attention deficit hyperactivity disorder. J Dev Behav Pediatr 20:106–110, 1999

Wysocki T, Harris MA, Greco P, et al: Randomized, controlled trial of behavior therapy for families of adolescents with insulin-dependent diabetes mellitus. J Pediatr Psychol 25:23–33, 2000

12

Pediatric Cancer, Bone Marrow Transplantation, and Palliative Care

Although pediatric cancers account for less than 2% of all malignancies, taken together they are the second leading cause of death for children, with as many as 12,400 new cases each year (American Cancer Society 2005). With a mean age of 5 years when first diagnosed and an average duration of treatment of 1–3 years, pediatric cancers have a particular impact on a family's early childrearing years. Pediatric cancers have an overall 5-year survival rate of 75%. National treatment trials organized by the Children's Oncology Group have led to significant advances in treatment approaches to the various pediatric cancers. Table 12–1 provides an overview of incidence and survival rates for specific pediatric cancers.

Psychiatric consultation to this population of patients is common. Specific areas for the consultant to examine in patients with pediatric cancers are outlined in Chapter 3, Table 3–2. The goal of assessment is a good biopsychosocial understanding of the patient from which the consultant can facili-

Table 12–1.   Overview of common pediatric cancers

Cancer	Incidence	Age	5-Year survival rate
Acute lymphoblastic leukemia (ALL)	4 per 100,000 30% of all pediatric cancers	2–3 years	80%
Acute myelogenous leukemia (AML)	25% of childhood leukemia	First 2 years of life and again in later childhood	40%
Central nervous system tumors	2.5 per 100,000 20% of all pediatric cancers	3–9 years	65%
Lymphoma	10% of all pediatric cancers	10% of cancers among children under age 15 years; more than 15% in those under age 20 years	70%–90%
Hodgkin's	0.5 per 100,000	Incidence increases throughout childhood	91%
Non-Hodgkin's	1 per 100,000	Slight increase in age 15–19 years	72%
Bone tumors	5%–6% of all pediatric cancers	Peak incidence age 15 years, which coincides with growth spurt	58%–63%
Retinoblastoma	11% in first year of life	80% of cases diagnosed before age 3 years	94%
Germ cell tumors	3.5% of cancers under age 15 years	15–20 years	88%
Soft tissue sarcoma	7% of cancers before age 20	15–19 years	71%
Hepatoblastoma	1%	First 18 months of life	59%
Wilms' tumor	>90% of childhood renal cancers	First 5 years of life	92%
Neuroblastoma	14% of pediatric cancers under age 5 years	Highest in first month of life and declines dramatically with age	64%

Source.   Adapted from American Cancer Society 2005.

tate clear communication between the family and medical team regarding the cancer and its treatment. The consultant must address emotional issues (e.g., anxiety and depression), behavioral issues (e.g., nonadherence and school re-entry), and physical symptoms (e.g., pain and vomiting).

Sequelae of Cancer

The consultant should be alert to the interrelated physical, emotional, and cognitive sequelae that pediatric cancers and their treatments have on children and adolescents.

Physical Sequelae

There are numerous physical effects of cancer, those that are a direct effect of the malignancy and those related to side effects of treatment. General effects that are almost universal include fatigue, malaise, weight loss, anorexia, physical limitations, and pain. Cosmetic effects (e.g., hair loss) are reported in two-thirds and functional limitations in one-third of cancer survivors. Patients can also develop mental status changes consistent with delirium and dementia related to the direct effects of their cancers as well as their treatment.

Pain is a particularly important issue in these youngsters and may be due to the direct effects of the disease, treatment procedures, or medication side effects (Slater 2002). The response can be complicated when patients minimize their pain complaints as a result of their association of pain with doctors' visits and hospitalizations or to avoid creating concern in their parents. Issues related to the assessment and treatment of pediatric pain are described in Chapter 9.

Direct Effect of Malignancy

The direct physical manifestations of cancer depend to a large degree on the location of the tumor (Granowetter 1994). Leukemia, for example, involves the bone marrow and generally presents with signs of anemia, bleeding, or infection. By contrast, solid organ tumors cause damage by local growth or metastases. The effects of brain tumors depend on their size and location such that patients may have headaches, vomiting, personality changes, or neurological symptoms.

Side Effects of Treatment

The side effects of chemotherapy include infection, bleeding, anemia, hair loss, nausea and vomiting, malaise, mouth sores, anorexia, and pain (Vannatta and Gerhardt 2003). Cardiac failure may result from treatment with anthracyclines, whereas pulmonary problems are associated with bleomycin (Granowetter 1994). Additional problems include growth delays, short stature, renal dysfunction, endocrine abnormalities, and neurotoxicity. Side effects of radiation include skin irritation, loss of appetite, diarrhea, headache, and the possibility of secondary malignancies. Cranial radiation in particular may cause acute anorexia, confusion, and somnolence as temporary, reversible effects, but late effects on memory and cognition may be both irreversible and progressive. Surgical treatment may include amputation and enucleation for specific tumors. There may also be interactions between chemotherapy and radiation, for example, cisplatin interacts with cranial radiation to cause progressive hearing loss and diffuse encephalopathy. Similarly, loss of fertility and delays in sexual maturation can result from irradiation and chemotherapy.

Emotional Sequelae

Early in their treatment recently diagnosed children report increased levels of distress related to hospitalizations, invasive procedures, and physical effects of their treatment (Vannatta and Gerhardt 2003). However, it is important to note that studies of long-term survivors of pediatric cancer have found that children appear to have good general adjustment, with only 25%–33% developing significant psychosocial problems (Eiser et al. 2000; Redd 1994). Risk and resiliency factors associated with general psychological adjustment are given in Table 12–2.

When problems do occur, social isolation and shyness as well as concern about body image and physical appearance are commonly reported. Although of varying intensity, most patients report fears about recurrence of their cancer. Psychosexual effects include delays in the onset of puberty, loss of fertility, reduced libido, or inability to have erections. Long-term survivors have been known to have difficulties with dating, identity development, and romantic relationships as well as experimentation with high-risk behaviors including sexual activity and substance abuse (Slater 2002; Vannatta and Gerhardt 2003). Attention has been given to the model of cancer as a traumatic event that is associated with symptoms of posttraumatic stress disorder in both pa-

Table 12–2.   Risk and resiliency factors in pediatric cancer

Category	Risk factors	Protective factors
Patient correlates	Avoidant coping style Premorbid psychiatric illness Concurrent social stressors	Repressive coping style High self-esteem Self-confidence
Family correlates	Parental psychiatric illness Marital conflict Divorce History of previous losses	Marital satisfaction Adaptability Cohesion Family support Communication/Expressiveness Flexibility Moral and religious emphasis Presence of social support Financial security

Disease correlates	Central nervous system
	  involvement
	Visibility of illness
	Long duration of illness
	Frequency of
	  hospitalizations
	Poor medical prognosis
	Degree of incapacitation
	Cranial radiation
	Intrathecal chemotherapy
	Severity of treatment side
	  effects	

tients and family members. Distress may be related to the diagnosis of cancer as well as to invasive procedures and treatment. Studies suggest that as many as 15% of patients meet full DSM-IV-TR diagnostic criteria for posttraumatic stress disorder, particularly in those patients that experience their treatment as being difficult or life threatening or who experience a relapse in their disease (Barakat et al. 1997).

Cognitive Sequelae

Cognitive and Learning Deficits

There is a large body of literature documenting the long-term cognitive development of pediatric cancer survivors (Slater 2002). In a study of patients with leukemia, 50% of children had academic problems at 5-year follow-up, 61% had attentional problems, and 33% had impaired cognitive functioning (Jannoun and Chessells 1987; Parsons and Brown 1998). Patients under 3 years of age and those treated with cranial radiation or intrathecal chemotherapy are at high risk for cognitive difficulties. These cognitive deficits may be the direct effect of the tumor, metastatic disease, hydrocephalus, or seizures or may be related to the indirect effects of infections, fevers, and medications. Problems with performance skills, arithmetic, perceptual motor skills, visual processing, visuomotor integration, sequencing abilities, and short-term memory have all been reported (Redd 1994).

School Adjustment

There is an increased risk of school-related difficulties, with many parents describing difficulties with school reentry in their children (Slater 2002). Barriers to successful reintegration into school include anxiety related to possible teasing and rejection or concerns about academic delays (Leigh and Miles 2002). In addition, patients may have continued intermittent school absences due to their illness that may compound difficulties keeping up with the demands of schoolwork.

Family Adjustment

Parents may experience even greater adjustment difficulties than their children (Slater 2002). Acute symptoms of separation anxiety, insomnia, and obsessive-compulsiveness are common in parents, along with more chronic depressive and anxiety symptoms (Brown et al. 1993). Reports of isolation, self-blame, and anxiety about relapse are common, as are concerns about the long-term emotional and educational needs of their child (Slater 2002). Nevertheless, the majority of parents report that they return to normal emotional functioning within the first year (Dahlquist et al. 1996; Vannatta and Gerhardt 2003).

Enskar et al. (1997) described categories of problems faced by parents in dealing with cancer in their children: 1) feelings of powerlessness associated with the child's suffering or reaction to disease; 2) the feeling that life has become governed by the child's illness, including work and finances; 3) significant changes in family dynamics related to the lack of privacy, the impact on the marital relationship, insufficient time for siblings, and a tendency to spoil the affected child; 4) change in parental self-image due to the shift in priorities, or feelings of despair or sadness; 5) attempts to cope with the demands of the illness and its treatment; 6) difficulties dealing with the reactions of others, including a need to take care of the emotional reactions of extended family members and friends; 7) efforts to find support from other friends, family members, and medical staff; and 8) problems encountered in the delivery and organization of health care.

Different models have been proposed to explain the nature of reactions in family members (Kupst 1994). The *anticipatory grief model* hypothesizes that parents go through a bereavement reaction at the time of diagnosis and early treatment. The response of the family has also been conceptualized as one of chronic sorrow related to the loss of the "complete" child (Buschmann 1988). In the *stress and coping model,* the focus is on the stresses of the situation and how the individual copes with these stresses (e.g., problem-focused vs. emotion-focused coping) (Lazarus and Folkman 1984). Koocher and O'Malley (1981) adapted this model for pediatric oncology and suggested the following family tasks: 1) learning to manage distress, 2) maintaining a sense of personal worth, 3) maintaining rewarding interpersonal relationships, and 4) using available resources to meet specific situational tasks. In this model, the expected outcome is adaptation to the stress of the illness rather than a pathological grieving process.

Different family tasks are associated with different stages in the child's cancer treatment, as shown in Table 12–3. Transitions between these phases require flexibility on the part of the family. In the early phases of diagnosis and treatment most families have a tendency to pull inward, with the goals of increasing cohesion and mobilizing resources and support. In time, after the family has integrated the illness into the daily routine, the need for increased cohesion may diminish, and the family may focus on efforts to resume normal developmental tasks and resolve conflicts between needs of the patient and other family members. In the rehabilitation phase, there may often be a paradoxical increase in psychological symptoms as pent-up emotions surface and the financial, interpersonal, and emotional difficulties incurred during the acute phase may need to be addressed.

Although siblings are frequently overlooked in pediatric oncology, up to 50% of siblings have adjustment difficulties that include feelings of guilt, loneliness, rejection, jealousy, anger, sadness, and depression (Carpenter and Levant

Table 12–3.   Family tasks associated with stage of cancer treatment

Stage of cancer treatment	Family tasks
Diagnosis of cancer	Temporary reassignment of family roles Shifts in power and responsibility Engaging family and social support
Acute phase of treatment	Adapting to physical changes in the child Grieving the loss of the family life prior to diagnosis Balancing the demands of treatment with the family's daily routine
Rehabilitation after initial treatment	Restoration of previous roles and responsibilities Reentry into school Reintegration with the peer group Adaptation to the functional limitations of the child Living with the uncertainty of relapse
Long-term survivors of cancer	Living with long-term disabilities caused by illness Mourning of losses such as fertility or career goals Adjusting to financial restrictions Living with uncertainty of relapse
Relapse of illness	Further readjustment of roles Anticipatory grief
Terminal phase of illness	Integrating and accepting the imminent loss of the child Anticipating permanent change in family structure and potential loss or alteration of parental role Planning for life after death of the child

1994). Parents often neglect to communicate clearly or adequately about the illness, and siblings are usually left out of aspects of the ill child's care. The following feelings, thoughts, and reactions can be experienced by siblings: 1) physical and emotional isolation, 2) inadequate emotional and social support, 3) blame and responsibility for the illness, 4) abandonment by the parents, 5) resentment about the loss of parental attention, 6) reluctance to further burden their parents with their own concerns, 7) guilt about their anger directed toward the affected sibling, 8) shame and embarrassment about the appearance of their sibling, 9) worries about contagion, 10) somatic preoccupations, and 11) increased risk of behavior problems (Carpenter and Levant 1994).

Bone Marrow Transplantation

Bone marrow transplantation has become the standard treatment for high-risk or relapsed leukemia. Ablation of the recipient's bone marrow is followed by replacement with donor bone marrow. For 3–6 weeks after the marrow transplantation, patients require protective isolation because of their high risk for infection and bleeding. Key tasks and common issues prior to transplantation, during the acute phase, and posttransplantation are summarized in Table 12–4 (Phipps 1994).

Psychological Issues

The consultant should be alert to the following issues when called to work with patients and families undergoing bone marrow transplantation (Phipps 1994): 1) response to protective isolation, 2) donor issues, 3) family issues, and 4) staff issues.

Response to Protective Isolation

Studies suggest that pediatric patients experience problems with concentration, anxiety, depression, and affective instability in response to the prolonged period of protective isolation (Phipps 1994). Children may exhibit regressed behaviors, including separation anxiety and increased dependency on their caregivers. It is not unusual for children to begin with feelings of optimism and motivation, only to become increasingly oppositional when experiencing continued isolation or as a result of complications of treatment such as graft versus host disease.

Donor Issues

Although there are few data on the psychological outcome of bone marrow donors, there is the potential for significant distress. Although feelings of increased intimacy often develop between the patient and the donor, there is the potential for feelings of guilt and increased responsibility, particularly if the transplant is unsuccessful. In comparison with nondonor siblings, sibling do-

Table 12–4. Key aspects of bone marrow transplantation

Phase	Key tasks	Common issues
Pretransplant	Blood typing of immediate family members to identify donor	Feelings of anxiety and ambivalence in compatible sibling
	Search of bone marrow registry if family donor not identified (1- to 6-month delay)	Feelings of disappointment in incompatible siblings
		Anxiety due to fear of relapse or medical complications while awaiting transplant
Acute (1–3 months)	Admission for transplant	Nausea and vomiting
	Pretransplant conditioning, including chemotherapy and possible total body irradiation (7–10 days)	Fatigue and malaise
		Fevers
		Mucositis
	Protective isolation	Risk of acute cardiorespiratory problems, organ toxicity, and seizures
	Infusion of donor marrow	Risk of graft versus host disease
	Waiting for engraftment (2–4 weeks)	Risk of latent infections due to immunosuppressants, including cytomegalovirus (10%–20% fatality rate)
	Total parenteral nutrition	
	Aggressive treatment of suspected infections	
Posttransplant	Discharge from hospital (3–6 weeks in uncomplicated cases)	Anxiety about leaving security of the hospital
		Period of elation frequently followed by depression
	Continued physical and social isolation due to immunocompromised state	Risk of chronic graft versus host disease
	Frequent readmissions for fever and neutropenia	Late effects including cognitive delays, infertility, delays in puberty, and frequent chronic medical complications

Source.   Adapted from Phipps 1994.

nors are more likely to develop internalizing symptoms (e.g., anxiety and posttraumatic stress symptoms) and less likely to have externalizing symptoms (i.e., behavioral difficulties) during treatment (Packman et al. 1997). It is important to carefully assess bone marrow donors prior to transplant to determine whether they have an appropriate understanding of the procedure, to assess their attitude toward being a donor, and to ensure that they are not being unduly coerced by their parents (Phipps 1994).

Family Issues

The multiple challenges presented by bone marrow transplantation may deplete the physical, emotional, and financial resources of the most resilient families. Geographical separation is common for families who live far away from transplant centers. It is not unusual for one parent to take on a primary caretaking role with the ill child while the other parent continues to work and manage the healthy siblings. The single-parent family may be faced with one person trying to handle all of these tasks. Patients often develop a particular closeness with the primary caretaking parent, who in turn may become isolated from healthy family members (Pot-Mees 1989). There is potential for increased levels of family tension along with feelings of guilt and alienation among family members, particularly when the transplant does not proceed smoothly.

Staff Issues

Given the high rates of morbidity and mortality in busy bone marrow transplant and oncology programs, the medical and nursing staffs face significant levels of stress. Serial deaths can take their toll on staff morale, particularly when there is an intense emotional involvement with patients and their families. The staff may experience a range of countertransference feelings, including sadness, sorrow, guilt, satisfaction (i.e., sense of accomplishment, inspiration, and sense of importance), and heightened altruism (Peteet et al. 1992). The stress can put the staff at risk for "burnout" or "compassion fatigue."

Medication Effects

Polypharmacy is the rule during bone marrow transplantation. In addition to the chemotherapeutic agents used during the conditioning phase of treatment, patients are frequently prescribed antiemetic medications, narcotic analgesics, and high-dosage corticosteroids or immunosuppressants to prevent the devel-

Table 12–5.   Common indications and side effects of medications used during bone marrow transplantation

Medication class	Indications	Side effects
Antiemetics		
Benzodiazepines	Nausea	Sedation
Cyproheptadine	Vomiting	Acute dystonic
Ondansetron		reactions
Granisetron		
Analgesics	Pain	Sedation
Opiates	Mucositis	
Antihistamines	Premedication for	Sedation
Diphenhydramine	transfusion	Hallucinations
Hydroxyzine	Antipruritics	Delirium
	Mild sedatives	Cholinergic rebound
	Nausea/Vomiting	
Immunosuppressants	Graft versus host disease	Delirium
Cyclosporine		Encephalopathy
		Renal failure
		Hepatic failure
		Hirsutism
Corticosteroids	Graft versus host disease	Affective instability
	Appetite stimulation	Steroid psychosis
	Nausea	Cosmetic effects
Benzodiazepines	Nausea	Sedation
Lorazepam	Anxiety	Cognitive slowing
Diazepam	Insomnia	
Clonazepam		

opment of graft versus host disease. Significant physical side effects include nausea, vomiting, mucositis, and sedation, and in many cases side effects may be cumulative as a result of the need to use several agents simultaneously (Table 12–5).

Late Effects

Survivors of bone marrow transplants are at risk of multiple complications affecting different organ systems, particularly those related to the conditioning treatment that usually includes total body irradiation (Phipps 1994). Endocrine effects include thyroid dysfunction and decreased growth velocity. Patients receiving total body irradiation may have delayed or absent sexual development and a greatly increased rate of infertility (Sanders et al. 1989). The development of cataracts is a common late toxicity, and careful ophthalmological monitoring is important. There is an increased risk of cognitive deficits related to chemotherapy, total body irradiation, and as a potential side effect related to immunosuppressant treatment. These issues may be reflected in poorer academic achievement (Pot-Mees 1989).

Palliative Care

Dying is defined as the end stage of an illness when treatment is no longer thought to offer the possibility of a cure. At this point, the focus for the oncology/bone marrow transplant team becomes that of comfort and care. It is estimated that 25% of children, or 1,700 children each year, die from cancer or the side effects of its treatment (American Cancer Society 2005). The sudden death of a patient with cancer is relatively rare, although it does occur in aggressive treatment regimens such as those involved in bone marrow transplant. Although many children die in the hospital, there has been an increasing trend toward children returning home during the terminal stages of their illness. This is further reflected in an increasing trend for hospitals to provide a specialized bereavement room in the hospital that creates a home-like atmosphere for the dying child and family.

End-stage cancers present many challenges for both the family and the oncology staff. Most oncology treatment centers have developed comprehensive palliative care protocols in which attention is paid to the physical, psychosocial, and spiritual interventions that are specifically aimed at alleviating patient suffering. During the terminal phase, families may become more directly involved in their child's day-to-day care. Care changes from the medical team's usual emphasis on cure to that of maximizing the quality of life, lessening pain, and assisting family members in preparing for their child's death.

Palliative Care Issues for the Consultant

The consultant who is well grounded in a developmental understanding of death can be enormously helpful in facilitating the grief process in children and families as well as the oncology staff. The following palliative care issues should be kept in mind by the consultant.

Conception of Death

A child's developmental level determines his or her understanding of death. Four major concepts related to death that are commonly cited include irreversibility, finality, causality, and universality. Inability to understand one or more of these concepts due to cognitive immaturity may interfere with the child's ability to go through the mourning process (Lewis and Schonfeld 2002). Preschool children (younger than age 2 years) tend to view death as reversible or even temporary. Death is experienced as a disruption in or separation from caretaking. There is no cognitive understanding of death at these younger ages. From ages 2 to 6 years, death is viewed as temporary or reversible. It is personified and often seen as punishment. Magical thinking, in which wishes become true, is a consistent finding. School-age children (ages 6–11 years) have a more concrete conception that allows an ability to see cause and effect relations. There is a general awareness of irreversibility and finality, although the specific illness or death of the self or a loved one is difficult to understand. Adolescents tend to "do their own thing" and characteristically may grieve more easily with peers than with family members. Adolescents understand that death is irreversible, universal, and inevitable, although generally only in the distant future. This age group is also capable of abstract and philosophical thinking. A universal concern, regardless of age, often involves the question, "Did it happen because of something I did?"

Range of Grief Manifestations

Table 12–6 lists the range of manifestations of childhood grief. Reactions fall along a spectrum from normal or variants of normal to problems or disorders.

Family Adjustment

The death of a child represents a reversal in the natural order of life, because parents have the expectation that their children will outlive them (Martinson and Papadatou 1994). They may experience profound and enduring symptoms of sadness, guilt, somatic symptoms, sleep difficulties, and anger (Vannatta and Gerhardt 2003). Significant family dysfunction and marital difficulties may also be precipitated by the loss. Bereaved family members may overlook the needs of their surviving children, creating feelings of abandonment and emotional isolation. McLowry et al. (1987) identified different patterns to describe parental efforts to come to terms with the death of a child: 1) getting over the

Table 12–6. Range of common grief manifestations in children and adolescents

Normal/Variant	Problem/Disorder*
Shock/Numbness	Long-term denial and avoidance of feelings
Crying	Repeated crying spells
Sadness	Disabling depression and suicidal ideation
Anger	Persistent anger
Feeling "guilty"	Believing "guilty"
Transient unhappiness	Persistent unhappiness
Keeping concerns "inside"	Social withdrawal
Increased clinging	Separation anxiety
Disobedience	Oppositional or conduct disorder
Lack of interest in school	School performance decline
Transient sleep disturbance	Persistent sleep problems
Physical complaints	Physical symptoms of deceased
Decreased appetite	Eating disorder
Temporary regression	Disabling or persistent regression
Being "good or bad"	Being "much too good or bad"
Belief still alive	Persistent belief still alive
Adolescent relates better to friends	Promiscuity or delinquent behavior
Behavior lasts days to weeks	Behavior lasts weeks to months

*Should prompt investigation by medical and nursing staff with probable mental health referral.
Source. Adapted from American Academy of Pediatrics Committee on Psychosocial Aspects of Child and Family Health: "The Pediatrician and Childhood Bereavement." *Pediatrics* 105:445–447, 2000. Copyright 2000, American Academy of Pediatrics. Used with permission.

child's death by accepting and giving a meaning to the loss, 2) filling the emptiness by efforts to keep busy, and 3) maintaining the connection with the child by integrating the empty space caused by the death into everyday living and cherishing recollections of the child.

Sibling Reactions

Siblings are also strongly affected during the dying process and may present with somatic symptoms, separation anxiety, school phobia, and poor school performance (Martinson and Papadatou 1994). Difficulties that are commonly reported by siblings include the experience of a major unanticipated change without adequate opportunity for preparation, disruption in peer relationships, absence of parents, concerns about physical changes in the sick sibling, and disturbance to the family routine (Iles 1979). Siblings also report fears about their own health as well as feelings of confusion, anger, depression, and guilt (Martinson and Papadatou 1994).

End-of-Life Strategies for the Consultant

The following principles may help inform the work of the psychiatric consultant with families of dying children (American Academy of Pediatrics 2000; DeMaso et al. 1997).

Be Open and Honest

Children benefit by knowing openly and honestly at an age-appropriate level about their own or their sibling's illness or death. Some families may be concerned that their children may be too young and that hearing about death may be too painful and increase their worry. However, children and adolescents generally know or suspect what is going on, and open discussion may reduce feelings of isolation from the rest of the family as well as correct irrational worries. The consultant can tell the family that the goal in telling patients or siblings is to help them gain family support by opening communication within the family as well as provide an opportunity to facilitate grief.

Be Age Appropriate

As mentioned earlier, the manifestation of grief varies according to the developmental level of the child. The consultant can educate the family about the child's developmental level and the expected responses to death.

Explain the Illness and Death

The consultant can help families and medical staff members tailor explanations to the child's developmental age. For instance, death can be explained to young children as the "body stops working." It can be helpful to draw on past experiences of loss (e.g., other family members or even pets). Euphemisms (e.g., death is like being asleep) should be avoided, particularly in the younger child who may concretely respond to such analogies.

Showing Feelings Is Normal and Helpful

It is reassuring for parents to know that they can let their children see their own feelings of sadness and anger. It is part of the child's learning experience in dealing with loss. Parental withdrawal may cause fear and may be experienced as another loss. The consultant can provide sanction for the expression of the parent's grief.

Be Alert to Behavior Changes

As noted earlier regarding siblings, behavioral changes are common. The consultant can advise the family to continue normal family routines and discipline as much as possible. Permission can also be given to use family, friends, and relatives for support and help during this time of loss.

Discuss the Funeral

The funeral gives family members an opportunity for connecting or grieving with each other as well as an opportunity to commemorate. Even young children can participate. It is helpful for the young child to know that there is someone nearby who can support them (i.e., close enough to put a "hand on the shoulder"). It is helpful to prepare and structure a younger child's involvement in the funeral process. This may include limiting the amount of time at the funeral, allowing special/private time, bringing stuff to do, or helping structure the time at the funeral.

Mention Grief as Process

Grief is a process that classically falls into three stages that may occur over weeks to months to years: 1) shock and denial, 2) protest and anguish, and 3) mourning and restitution. Children tend to "dose themselves" in their mourning (i.e., a young child can be crying one minute then be right back into play the next). Childhood bereavement tasks for siblings include understanding, grieving, commemorating, and going on. The consultant can emphasize the importance of parents taking care of themselves as a way of helping their other children. The consultant may recommend support from friends, pediatricians, religious leaders, hospice programs, support groups, and psychotherapy.

References

American Academy of Pediatrics: Committee on Psychosocial Aspects of Child and Family Health: The pediatrician and childhood bereavement. Pediatrics 105:445–447, 2000

American Cancer Society: Cancer Facts and Figures 2005. Available online at http://www.cancer.org/docroot/STT/stt_0.asp. Accessed April 23, 2006.

Barakat L, Kazak EA, Meadows A, et al: Families surviving childhood cancer: a comparison of posttraumatic stress symptoms with families of healthy children. J Pediatr Psychol 22:843–859, 1997

Brown RT, Kaslow NJ, Madan-Swain A, et al: Parental psychopathology and children's adjustment to leukemia. J Am Acad Child Adolesc Psychiatry 32:554–561, 1993

Buschmann PR: Pediatric orthopedics: dealing with loss and chronic sorrow. Loss Grief Care 2:39–44, 1988

Carpenter PJ, Levant CA: Sibling adaptation to the family crisis of childhood cancer, in Pediatric Psychooncology: Psychological Perspectives on Children with Cancer. Edited by Bearison DJ, Mulhern RK. Oxford, England, Oxford University Press, 1994, pp 122–142

Dahlquist LM, Czyzeweski DI, Jones CL: Parents of children with cancer: a longitudinal study of emotional distress, coping style, and marital adjustment to and 20 months after diagnosis. J Pediatr Psychol 21:541–554, 1996

DeMaso DR, Meyer EC, Beasley PJ: What do I say to my surviving children? J Am Acad Child Adolesc Psychiatry 36:1299–1302, 1997

Eiser C, Hill JJ, Vance YH: Examining the psychological consequences of surviving childhood cancer: systematic review as a research method in pediatric psychology. J Pediatr Psychol 25:449–460, 2000

Enskar K, Carlsson M, Golsater M, et al: Parental reports of changes and challenges that result from parenting a child with cancer. J Pediatr Oncol Nurs 14:156–163, 1997

Granowetter L: Pediatric oncology: a medical overview, in Pediatic Psychooncology: Psychological Perspectives on Children with Cancer. Edited by Bearison DJ, Mulhern RK. Oxford, England, Oxford University Press, 1994, pp 9–34

Iles JP: Children with cancer: healthy siblings' perceptions during the illness experience. Cancer Nurs 2:371–377, 1979

Jannoun L, Chessells JM: Long-term psychological effects of childhood leukemia and its treatment. Pediatr Hematol Oncol 4:293–308, 1987

Koocher GE, O'Malley JE: The Damocles Syndrome: Psychological Consequences of Surviving Childhood Cancer. New York, McGraw-Hill, 1981

Kupst MJ: Coping with pediatric cancer: theoretical and research perspectives, in Pediatric Psychooncology: Psychological Perspectives on Children With Cancer. Edited by Bearison DJ, Mulhern RK. Oxford, UK, Oxford University Press, 1994, pp 35–60

Lazarus R, Folkman S: Stress, Appraisal, and Coping. New York, Springer Publishing Company, 1984

Leigh LD, Miles MA: Educational issues for children with cancer, in Principles and Practice of Pediatric Oncology, 4th Edition. Edited by Pizzo PA, Poplack DG. Philadelphia, PA, Lippincott Williams & Wilkins, 2002, pp 1463–1476

Lewis M, Schonfeld DJ: Dying and death in childhood and adolescence, in Child and Adolescent Psychiatry: A Comprehensive Textbook, 3rd Edition. Edited by Lewis M. Philadelphia, PA, Lippincott Williams & Wilkins, 2002, pp 1239–1245

Martinson ID, Papadatou D: Care of the dying child and the bereaved, in Pediatric Psychooncology: Psychological Perspectives on Children with Cancer. Edited by Bearison DJ, Mulhern RK. Oxford, England, Oxford University Press, 1994, pp 193–214

McLowry SG, Davies EB, May KA, et al: The empty space phenomenon: the process of grief and the bereaved family. Death Stud 11:361–374, 1987

Packman WL, Crittenden MR, Schaeffer E, et al: Psychosocial consequences of bone marrow transplantation in donor and nondonor siblings. J Dev Behav Pediatr 18:244–253, 1997

Parsons SK, Brown AP: Evaluation of quality of life of childhood cancer survivors: a methodological conundrum. Med Pediatr Oncol Suppl 1:46–53, 1998

Peteet JR, Ross DM, Medeiros C, et al: Relationships with patients in oncology: can a clinician be a friend? Psychiatry 55:223–229, 1992

Phipps S: Bone marrow transplantation, in Pediatric Psychooncology: Psychological Perspectives on Children with Cancer. Edited by Bearison DJ, Mulhern RK. Oxford, England, Oxford University Press, 1994, pp 143–170

Pot-Mees CC: The Psychosocial Effects of Bone Marrow Transplantation in Children. Delft, The Netherlands, Eburon, 1989

Redd WH: Advances in psychosocial oncology in pediatrics. Cancer 74:1496–1502, 1994

Sanders J, Sullivan K, Witherspoon R, et al: Long-term effects and quality of life in children and adults after marrow transplantation. Bone Marrow Transplant Suppl 4:27–29, 1989

Slater JA: Psychiatric aspects of cancer in childhood and adolescence, in Child and Adolescent Psychiatry: A Comprehensive Textbook, 3rd Edition. Edited by Lewis M. Philadelphia, PA, Lippincott Williams & Wilkins, 2002, pp 1135–1147

Vannatta K, Gerhardt CA: Pediatric oncology: psychosocial outcomes for children and families, in Handbook of Pediatric Psychology, 3rd Edition. Edited by Roberts MC. New York, Guilford, 2003, pp 342–357

13

Individual Psychotherapy in the Pediatric Setting

The psychological reaction to any physical illness or disability can be viewed as a transitional process that begins with shock and disbelief and proceeds through feelings of anguish (sadness) and protest (anger) toward the gradual assimilation of illness information and adjustment to the implications of the disease. Tailored to the patient's individual developmental level, psychotherapy in the pediatric setting can help patients understand the meaning of and responses to their illnesses. Treatment can be targeted at assisting children or adolescents at various points along this grieving process by enhancing the use of adaptive coping mechanisms that promote patients' continued psychological development and adaptation to their illnesses.

Models of Psychotherapy

Psychotherapy can provide a time and place where patients can effectively vent feelings of fear, anger, or sadness. Common elements of the interaction include support, reassurance, suggestion, explanation, and introspective exploration of the causes of a patient's feelings of demoralization (Goldberg and Green 1985). There are a number of different models of psychotherapy that may be applicable in the inpatient setting.

Supportive Psychotherapy

Supportive psychotherapy aims to minimize levels of emotional distress through ego support, enhancement of coping mechanisms, and protection of self-esteem (Green 2000). In the pediatric setting, support may be brief (i.e., during a single visit) or more prolonged and ongoing. The treatment is focused on the "here and now," providing the patient symptomatic relief by dissipating the powerful emotions that may have emerged in the context of the illness. The consultant is active and helpful in ways that work to contain anxiety and allow the patient to function (Green 2000). The goal is not to help uncover unconscious motivations and conflicts but to provide education, encouragement, and support. Reassurance and explanation are provided by pointing out the patient's strengths and by removing misconceptions about the illness or its treatment. The consultant aims to support and strengthen existing defenses to better facilitate patients' response to physical illnesses.

Insight-Oriented Psychotherapy

Insight-oriented psychotherapy attempts to promote psychological maturation by exploring the turmoil of emotional upheaval caused by the illness. The therapeutic task is to help patients acknowledge and put into perspective painful feelings of loss that are brought up in the context of their lives (Green 2000). Patients are made aware of previously unrecognized emotions that are blocked from consciousness by their defense mechanisms. By recognizing the intensity of these feelings, patients hopefully come to achieve some resolution of their personal conflicts. Insight-oriented psychotherapy depends to a significant degree on the patient's ability to tolerate the anxiety that goes along with exploratory work. However, insight-oriented therapy is generally of limited applicability in the inpatient setting for several reasons: 1) acutely ill pediatric patients usually have a diminished capacity of self-expression or self-examination because of the direct effects of their illness; 2) younger patients may not be at a cognitive level to participate in this type of approach; 3) patients may already be overwhelmed emotionally by the constraints of their illness such that they cannot tolerate additional anxiety that might be generated in an insight-oriented approach; and 4) the brief time available to intervene in a pediatric setting does not readily lend itself to this more reflective and emotion-generating treatment.

Narrative Therapy

Narrative therapy emphasizes the construction of meaning as a central concept and goal. In this approach the consultant allows patients to tell their stories, which in the pediatric setting are generally the stories of their physical illness. The consultant helps patients to "make meaning" of their stories and thereby increases self- and other-understanding. Studies have shown positive effects in patients who have the opportunity to narrate their stories (Suedfeld and Pennebaker 1997). For instance, Pennebaker (1997) had participants write about a traumatic or stressful event for 15–20 minutes each day for 3–4 days. This writing task is thought to improve emotional regulation by facilitating attention and habituation to uncomfortable emotional experiences. When patients feel a sense of control over their emotions, they are better able to integrate difficult experiences and experience distress (Schwartz and Drotar 2004).

Cognitive-Behavioral Therapy

Cognitive-behavioral therapy is problem-oriented treatment that seeks to identify and change maladaptive beliefs about the self, world, and future and to modify behavior. In the physically ill pediatric patient this therapy is based on the premise that patients can develop cognitive distortions that have an adverse impact on their treatment (Table 13–1). For example, an erroneous belief that important medical information is being withheld could lead to the belief that the prognosis is hopeless, which may undermine patients' willingness to cooperate with treatment. Cognitive-behavioral therapy can be used to address specific emotional responses that result in distress about illnesses or interfere with their treatment. It can be applied to counterbalance negative cognitions about physical symptoms and irrational thoughts of being physically ill as well as treat disabling comorbid mood or anxiety symptoms. It has been used with a variety of conditions, including irritable bowel syndrome, somatoform disorders, functional dyspepsia, inflammatory bowel disease, fibromyalgia syndrome, and juvenile rheumatoid arthritis (Szigethy et al. 2004, 2006).

Table 13–1.   Common cognitive distortions in pediatric illness

Belief that

   Nothing will change the outcome of my illness

   Minor physical symptoms herald the return of my illness

   My illness is a punishment for bad behavior

   I will not be able to resume school or social activities

Fear about

   Inevitable progression of my illness

   Inevitability of pain

   Becoming a burden to my family

   Friends not wanting to associate with me

   Medical information being withheld

Group Therapy

Group therapy has been found to be useful in physically ill patients who have shared diagnoses or illness-related issues (Gore-Felton and Spiegel 2000; O'Dowd and Gomez 2001). Table 13–2 outlines the functions that group therapy may serve in physically ill patients. The targets of group interventions are attitude and behavior changes that will result in better self-care and, as a result, improved overall health. The heightened social support and reduced feelings of isolation afforded by a peer group with a similar illness or experience are the foundation of group therapy.

Educational groups disseminate information as well as provide a forum in which patients do not feel like they are the only ones with their illness. These groups can be used to educate and introduce preventive health care (e.g., to adolescents with high-risk sexual behaviors) (Gore-Felton and Spiegel 2000). Although there are few data on the efficacy of these interventions, their popularity would seem to support their value to participants. Although similar, cognitive-behavioral–oriented groups more typically use problem-focused skills to help build patient coping skills. Groups for physically ill children must have activities that are developmentally appropriate (i.e., young children may have art projects, storytelling, or therapeutic play as opposed to conventional verbal techniques). Adolescents may be particularly receptive to group therapy with peers who have similar medical diagnoses.

Table 13–2. Functions of group therapy for physically ill patients

Social support

Establishment of a new social network with common underlying medical issues

Decreased feelings of stigma and difference

Emotional expression

Facilitation of the expression of common emotions of sadness, anger, and fear

Discussion of issues of loss

Increased understanding of illness

Education about illness and treatment

Detoxification of death

Facilitation of discussion of issues related to dying

Exploration of fears associated with the process of dying

Reordering of life priorities

Accomplishing important life projects

Family support

Identification and communication of needs to parents and family members

Facilitating communication with health care providers

Mutual encouragement to participate in health care decisions

Symptom control

Cognitive techniques to help manage anticipatory anxiety, nausea, and pain

Source. Adapted from Gore-Felton and Spiegel 2000.

Selecting a Psychotherapeutic Strategy

Factors that may influence the choice of psychotherapy approach include the level of personal functioning along with stability of interpersonal functioning. The assessment should take into account a patient's level of emotional development, intellectual capacity, and ability to assume responsibility. Patients who are more flexible or have a variety of coping responses with more apparent resilience in their functioning are more likely to tolerate insight-oriented treatment. Patients who have a greater tendency to use denial, avoidance, or distortion or who have trouble relating with others are more likely to respond to more supportive or concrete behavioral approaches. The consultant should strike a balance between the different models of psychotherapy, targeting the pragmatic integration of the diverse approaches into an effective treatment approach. Children and adolescents with chronic physical illnesses may be at different phases of their treatment and thus different therapy models may be more effective. For instance, treatment at diagnosis may require a more supportive approach, with a transition to more insight-oriented goals as the illness progresses and as patients are more able to tolerate exploration of their illnesses. Supportive treatment may be especially necessary to prevent maladaptive emotional responses during acute exacerbations of an illness or at times of relapse.

Therapeutic Use of Play

In childhood, play is a major means of communication. The direct and indirect (reactive) effects of a physical illness can interfere with the ability to play, whereas restoration of the ability to play may indicate improvement in the illness or response to psychotherapy. Play can provide a medium in which the experience of the illnesses can be more easily understood and mastered. Play materials, including stuffed animals or dolls, art materials, and medical supplies, are needed. Real medical objects may be introduced to help desensitize the child and provide a sense of mastery. Sourkes (1998) described several play therapy techniques that can be used with physically ill children. The consultant can make lists of things that the child does not like about being sick (e.g., medical procedures, nausea, hair loss, hospitalization). In letter writing, the patient and the consultant jointly write a letter to a parent, a friend, a physician, or even a stuffed animal. The child and the consultant may also elect to write an illustrated book about the illness and hospitalization. Even during play, Sourkes (1998) suggested that the consultant may make use of what she calls the "therapist monologue." In this technique, the consultant articulates hypothesized feelings or fears that the child may experience. These emotions are introduced to the child in general terms such as "some children feel…" without the expectation that the child respond to the comments. Nonverbal art techniques may be useful in helping gain access to and understanding of a patient's inner world. Techniques such as a feelings mandala project and feelings pie project (described in Chapter 3) can prove useful in facilitating the expression of emotional responses and cognitive misunderstandings. The kinetic family drawing technique, in which the child is asked to draw the change in the family following the diagnosis of his or her illness, is a similar approach to facilitate dialogue.

Selected Psychotherapy Issues in Pediatric Illness

There are several important issues to consider in psychotherapy with the physically ill child.

Setting

Individual therapy in the hospital may occur at the patient's bedside or in a hospital conference room or hallway, often without the degree of privacy that is expected in the outpatient setting. Patients may be wearing hospital gowns or be attached to intravenous lines. The consultant has essentially little or no control over the patient's schedule. It is not unusual for the consultant and patient to be interrupted numerous times at the bedside. The length of the session may be unpredictable, sometimes as short as only a few minutes. Despite these impediments, it is common for a solid therapeutic alliance or relationship to develop rapidly. This has been attributed to the fact that hospitalized patients are in a more vulnerable emotional state with relatively fewer defense mechanisms and coping strategies (O'Dowd and Gomez 2001).

Duration

Lengths of hospital stays have dramatically decreased over the past several years, with the result being that the hospital consultant generally has time-limited involvement with most patients. This is best reflected in the consultant's frequent use of brief supportive therapy techniques aimed at building and supporting coping strategies. Brief treatment approaches, however, are well suited to youngsters who are dealing with the trauma of pediatric illness as well as the attendant feelings of loss and grief. O'Dowd and Gomez (2001) suggested that patients who are dealing with the stress of a life-threatening illness may be more open to utilizing psychotherapy because illness may prompt patients to reevaluate their life circumstances. However, the consultant will generally find that hospitalized patients are not interested in exploring deep-seated psychological issues but may be open to exploring the current issues related to their physical illness.

Consistency

Fluctuations in a patient's health may significantly limit the consistency of treatment. Youngsters receiving stressful and intense treatment regimens may be unable to participate in therapy either while in the hospital or as an outpatient. They may also be reluctant to give up what available free time they have for something that is seen as dispensable. Children and adolescents in the terminal phases of their illness similarly have difficulties keeping appointments. In addition, patients often prefer to minimize or ignore their emotional reactions during periods of relatively good health and become more engaged in catching up on missed school and peer activities. The consultant requires flexibility (e.g., changes in appointment times at short notice) and creativity (e.g., home visits) to maintain treatment consistency.

Illness as a Grieving Process

The bereavement model has been used to help conceptualize the process of adaptation to physical illness and to guide treatment intervention. Schneider (1984) emphasized the need to discover and accept what has both been lost and what has been left, in addition to what is possible that would not have been possible if the loss of health had not occurred. It is important to realize that the acceptance of illness is a process and that numerous events (e.g., relapse or developmental transitions) may trigger the grieving process. Ongoing losses in a chronic illness can complicate the process and extend the time needed to grieve.

Physical illness may involve loss in the following areas: independence, sense of control, privacy, body image, relationships, roles inside and outside the family, self-confidence, self-esteem, productivity, self-fulfillment, future plans, fantasies of immortality, unhindered movement, familiar daily routines, uninterrupted sleep, ways of expressing sexuality, and pain-free existence (Lewis 1998). Many of the assumptions of the child's daily life, including the sense of future, can be shattered by the diagnosis of an illness. Children and adolescents may experience overwhelming threats and fears, including threats to narcissistic integrity and self-esteem, regressive fear of strangers on whom the patient must rely, separation anxiety, fears of loss of love and approval, fear of loss of control of bodily functions, and fear of pain and humiliation as well as guilt and the fear of retaliation reflecting the unconscious belief that illness may be a punishment for past behavior (Lipsitt 1996; Strain and Grossman 1975).

As already noted, the emotional responses to physical illness or disability can be viewed as a process that begins with shock or denial and proceeds through feelings of anguish and protest toward the assimilation of illness information and adjustment. Emotional adjustment is also shaped by the developmental capacity of children to understand their illness (Table 13–3).

Denial

Denial is generally the first response to an illness as well as a common reaction in patients who have difficulty accepting distressing feelings or emotions. Denial serves an adaptive function in helping a patient at least temporarily ignore or minimize the overwhelming impact of stress that might otherwise threaten his or her psychological integrity. Denial is common during periods of illness quiescence when patients do not face the direct effects of their illness (e.g., pain). Denial becomes problematic when its use prevents acceptance of the realities of the illness. For example, denial may interfere with the acceptance of the diagnosis, delay the search for medical treatment, and interfere with treatment adherence. Denial has the potential to affect the child's motivation for psychotherapy and make psychotherapeutic work difficult or even impossible.

Anxiety

Anxiety may accompany an illness, particularly when the prognosis is uncertain or unresolved. Depending on their developmental level, patients may have fears of being abandoned or physically harmed. Fear of dying is not unusual for school-age children and adolescents in the midst of illness flares. Anxiety can interfere with a child's willingness or ability to disclose symptoms, resulting in treatment delays. In contrast, anxiety may lead children to over-interpret physical symptoms, leading to unnecessary medical investigations.

Anger

Anger is routine, although patients are generally more apt to use the word *frustration* when asked to name their feelings. Patients develop strong feelings of frustration, resentment, and hostility in the context of the losses (e.g., being with peers, being physically active) engendered by their illnesses. Patient anger can be directed internally, toward family members, at the pediatric team, or toward all three. Children may judge family members or their peers as being insensitive or unsupportive or even blame ancestors for illnesses that are thought to have a genetic component. The pediatric team members may be

Table 13–3.   Children's conceptions of illness

Age	Concepts and beliefs about illness
< 7 years	Preoperational stage of cognitive development Belief in the power of magical thinking Limited ability to understand functions of organs Inability to understand processes and mechanisms of illness Tendency to define illness as occurring only when they are told they are ill Belief that illnesses are caused by concrete actions Believe that illness can be avoided by obeying a rigid set of rules Inability to explain why or how these rules prevent illness Expectation that recovery from illness occurs either automatically or by rigid adherence to rules
8–10 years	Stage of concrete operational thinking Beginning ability to explain complex mechanisms of physical causality Immature understanding of the mechanisms of illness Belief that outside factors both cause and cure illness Belief that illness is caused primarily by germs or contagion Inability to explain the mechanism by which germs cause illness Expectation that recovery from illness occurs by "taking care of themselves" and allowing medicines to act on the illness Limited understanding of how the body heals itself Tendency to be more passive about health care
10–12 years	Stage of formal operations Ability to think hypothetically and to fill gaps in knowledge with generalizations from prior experience More sophisticated notion of concepts of illness Greater ability to understand physiological functions of the body Understanding that there are many interrelated causes of illness Understanding that illnesses are caused and cured as a result of the complex interaction between host and agent factors Understanding that the body's response is critical if treatment is to be effective No longer believes in the mere existence of things or events as being sufficient to cause, treat, or prevent disease Ability to see how diverse factors actively interact to affect health Very limited ability to understand concepts of prevention

Source.   Adapted from Bibace and Walsh 1981; Perrin 1984.

blamed for a wide range of problems, including poor communication, insensitivity, lack of time with patient, medication side effects, school absences, or adverse outcomes. Wherever the anger is directed, it is often shown by means of oppositional behaviors, including disobedience, self-defeating behaviors, refusal to cooperate with procedures, or nonadherence with treatment.

Depression

Sadness commonly accompanies pediatric illnesses. As with anger, the intensity of this feeling ranges from an expected normal response to a change in one's life to clinical depression. It can be difficult to tease out the symptoms of reactive sadness from those of the direct physical effects of an illness (e.g., malaise) in physically ill youngsters (see Chapter 6). Nevertheless, pediatric patients can manifest their sadness through both their mood and their behavior. They may be less active than expected, whether in the hospital or at home. They may become more focused on somatic concerns and be unwilling or unable to participate in daily activities.

Although most patients will emerge from this cycle of emotions and reestablish a healthy emotional equilibrium, an abnormal response occurs when the child is unable to effectively grieve the losses caused by the illness. Patients may be unable to recognize, experience, or put into perspective the feelings precipitated by the illness. Often the child may deny all emotions or may experience a specific mood to the relative exclusion of others, thus preventing emotional resolution regarding the loss of health. There may also be pathological grief manifestations that include excessive mood disturbances or behavioral problems.

Anticipatory Bereavement

The death of the child marks a tragic and dramatic intrusion into the normal order of the family life cycle. Children are supposed to outlive their parents, not the other way around. Decisions related to treatment during the terminal phase of an illness can be excruciating for parents who, on one hand, do not wish for their child to suffer but, on the other hand, cannot tolerate thoughts of ending treatment. Psychotherapy with the dying child is differentiated from more routine psychotherapy by the simple fact that the patient is confronting the concrete reality of death and loss rather than unrealistic fears and fantasies. Patients are generally aware that death is approaching, with the only unknown being its time of occurrence. Nevertheless, awareness of death is a fluid rather than static state (Sourkes 1998, 2000). Children tend to "dose themselves" regarding the degree to which they can discuss their illness (e.g., one minute crying and the next minute playing a game). The level of awareness may fluctuate depending on their medical status. Therapy provides the opportunity for the expression of grief and integration of life experiences. It provides an opportunity for discussion of quality-of-life issues as well as facilitating the child's expression of his or her own wishes for what is left of his or her life.

Children and adolescents can derive great comfort from the safety of a therapeutic relationship in which there is the opportunity to discuss their awareness of impending death. The consultant bears witness to the child's extraordinary situation and responds within the context of that reality (Lindemann 1990). A shared "knowledge" of the fine line that separates living from dying, whether implicit or explicit, becomes the containment of the psychotherapy (Sourkes 1992).

The development of anticipatory bereavement suggests a patient's greater recognition of his or her poor prognosis. The grief related to the impending loss of important relationships becomes manifest in an increased sensitivity to separation without specific references to death or in the form of direct and explicit discussion about death (Sourkes 1992). There may be themes of presence and absence or disappearance and return. Patients can project their concerns onto significant adults as well as show concern about the emotional well-being of their parents or loved ones after their death. There may be fears about being replaced and resentment of healthy siblings. As death draws near, children often turn inward and withdraw from the external world. Normal responses at this time can include retreat from physical contact, quietness, and irritability. It is common for the patient to withdraw from the therapeutic relationship. In the terminal phase, the consultant may only get to see the child in the presence of the parents. This may, however, be a time when important disclosures are made by the child.

Countertransference Issues for the Consultant

In work with physically ill patients the consultant must possess a high threshold for witnessing and tolerating pain, particularly pain involving separation and loss (Sourkes 1992). The consultant is in the position of witnessing the patient's experience of his or her illness. This requires an ability to contain and process intense emotional feelings in order to allow the child to have access to his or her own feelings and reactions. This is all the more salient because children and adolescents often try to protect their parents by not disclosing the full extent of their own awareness of their illness and may not have another place to share their painful feelings.

Working with children can elicit issues from the consultant's own childhood. It is important to be aware of these reactions, particularly if the consultant has his or her own history of childhood loss. The consultant may also have feelings of guilt about his or her own health or that of loved ones in relation to the patient's illness. Guilt about being healthy may develop unexpectedly and intrude on the therapeutic process, causing the consultant to withdraw instead of focusing on the patient's feelings of anger and isolation. It is common for consultants to develop a heightened appreciation for their own health and that of their families.

There is the potential for the therapist to over-identify with the patient or the family. This is particularly true when an endearing patient and family are facing severe debilitating or chronic illness. This reaction may be intensified if the consultant is also a parent. The consultant must be alert to "rescue fantasies" that result in a failure to maintain appropriate therapeutic boundaries. It is possible for the therapist to develop competitive or angry feelings directed toward the parents. Parents similarly may harbor feelings of resentment about the special relationship that can develop between a child and the consultant at this critical time in the child's life.

Awareness of these issues is important for the therapeutic relationship. Children who become aware of negative feelings between the consultant and their parents may withdraw from the therapeutic relationship. A strong alliance between the consultant and the parents diminishes this threat and facilitates the therapeutic work. The consultant's role as a therapist is to enhance the parents' understanding of their child's experience so that they can provide effective support to the child. Children may also be helped by the knowledge that the consultant can provide support to their parents.

Sourkes (1992) outlined a number of key aspects of therapeutic work with dying children and their potential implications for the countertransference; these are discussed in the following sections.

Tolerance for Physical Pain

The consultant must be prepared to witness firsthand the realities of the child's illness. The consultant must be able to tolerate the physical aspects of the child's treatment, including disfigurement or extreme pain. The consultant will often have to endure feelings of profound helplessness involved in watching suffering and yet still feel that he or she has something useful to offer. Adolescents in particular may heighten these doubts by making explicit accusations, directed toward the consultant, expressing their anger about the injustice of their illness. The consultant's credibility with the patient is partially based on his or her ability to tolerate the physical and emotional aspects of the patient's illness. Any unprocessed feelings of anxiety or discomfort have the potential of intruding into the therapeutic work.

Disclosure of Personal Information

The consultant must be prepared to disclose more personal information than may be typical in other types of treatment. Psychotherapy with a patient that has a life-threatening illness makes demands on the consultant to use him- or herself to an extraordinary degree. As anxiety, anger, and sadness emerge, the consultant may need to join the patient in expressing and exploring these emotions in a way that is linked to the patient's experience. For example, the consultant may need to acknowledge that he or she also would be frightened or angry if faced with similar circumstances. The ability to share these emotions allows the patient to feel less alone and can strengthen the patient's sense of safety.

Consistency and Continuity

The consultant must recognize the importance of his or her presence in the patient's life as one of the key consistent and reliable figures. Although important in any form of psychotherapy, continuity is an absolute prerequisite in working with physically ill children. The work requires an ongoing availability and accessibility to the patient that is more pronounced than in routine psychotherapy. The consultant must accept the potential need for increased contact such that careful planning occurs around vacations and absences. A failure to acknowledge and confront these issues may result in countertransference feelings of irritation and resentment as well as feelings of guilt in relation to the patient's needs. There is the potential that the consultant may withdraw at critical times from the patient (e.g., close to the time of the child's death).

Processing of Personal Losses

The consultant needs to develop ways to process and mourn the losses involved in the work. Without an outlet for these feelings, the consultant is at risk of harboring his or her own feelings of unresolved grief that may affect work with subsequent patients. Consultants should have access to ongoing support and consultation from peers and supervisors and engage in ongoing, honest appraisals of their capacity for repeated cycles of attachment and loss. Consultants may develop their own personal rituals regarding the death of their patients that can be helpful to facilitate further engagement in their work.

References

Bibace R, Walsh ME: Children's conceptions of health, illness, and bodily functions, in New Directions in Child Development. Edited by Bibace R, Walsh ME. San Francisco, CA, Jossey-Bass, 1981, pp 31–65

Goldberg RI, Green S: Medical psychotherapy. Am Fam Physician 31:173–178, 1985

Gore-Felton C, Spiegel D: Group psychotherapy for medically ill patients, in Psychiatric Care of the Medical Patient. Edited by Stoudemire A, Fogel BS, Greenberg DB. Oxford, England, Oxford University Press, 2000, pp 41–49

Green SA: Principles of medical psychotherapy, in Psychiatric Care of the Medical Patient. Edited by Stoudemire A, Fogel BS, Greenberg DB. Oxford, England, Oxford University Press, 2000, pp 3–15

Lewis KS: Emotional adjustment to a chronic illness. Prim Care Prac 2:38–51, 1998

Lindemann E: Quoted in Coles R: The Spiritual Life of Children. Boston, MA, Houghton-Mifflin, 1990, p 101

Lipsitt DR: Psychotherapy, in Textbook of Consultation-Liaison Psychiatry. Edited by Rundell JR, Wise MG. Washington, DC, American Psychiatric Press, 1996, pp 1053–1079

O'Dowd MA, Gomez MF: Psychotherapy in consultation-liaison psychiatry. Am J Psychother 55:122–132, 2001

Pennebaker JW: Opening Up: The Healing Power of Expressing Emotions. New York, Guilford Press, 1997

Perrin EC: The development of concepts about illness, in Child Health Care Communications. Edited by Thornton SM, Frankenberg WK. New York, Praeger, 1984, pp 17–30

Schneider J: Stress, Loss, and Grief. Baltimore, MD, University Park Press, 1984

Schwartz L, Drotar D: Effects of written emotional disclosure on caregivers of children and adolescents with chronic illness. J Pediatr Psychol 29:105–118, 2004

Sourkes B: The child with a life-threatening illness, in Countertransference in Psychotherapy With Children and Adolescents. Edited by Brandell J. Northvale, NJ, Jason Aronson, 1992, pp 267–284

Sourkes B: Psychotherapy, in Psycho-Oncology. Edited by Holland J. New York, Oxford University Press, 1998, pp 946–953

Sourkes B: Psychotherapy with the dying child, in Handbook of Psychiatry in Palliative Care. Edited by Chochinov H, Breitbart W. New York, Oxford University Press, 2000, pp 265–272

Strain JJ, Grossman S: Psychological Care of the Medically Ill. New York, Appleton-Century-Crofts, 1975

Suedfeld P, Pennebaker JW: Health outcomes and cognitive aspects of recalled negative life events. Psychosom Med 59:172–177, 1997

Szigethy EM, Whitton SE, Levy-Warren A, et al: Cognitive-behavioral therapy for depression in adolescents with inflammatory bowel disease: a pilot study. J Am Acad Child Adolesc Psychiatry 43:1469–1477, 2004

Szigethy ES, Carpenter J, Baum E, et al: Longitudinal treatment of adolescents with depression and inflammatory bowel disease. J Am Acad Child Adolesc Psychiatry 45:396–400, 2006

14

Family Therapy

The psychiatric consultant in the pediatric setting is often called upon to intervene directly with families of physically ill children. Requests for counseling are commonly made for issues such as 1) difficulties with emotional adjustment in family members, 2) family conflict related to the issues of parenting and responsibility for the medical treatment, and 3) conflict between the family and the pediatric team. Chronic physical illness commonly leads to alterations in the structure and functioning of the family system. From a family systems perspective, rules that have traditionally governed patterns of family interaction and the definition of roles within the family may be challenged by the demands of the illness. The quality of the marital relationship may be altered if one parent takes on a primary role in the management of the child's illness with the potential for exclusion of the less involved parent. Similarly, an overly close relationship between the ill child and one of the parents has the potential to interfere with important developmental tasks, such as the need for increased autonomy in the adolescent. Successful families maintain their integrity in the face of chronic illness provided they are able to demonstrate the flexibility to make necessary changes to facilitate effective childrearing in affected and healthy children as well as supporting the goals of all family members.

Medical family therapy describes the biopsychosocial treatment of individuals affected by medical illness (McDaniel et al. 1992). It emphasizes the collaboration between physicians, health care professionals, and family therapists. Medical family therapy provides a conceptual way to understand and promote the relationship among individuals involved in the treatment of the physically ill child. Sholevar and Sahar (2003) defined the main goals of medical family therapy as follows: 1) provide a framework for working with chronic illness, 2) recognize the impact of illness on the family, 3) promote collaboration with health care professionals, and 4) promote active involvement of the patient and family member in the management of the illness. This approach starts with a focus on the patient and often utilizes psychoeducational techniques to explain medical and psychological concepts related to the illness. It is enhanced by recognition of the developmental issues of the family.

Illness Course

Rolland (1987) was one of the first theorists to conceptualize the life cycle of an illness. This notion implies that there is an expected basic sequence or unfolding that may occur in the domains of individual and family life as well as in the life cycle of the illness. The onset, course, prognosis, and illness phases should be considered in the context of the illness (Newby 1996; Figure 14–1).

Pediatric physical illnesses can be classified as either acute or chronic onset. Acute-onset illnesses (e.g., meningitis) require more rapid mobilization of family crisis-management skills, whereas a chronic-onset illness (e.g., rheumatoid arthritis) allows for a more protracted period of adjustment. Illnesses may be characterized as being progressive, constant, or relapsing/episodic in terms of their chronological course. Progressive diseases are continuous and generally symptomatic with a progression in illness severity (e.g., cystic fibrosis). Disability increases in a stepwise or progressive fashion, with minimal periods of relief from the demands of the illness. In a constant-course illness there is a period of stabilization after the initial diagnosis (e.g., head injury). Recurrence can occur, but in general there are stable and predictable changes to which the family must adapt. Relapsing/Episodic illnesses are characterized by alternating periods of stability during which there is an absence of symptoms with flare-ups and exacerbations (e.g., ulcerative colitis). The extent to which the illness is likely to shorten the child's life is another critical variable.

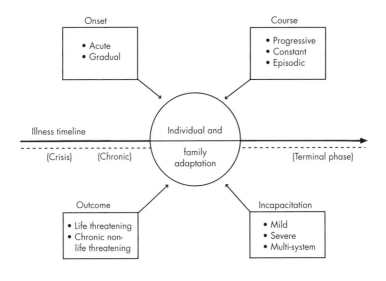

Figure 14–1. Family life cycle.

Source. Newby NM: "Chronic Illness and the Family Life-Cycle." *Journal of Advanced Nursing* 23:786–791, 1996. Copyright 1996, Blackwell Science Ltd. Used with permission.

Illnesses may be progressive and terminal in nature or of minor severity. Prognosis can be defined in terms of the degree of incapacitation as a result of impairments in cognition, physical mobility, or disfigurement.

Finally, it is helpful to determine the phase at which the family is located in terms of the longitudinal course of their child's illness. Rolland (1987) differentiated crisis, chronic, and terminal phases of the illness, each of which requires different responses on the part of family members. Periods of transition from one phase to another often require family members to reevaluate their circumstances and make changes to accommodate to the new demands of the illness. Issues that are not resolved in one phase have the potential to create difficulties in subsequent stages. For example, parents who are unable to agree upon career or work changes that are needed during the crisis phase may experience significant conflict or feelings of resentment that interfere with later adjustment.

Family Life Cycle

The family has been conceptualized as having its own life cycle with characteristic developmental stages that include the single adult, the new couple, the family with young children, the family with adolescent children, the family launching young adult children, and the family in later life (Carter and McGoldrick 2005). Similar to theories of individual development, in the family model, families are thought to have different developmental tasks associated with each phase of the family life cycle that include adjustments in the structure and nature of relationships to allow for the entry and exit of family members from the immediate family system. Specific hypotheses have been developed to conceptualize the particular psychological issues facing the family at each stage of development (Table 14–1).

Pediatric illness occurring at any one of these phases may interfere with the accomplishment of important developmental tasks. Carter and McGoldrick (2005) differentiated *vertical stressors,* which are the stressors related to historical issues in the family of origin, from *horizontal stressors,* which include the stressors associated with developmental life cycle transitions and external factors such as physical illness (Figure 14–2). Illness in an adolescent may result in the need for increased caretaking and supervision by parents at a time when the adolescent has normal developmental needs for greater autonomy and independence. The outcome may be a power struggle and oppositional behavior that is expressed in the form of treatment nonadherence. Similarly, the arrival of grandparents in the home to provide help may be more problematic for the family with a new infant at a time when the parents have yet to figure out their new parental roles.

The concept of centripetal and centrifugal forces has been used to explain how medical illness may interfere with family development (Rolland 1987). Family systems commonly oscillate between periods of family closeness (centripetal period) and periods of family disengagement (centrifugal period). During a centripetal period (e.g., childrearing), external boundaries around the family are tightened while personal boundaries between members are relaxed to facilitate the focus on childrearing responsibilities. By contrast, in the transition to a centrifugal period (e.g., young adult children leaving home), the family structure shifts to support a loosening of the relationship between the child and the parents and a greater connection to the outside world.

Table 14–1.   Illness and the family life cycle

Family life cycle stage	Psychological issues	Potential adverse impact of medical illness
Family with young children	Focus on the developmental issues of the child Develop confidence in parenting skills Preserve the intimacy of the couple Establish the role of extended family members	Parental difficulties in setting appropriate limits with consequent tendency to foster oppositional behavior in the child Disagreement about parenting issues Negative impact on the marital relationship Intrusion of extended family in caretaking role
Family with adolescent children	Support increased autonomy of the adolescent while maintaining appropriate levels of supervision Gradual transition to a greater level of adolescent responsibility for the medical treatment	Illness to interfere with appropriate adolescent needs for greater autonomy Increased feelings of insecurity in the adolescent and failure of individuation Acting out and oppositionality by the adolescent in response to constraints of medical illness Nonadherence with treatment
Family preparing for children to leave home	Support efforts of the young adult to leave home Young adult to develop romantic and social relationships outside of the family	Illness may limit or restrict academic and vocational plans of the young adult Interference with romantic and sexual relationships Ongoing financial dependency of the young adult on parents

Source.   Adapted from Carter B, McGoldrick M: "Overview: The Expanded Family Life Cycle," in *The Expanded Family Life Cycle: Individual, Family, and Social Perspectives,* 3rd Edition. Edited by Carter B, McGoldrick M. Boston, MA, Allyn and Bacon, 2005, p. 2. Copyright 2005, Pearson Education. Used with permission.

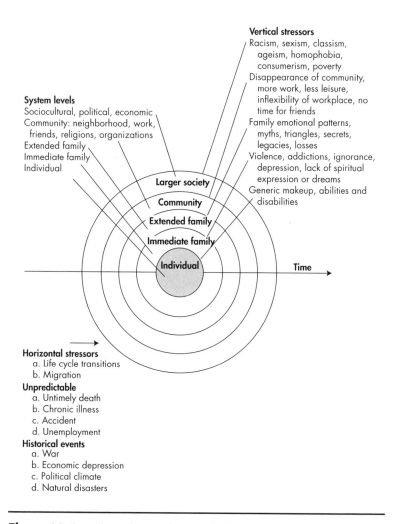

Figure 14–2. Flow of stress through the family.

Source. Reprinted from Carter B, McGoldrick M: "Overview: The Expanded Family Life Cycle," in *The Expanded Family Life Cycle: Individual, Family, and Social Perspectives*, 3rd Edition. Edited by Carter B, McGoldrick M. Boston, MA, Allyn and Bacon, 2005, p 6. Copyright 2005, Pearson Education. Used with permission.

Medical illness exerts a centripetal force on the family system. The demands of the medical treatment as well as the need to adjust to changes in the child's level of functioning may result in an inward family focus. Extended family members may be temporarily drawn back into the nuclear family to provide emotional and logistical support. Difficulties arise when the centripetal influence of the illness occurs at a time when the family is at a centrifugal stage of development. Developmental transitions that involve children leaving home may be prevented by the greater dependency that occurs in the context of the illness. Parents may also have to relinquish interests outside of the family to focus on caretaking for a sick child.

Factors Affecting Family Adjustment

More than 50% of families with a physically ill child manage to establish a healthy level of functioning, although individual family members may be prone to symptoms of anxiety, depression, anger, and somatic complaints (Jacobs 2000). This positive response occurs across the wide range of illness factors as well as at different stages of the family life cycle. To more fully understand family adjustment to a child's physical illness the following factors must be considered: illness factors, family belief system, and family structure.

Illness Factors

Degree of Predictability

The degree to which family members can anticipate acute exacerbations of the illness may affect their ability to make short- and long-term plans. The ability to plan for meaningful events (e.g., school attendance) for both ill and healthy siblings and even smaller daily routines (e.g., carpooling) are critical to the quality of family functioning. Unpredictability can create a cycle of anxiety and anger, particularly in families that have a history of early trauma or loss.

Degree of Disability

The extent of the child's physical disability has important implications for the way roles are allocated in the family. It may be necessary to engage additional childcare on a long-term basis in order for work and family routines to continue. Mothers are more likely to give up employment or career aspirations to care for ill children. The loss of income may affect the family's financial resources.

Stigma

Disorders with significant social stigma, such as AIDS, bring up some unique issues. Family members may be reluctant to share information about the child's illness with friends, family members, or professional colleagues. There may be a reluctance to have friends or friends of healthy siblings visit the home. This tendency toward collective shame may isolate family members from critical sources of social support.

Degree of Monitoring

The degree of supervision and monitoring required for specific illnesses, such as diabetes mellitus or cystic fibrosis, may have a significant impact on the autonomy of individual family members. Adolescents are particularly prone to resist these efforts and may fail to adhere to their treatment. Increased demands for adult supervision may also have an adverse impact on the parents' ability to work and participate in non–illness-related family events.

Prognosis

An uncertain prognosis can leave the family struggling with fears of relapse or death and can be a major source of stress in the family (Jacobs 2000). Illnesses with a poor prognosis (e.g., acute myelogenous leukemia) are often characterized by the experience of anticipatory grief in family members as they imagine the child's death. There is the potential for isolation of family members in families that are not able to discuss these concerns.

Family Belief System

Family behavior cannot be understood in isolation from its history. Family coping patterns are transmitted across generations as family myths, taboos, expectations, and belief systems. Stressors occurring as a result of the diagnosis of a pediatric illness may be intensified based on long-held family beliefs and prior experiences of illness and loss. Family members may have particular assumptions about illness and its prognosis as well as traditions and expectations regarding caretaking behaviors during times of illness (Shaw and Halliday 1992). Generally, family beliefs are related to illness permanence, commitment, and connectedness. Family beliefs assist the family in preserving a sense of competence and mastery during a time of crisis. For example, some families may see illness as a test of the family strength and as a challenge to be worked through to strengthen the family. There is often a polarity between the family's belief in their ability to master issues versus a fatalistic position in which the family believes they have no control over the outcome. The family's place on this continuum often determines how well the family is able to adapt.

Family Structure

Family adaptation is influenced by unique family characteristics that shape and influence children's behavior. Minuchin (1974) described a structural family approach to explain how families function (Table 14–2). Families are conceptualized as comprising different subsystems that are separated from each other by boundaries and levels of authority. Healthy families have a wide range and flexibility in the way that subsystems interact with one another, but under conditions of stress they may develop more rigid interactional patterns. Childhood physical illness stresses the family structure and can result in family members having to negotiate new patterns of interaction. Boundary regulation, enmeshment, overprotectiveness, role allocation, hierarchy, rigidity, and communication problems are concepts that have been used to explain family behaviors in response to a medical illness (Minuchin et al. 1978).

Impact of Illness on Family Functioning

Emotional, cognitive, and behavioral responses on the part of the family are set in motion when a child develops a medical illness. The family experiences the vulnerability of their child along with their inability to control and protect the child from the illness. Successful adaptation requires that the family develop a good understanding of the illness and recognize its potential complications and treatment. The family must continue to acknowledge their child's skills and abilities while at the same accommodating to changes in the child's health and ability. Parents must maintain discipline and encourage the active contribution of their child and his or her siblings. Rolland (1987) described three developmental phases (crisis, chronic, and terminal) that are helpful in understanding the impact of the illness on family functioning.

Crisis Phase

The crisis phase is the period immediately before and after the diagnosis of a pediatric illness. Medical activities are directed toward controlling the symp-

Table 14–2. Family structure and physical illness

Concept	Definition	Relationship with physical illness
Boundary regulation	The management of space and privacy among individuals in the family, between generations, and between the family and the outside world	Boundaries are vulnerable to disruption in chronic illness. Individual family members may feel they have no right to private time when a sick family member needs emotional support. There is a potential for coalitions between one of the parents and the sick child or between one parent and a healthy sibling. Boundaries with the outside world may become more rigid, particularly if the illness carries a social stigma.
Enmeshment	A situation in which there is a high degree of involvement and lack of appropriate boundaries between family members	There is a potential for increased risk of enmeshment between the child and parent due to the child's increased need for emotional support. There is a potential for exclusion of the less involved parent and unaffected siblings. There is a potential for interference with the child's developmental needs for autonomy and privacy.
Overprotectiveness	An overly high degree of concern that family members show toward each other	Overprotectiveness is a common consequence of chronic illness. Excessive parental protective and nurturing responses may accompany even minor signs of emotional distress in the child. Parents may excuse their child from normal responsibilities or fail to set appropriate limits, fostering maladaptive patterns of behavior (e.g., nonadherence with treatment).

Table 14–2.   Family structure and physical illness *(continued)*

Concept	Definition	Relationship with physical illness
Role allocation	The assignment of roles within the family structure	The ill child may assume a position of centrality within the family. Healthy siblings may be asked to take on caretaking roles or responsibilities that are not appropriate for their age. There may be a potential pressure on one of the parents to take on a full-time caretaking role while the other parent attempts to find new ways to increase the family's income.
Family hierarchy	The level of authority that exists in the family Healthy families are defined by having parents at the top of the hierarchy with appropriate delegation of responsibilities to siblings and extended family members.	Families with a strict generational hierarchy may have difficulty in allowing healthy siblings assume appropriate caretaking roles for an ill child. There is a potential for inversion of the traditional power hierarchy, with the child using the physical illness to take on an unhealthy position of emotional dominance.
Rigidity	The family's generally appropriate tendency to maintain the status quo	The threat to a family's stability caused by a physical illness may lead the family to persist with rigid patterns of behavior. Attempts to maintain pre-illness routines that are no longer realistic may increase family stress. Families with rigid boundaries may have difficulties in mobilizing social support and allowing the entry of extended family members, pediatric staff, and outside agencies.

Table 14–2.   Family structure and physical illness *(continued)*

Concept	Definition	Relationship with physical illness
Communication problems	Lack of transmitting information within the family	There is a potential for the gradual restriction of affect among family members. There is a potential to minimize discussion of important issues because of fears that tension may trigger episodes of the illness. There may be fears that strong emotional expression may worsen the patient's prognosis.

Source.   Adapted from Minuchin 1974.

Table 14–3. Family coping tasks during the crisis phase of the illness

- Obtain and retain information about the disease
- Explain the illness to healthy siblings and family members
- Mobilize support from friends and extended family
- Manage the emotional reactions to the illness (e.g., anxiety and depression)
- Temporarily reallocate family resources

Source. Adapted from Jacobs 2000.

toms and progression of the illness. This phase is characterized by shock and bewilderment, closely followed by feelings of grief regarding the potential loss of the healthy child (Sholevar and Sahar 2003). This is a time when there may be an oscillation between denial of the illness and acceptance of permanent change. Rowland (1989) described the "five Ds" to summarize the concerns and worries about the patient's (and family's) reaction to a new diagnosis of cancer: distance, dependence, disability, disfigurement, and death.

The crisis phase represents an existential crisis during which a family may search for meaning in an effort to obtain a sense of mastery. This can be a time when families may turn to religious and spiritual support. Families may respond to their "need for meaning" in different ways, including resignation (assuming a passive role in the search for meaning by resigning oneself to circumstances), reconciliation (a more active approach in which the patient or family may believe there is a reason for the illness of which they are not aware but are able to accept), and remonstration (in which there is a continued search for meaning throughout the course of the illness) (Taylor 1995). Table 14–3 outlines family coping tasks during the crisis phase. Anxiety levels are generally so high that it may be difficult for family members to integrate all of the new medical information. Additional tasks may include learning how to live with pain and disability and adapting to the pediatric hospital setting.

The central role of the illness in the family necessitates other family problems being temporarily placed on hold. If these issues have previously been problematic or difficult to negotiate, the centrality of the illness may serve the role of helping the family avoid having to deal with other issues. This is particularly true in parents who have unresolved marital issues. Illness may be used to regulate marital distance or parental conflict. Parenting may become an adversarial process because the illness tends to polarize and fragment the family such that opposing sides are taken regarding issues related to the illness.

Chronic Phase

The chronic phase unfolds after the initial diagnosis of and readjustment to a pediatric illness. In many ways this is a maintenance period characterized by the goal of minimizing the risk of relapse through appropriate medical care. Social support and rehabilitation are important in this phase to reduce disability and maximize functioning. Illnesses can have stable, progressive, and episodic courses of varying time length. In the treatment of cancer, for example, families enter a phase in which they hope for long-term remission but remain aware of the potential for recurrence. As fears about recurrence lessen, patients may be defined as long-term survivors. If the illness is fatal, the chronic phase becomes a period of "living in limbo."

Children and their families may have delayed emotional reactions to their illness. It is not unusual for an ill child to be at a different phase in his or her reaction to the illness after treatment ends, with family members wanting to move on and to restore a sense of normalcy that may not be possible for the child. Families may experience a sense of abandonment by the health care team due to the reduction in frequency of medical appointments. Common concerns in the chronic phase include fears of recurrence, body image concerns, school and academic difficulties, peer problems, and awareness of longer-term illness complications. Family members may also mourn the loss of past and future opportunities for the ill child or maintain crisis patterns of behavior from the crisis phase that have the potential to reinforce the child's sick role. The term *illness-maintaining behaviors* has been used to describe patterns of poor treatment adherence, excessive dependency on the sick role, behavioral problems, and depression (Frey 1984).

Families with adaptive coping mechanisms during the chronic phase of the illness are able to contain the impact of the illness and prevent it from dominating family life. The goal should be one of restoring a sense of normalcy and reestablishing important family routines that accommodate the demands of the child's illness. It is important wherever possible for the family to accept the permanent changes brought about by the illness and to positively redefine the developmental trajectory of both the child and the family.

Terminal Phase

In the terminal phase of the illness, the inevitability of death becomes apparent and dominates family life. The major task for the family during the terminal phase is for family members to process their emotional feelings and make preparations for the loss of the child. This is the phase in which anticipatory bereavement and preparation for death occurs. It is a time for the family to review their child's life, address family conflicts, communicate important messages, and prepare to say good-bye. Adjustments in the family's daily routine become necessary as the child's health deteriorates. The most common problem that arises is disagreement between parents when their respective treatment goals are different from each other or from those of the child. In some circumstances families will attempt to push for or seek out increasingly aggressive or unrealistic treatment options.

Reactions of Siblings

In general there is an increasing psychosocial dysfunction in siblings of chronically ill children. Some studies have found siblings to have a greater likelihood of behavioral and school difficulties, whereas others have shown them to be both more shy and more anxious compared with control subjects. Siblings who have poor relationships with their parents or those who are in the middle of an important developmental transition appear to have a decreased ability to tolerate the stresses related to the diagnosis of an illness in a family member (Stewart et al. 1992).

Families generally have limited emotional and financial resources, and their priorities may need to be reordered following the diagnosis of a major medical illness. These changes have the potential of interfering with the goals and routines of healthy siblings. Parents, for example, may have to struggle with how to distribute the available resources and balance the good of one child against the other. Siblings are particularly vulnerable to the absence of their parents, who are pulled into caretaking responsibilities for the ill child. Siblings may be pulled into situations of early responsibility at the expense of their own developmental needs. Parents often experience feelings of guilt or believe that they have failed their children in fundamental ways by burdening them with additional stress. Siblings are often aware of these concerns and may further suppress their reactions in an effort to avoid further burdening their parents.

Siblings may have feelings of confusion about the illness (Table 14–4). Although siblings often overhear information from conversations between parents and with physicians, they are often not given adequate explanations about the illness. As a result, siblings arrive at theories of illness based on their own fears and immature perceptions and may have inappropriate feelings of responsibility or concerns about their own health. Siblings may struggle with conflicting emotions regarding their ill sibling. There can be strong feelings of resentment and complaints about unfairness regarding special treatment or privileges afforded the ill child. Siblings are often called upon to explain and defend the ill sibling and to protect him or her from being rejected or teased. Siblings may feel embarrassed or ashamed about the illness and the way it reflects on their family. Normal sibling rivalry may become associated with feelings of guilt in siblings who do not feel justified in having negative thoughts.

Relationship With the Pediatric Team

Although strong relationships develop between the family and the pediatric team, the impact of these relationships on the course of the illness is often underestimated. Interactions between the family and the medical team directly influence the family's experience of their child's illness. The large number of health care providers generally involved in giving complex pediatric care increases the opportunities for breakdowns in communication and conflict around care. Some families welcome the entry of outside caretakers, whereas others are more apprehensive and may want to limit access of medical providers to their children. Problems arise most often when parents and the pediatric team are in conflict over the treatment plan. Pediatric team members may experience pressures to join in a coalition with one parent against the other regarding the treatment planning decisions. Providers and family members must be able to work through the grieving process in a terminal illness to prepare for the death of the child. Family members may avoid dealing with these feelings by failing to integrate information from the pediatric team, by maintaining unrealistic expectations of the team, and by taking out their feelings of anger on the health care providers. Physicians in turn may experience feelings of failure, sadness, and anger related to their inability to cure the child and may withdraw emotionally at critical points during the child's treatment.

Table 14–4. Questions siblings have

About causation/prognosis

What caused my brother's/sister's illness/disability?
Will it get worse?
Will she/he ever get well?
Will she/he die?
Will I catch what my brother/sister has?
Has my own health been bought at the cost of my brother's/sister's health?
Is my brother/sister somehow defective or less of a person?
Why didn't my parents stop this from happening?
How can I explain this to other people?

About their own health

Am I ill/handicapped too?
How many of my brother's/sister's characteristics do I share?
Will the same thing happen to me sometime or am I safe?

About the unfairness

Why did this happen to our family?
What did we do to deserve this?
Why should I have to live with this when my friends don't?
Why are there different rules for my brother/sister than for me?
Am I not as important as my brother/sister?

About feelings

Do I have the right to be mad at someone who is ill/helpless?
How come all the money (time, love, etc.) goes to my brother/sister?
Doesn't anyone know that what I need is important, too?
How can I help my brother/sister and still have other kids like me?
Do I have to love him/her when she/he makes me so unhappy?
Whom do my parents love most?

About the future of their brother/sister

I hear a lot about ill/handicapped children, but I never hear about grown-ups.
What happens to ill or handicapped children when they grow up?
Do ill/handicapped children grow up at all?

About their own future

Will I be able to have my own children?
Do I carry a defective gene that I will pass on to other generations?
Will I have a defective child?
Will some accident or disease strike my life unexpectedly as it did with my parents?
Will this brother/sister compromise what I want to do with my own grown-up life?

Table 14–4.   Questions siblings have *(continued)*

About responsibility

How much do I own my brother/sister?

How much can I leave to others?

Where does ultimate responsibility lie for my brother/sister?

Will I be responsible for my sister/brother when she/he grows up?

Do my parents expect me to take charge when they no longer can?

Will I be able to do a good job in caring for my brother/sister?

Will I find a spouse who will want to share this job?

How much of what I need and want am I supposed to give up so my brother/sister can be happy, included, well?

Do I have to achieve twice as much to make up for what my brother/sister lacks?

Am I responsible for the care of my parents; to support and comfort them?

Source.   Reprinted from Siemon M: "Siblings of the Chronically Ill or Disabled Child." *Nursing Clinics of North America* 19:302, 1984. Copyright 1984, Elsevier Inc. Used with permission.

Family Intervention Guidelines

The psychiatric consultant aims to facilitate a system of support for the ill child. This requires collaboration with the child, the family, and the pediatric team. In this context, the goals of family therapy are to help the family acknowledge the extent of the illness, manage their emotional reactions, and adjust to the demands of the illness and its treatment. These goals are often achieved by putting the parents in charge of the management of the illness, encouraging the involvement of less-involved parents, reaching consensus regarding parenting tasks, supporting cooperation among the siblings, and addressing individual concerns of the child.

Assessment Phase

Effective consultation to any family requires an ability to understand the challenges brought about by the illness. The previous discussions regarding illness factors, the family life cycle, factors affecting family adjustment, illness impact on the family functioning, sibling reactions, and relationship with the pediatric team provide the consultant with a theoretical foundation for this assessment. It is important to have an understanding of previous psychiatric consultations and intervention efforts so that the consultant can understand what has worked and what has not worked well in the past.

Assessing the Family's Reaction to the Referral

Referrals regarding the family are generally made when the relationship between the family and the pediatric team is showing signs of tension. It is important for the consultant to demonstrate empathy and understanding of the concerns of the pediatric team. From the start, the consultant should attempt to understand any systems issues involving the medical team, including feelings of anger or blame on the part of either the family or the pediatric team. In the initial contact with the family, it is important to assess their attitudes toward both the referral and the physician making the referral. The referral is often prompted by a breakdown in the relationship between the family and the medical team for several reasons that may include poor communication, lack of trust, or frustration related to failures in making a diagnosis or in implementing effective treatment interventions.

Engaging the Family

Rather than focusing on chronic family issues, it is more helpful to focus on the current problems that are directly related to the illness. Even if difficulties in managing illness reflect more long-standing problems, the family's focus at the time of referral is usually on the illness. Treatment that results in a successful experience in managing the illness will reinforce confidence in the consultant. The objective can be conceptualized as maintaining a successful balance between managing the illness and maintaining family priorities. The following assessment methods may be useful in engaging the family:

- The *Family APGAR* (Smilkstein 1978) is a five-item instrument that assesses the patient's perceptions of his or her family relationships. These perceptions include adaptation, partnership, growth, affection, and results (Figure 14–3).
- The *family circle method* consists of asking family members to draw a circle and place their family members and other important people inside the circle. This technique helps assess closeness between individual family members as well as particular coalitions or subgroups.
- The *family genogram* is a helpful way to assess family genetic relationships, relationship issues, and the family's past experience of medical issues. The family genogram can also be used to note important life events in the family.
- The *family timeline* is a chronological description of the important life events within the immediate and extended family.

Family APGAR Questionnaire

Introduction: To be read to the family.
"The following questions have been designed to help us better understand you and your family. You should feel free to ask questions about any item in the questionnaire. Answer each question as 'almost always,' 'some of the time,' or 'hardly ever.' Add any additional comments you want. *Family* is defined as the individual(s) with whom you usually live."

For each question, check only one box.

	Almost always	Some of the time	Hardly ever
1. I am satisfied that I can turn to my family for help when something is troubling me. Comments:_____	☐	☐	☐
2. I am satisfied that my family talks things over with me and shares problems with me. Comments:_____	☐	☐	☐
3. I am satisfied that my family accepts and supports my wishes to take on new activities or directions. Comments:_____	☐	☐	☐
4. I am satisfied that my family expresses affection and responds to my emotions, such as anger, sorrow, and love. Comments:_____	☐	☐	☐
5. I am satisfied with the way my family and I share time together. Comments:_____	☐	☐	☐

Scoring: The patient checks one of three choices, which are scored as follows: "Almost always" (2 points), "Some of the time" (1 point), or "Hardly ever" (0 points). The scores for each of the five questions are then totaled. A score of 7–10 suggests a highly functional family. A score of 4–6 suggests a moderately dysfunctional family. A score of 0–3 suggests a severely dysfunctional family.

According to which member of the family is being interviewed, the physician may substitute for the word *family* either *spouse, significant other, parents,* or *children.*

Figure 14–3.   Family APGAR questionnaire.
Source.   Adapted from Smilkstein G: "The Family APGAR: A Proposal for Family Function Test and Its Use by Physicians." *Journal of Family Practice* 6:1234, 1978. Copyright 1978, Appleton and Lange, Inc. Used with permission.

Education and Normalization of Reactions to the Illness

Although it is the task of the pediatric team to educate the family about the illness, it is important for the consultant to evaluate the family's understanding of illness. It is not unusual, given the shock and anxiety that accompany a new physical illness diagnosis, that parents have difficulty integrating complex medical concepts and treatments. The consultant should take an active role in educating the family about developmental issues that may interfere with the child's ability to understand his or her illness and to take responsibility for treatment. The family may need guidance about the need to talk openly with their child about the illness as well as the importance of encouraging and answering questions in a direct yet age-appropriate manner. Normalization of the illness experience is an important therapeutic intervention. Families generally respond well to information that validates their own experience of and reactions to their child's illness. The family may need permission to place normal plans and activities on hold or encouragement to solicit and utilize support from extended family and outside agencies.

Identifying Major Family Concerns

The initial assessment should include an itemization of the major concerns of the family. The therapist may assist by listing common family concerns and by asking each family member to comment on the relevance to their own family (Table 14–5). Van Horn et al. (2001) were able to meaningfully and reliably categorize concerns of mothers of children with pediatric heart disease into medical prognosis, quality of life, psychosocial functioning, effects on family, and financial issues. An awareness of such concerns will improve clinical care by enabling the consultant to anticipate and address concerns in a proactive way. The results may inform the development of supportive mental health interventions for families dealing with a major medical illness.

Treatment Phase

After the initial assessment, the consultant moves into the treatment phase. This may range from support and education within the role of consultant to a more defined role as a family therapist. The following intervention principles are critical to employ when working with families facing pediatric illness.

Delegating Responsibility for Treatment

The therapist can assist the family in delegating responsibility for different components of a child's treatment. It is common to find that one family mem-

Table 14–5.   Common family concerns regarding illness diagnosis

- How to discuss implications of the illness with the affected child
- How to discuss the illness with healthy siblings
- Emotional impact of the illness on the child
- Emotional impact of the illness on healthy siblings
- How to manage involvement of extended family members and friends
- Educational impact of illness on the affected child
- How to delegate and manage treatment responsibilities
- Conflict or disagreement between parents regarding the medical treatment plan
- Increased risk of marital conflict
- Impact of illness on parents' work schedule and career goals
- How to manage limit setting and expectations of responsibilities in the affected child
- Tendency of children to protect their parents due to their concerns about the burden of the illness

ber takes on a disproportionate share of responsibility, with the most common dynamic in two-parent families being maternal overload and paternal distance. Common interventions include involving peripheral family members, delegating limited responsibilities to other family members, and giving increased self-care responsibility to the child. Lack of communication between parents regarding these issues may result in significant tension or marital conflict. Single-parent families struggle with not having someone with whom to share treatment responsibilities, and creative efforts are required to increase social support.

Establishing Appropriate Parental Authority

Parents are often reluctant to set limits or to discipline the ill child, particularly during the early phases of the illness. The natural tendency to overcompensate early in an illness, if not corrected, may result in behavior problems and feelings of vulnerability in the child as well as anger and resentment among siblings. The therapist can empower parents to resume their practice of setting age-appropriate limits, which is beneficial for all children in the family. Parents are encouraged to be consistent in their expectations of responsible behavior in both healthy and affected children.

Processing the Impact of the Illness on Family Life

Life-threatening illness introduces issues of uncertainty and potential loss into the family system. To some degree, the impact depends on the nature of the specific illness, its timing in the family life cycle, and family coping mechanisms. In addition to its effect on physical health, chronic illness may result in significant changes in a child's role and lifestyle. Role reversals, for example, may result in the delegation of responsibilities to healthy siblings and reduced responsibility for the ill child. There can be a progressive organization of family life around the ill child to the detriment of the developmental needs of the family. The first step in the treatment is recognition by the family of the profound and pervasive consequences of the disability. All family members should be given an opportunity to openly discuss the impact of the illness on their respective lives.

Intervening With Siblings

Siemon (1984) proposed several ways to help meet the needs of siblings of ill children. These include education about the illness, encouragement to express feelings, and opportunities for experiences separate from their sibling's illness. Open and clear communication about the illness is strongly encouraged, because efforts to protect healthy siblings from this information usually leads to increased feelings of loneliness and anxiety (Siemon 1984). Siblings appreciate being involved in decision making and responsibilities that are appropriate for their developmental age. Although it is impossible to completely shield siblings from the impact of the illness, the family should strive to strike a balance such that no one individual in the family is overwhelmed by the demands of the illness. Siblings need to know that their parents can understand their feelings of embarrassment, anger, and confusion. Siblings who feel confident in their parents' resilience are more able to express their own thoughts and feelings and feel secure in their parents' ability to protect the ill child. Parents may need to anticipate questions and concerns and not assume the siblings will independently raise these issues. Table 14–6 lists some general approaches that may be helpful to siblings.

Reestablishing the Family Balance

Families generally respond well to interventions that help reestablish a balance so that the illness does not continue to consume family life. In the

Table 14–6. How to assist siblings with adjustment to a family illness

- Speak directly in an age-appropriate manner about the illness.
- Encourage questions about their sibling's illness.
- Have scheduled family meetings to discuss new information and check in on how individual family members are coping.
- Spend time alone with each sibling.
- Encourage attention to healthy siblings when people are focusing on the illness.
- Include siblings in decision making.
- Anticipate behavior problems and regression in healthy siblings.
- Alert teachers to the stress of the illness at home.
- Facilitate participation of siblings in camps and social support groups.

chronic phase of the illness, the therapist can help the family gain perspective on the illness. Family members can be prompted to recall priorities and routines that were present before the illness. During the chronic phase the therapist can support a shift of attention away from the ill child. Narrative family therapy is useful in helping understand the family's definition of the illness and its impact (White and Epston 1990). Treatment techniques using this model include those of externalizing the problem and enlisting the family's ability to minimize the impact of the illness on the family's experience. Families may develop rigid or even incorrect narratives about the illness or specific family members that can be revised to allow for greater flexibility and appreciation of different future outcomes. Family therapy can help families take on a broader perspective and reduce the tendency to become overly focused on the illness. The therapist can help the family acknowledge constraints caused by the illness, normalize their emotional responses, increase family support, and reinforce the continuance of normal family rituals.

The therapist should be alert to dysfunctional family dynamics when there is resistance to establishing balance within the family. The resistance may lie in the need to resume normal family tasks that involve greater degrees of separation between family members and may also be present when the illness diverts attention away from problematic family conflicts. For instance, the ill child may have a central role in protecting the parents, including hiding legitimate physical and psychological needs. Minuchin et al. (1978) described the "psychosomatic family" whereby family processes predispose individual family members to have somatic responses to stress.

References

Carter B, McGoldrick M: Overview: the expanded family life cycle, in The Expanded Family Life Cycle: Individual, Family, and Social Perspectives, 3rd Edition. Edited by Carter B, McGoldrick M. Boston, MA, Allyn and Bacon, 2005, pp 1–26

Frey J III: A family/systems approach to illness-maintaining behaviors in chronically ill adolescents. Fam Process 23:251–260, 1984

Jacobs J: Family therapy in chronic medical illness, in Psychiatric Care of the Medical Patient, 2nd Edition. Edited by Stoudemire A, Fogel BS, Greenberg DB. Oxford, England, Oxford University Press, 2000, pp 31–39

McDaniel SH, Hepworth J, Doherty W: Medical Family Therapy. New York, Basic Books, 1992

Minuchin S: Families and Family Therapy. Cambridge, MA, Harvard University Press, 1974

Minuchin S, Rosman BL, Baker L: Psychosomatic Families: Anorexia Nervosa in Context. Cambridge, MA, Harvard University Press, 1978

Newby NM: Chronic illness and the family life-cycle. J Adv Nur 23:786–791, 1996

Rolland JS: Chronic illness and the life cycle: a conceptual framework. Fam Process 26: 203–221, 1987

Rowland JH: Developmental stage and adaptation: adult model, in Handbook of Psychooncology: Psychological Care of the Patient with Cancer. Edited by Holland JC, Rolland JH. New York, Oxford University Press, 1989, pp 25–43

Shaw MC, Halliday PH: The family, crisis and chronic illness: an evolutionary model. J Adv Nurs 17:537–543, 1992

Sholevar GP, Sahar C: Medical family therapy, in Textbook of Family and Couples Therapy: Clinical Applications. Edited by Sholevar GP, Schwoeri, LD. Washington, DC, American Psychiatric Publishing, 2003, pp 747–767

Siemon M: Siblings of the chronically ill or disabled child: meeting their needs. Nurs Clin North Am 19:295–307, 1984

Smilkstein G: The Family APGAR: a proposal for family function test and its use by physicians. J Fam Pract 6:1231–1239, 1978

Stewart DA, Stein A, Forrest GC, et al: Psychosocial adjustment in siblings of children with chronic life-threatening illness: a research note. J Child Psychol Psychiatry 33:779–784, 1992

Taylor EJ: Whys and wherefores: adult patient perspectives of the meaning of cancer. Semin Oncol Nurs 11:32–40, 1995

Van Horn M, DeMaso DR, Gonzalez-Heydrich J, et al: Illness-related concerns of mothers with congenital heart disease. J Am Acad Child Adolesc Psychiatry 40:847–854, 2001

White M, Epston D: Narrative Means to Therapeutic Ends. New York, WW Norton, 1990

15

Psychopharmacological Approaches and Considerations

The psychiatric consultant in the pediatric setting is often called upon to make recommendations about the use of psychotropic medications, including assistance in interpreting medication side effects and potential drug interactions. There may be requests for medication evaluations for distressed parents and family members. Effective pharmacological interventions can help patients relieve emotional and behavioral distress related to their illness or treatment as well as support the pediatric team in its care of patients.

A target symptom approach works well in the pediatric setting. Although medication use considerations by physicians frequently center on the presence or absence of a psychiatric disorder, medications target specific clinical symptoms as opposed to specific diagnostic entities. In the pediatric setting, these target symptoms generally fall into one or more of the following categories: agitation, anxiety, delirium, depression, fatigue, insomnia, pain, psychosis, or withdrawal. Table 15–1 is an outline of medications that the consultant can consider for these target symptom categories when formulating recommendations.

Table 15–1.   Target symptom approach in pediatric consultation

Target symptom	Medication considerations
Agitation	Atypical antipsychotic agent
	Typical antipsychotic agent
	Benzodiazepine
	Diphenhydramine (younger children)
Anxiety	Benzodiazepine
	Antidepressant
	Buspirone
	Gabapentin
	Clonidine
Delirium	Antipsychotic agent
Depression	Selective serotonin reuptake inhibitors
	Norepinephrine selective reuptake inhibitors
	Stimulant
Fatigue	Stimulant
	Selective serotonin reuptake inhibitors
	Modafinil
Insomnia	Diphenhydramine
	Benzodiazepine
	Trazodone
	Hypnotics (e.g., zolpidem or zaleplon)
	Amitriptyline
	Mirtazapine
Pain	Tricyclic antidepressants
	Norepinephrine selective reuptake inhibitors (e.g., duloxetine)
	Analgesic
	Anticonvulsants
Psychosis	Atypical antipsychotic agent
	Benzodiazepine
Withdrawal	Benzodiazepine
	Clonidine

Pharmacokinetics

Pharmacokinetics describes the absorption, distribution, metabolism, and elimination of medications (Robinson and Owen 2005).

Absorption

Medications can be administered by several routes, including oral, intravenous, intramuscular, subcutaneous, rectal, transdermal, or sublingual. Drug bioavailability is the rate and extent to which a drug's active ingredients are absorbed and made available for therapeutic action. The rate of absorption is influenced by drug formulation, drug interactions, and gastric motility, which all become important factors when rapid onset of action is required.

The extent of drug absorption is more relevant in the chronic administration of medications. Properties that affect absorption include the surface area, mucosal integrity/function, gastric pH, and local blood flow. In general, gastric absorption is increased when the stomach is empty, although gastrointestinal side effects are often increased when medications are taken without food. Drugs given orally that are absorbed through the gastrointestinal tract may be altered by first-pass hepatic metabolism. Sublingual and topical administration of drugs minimizes the first-pass effect, and rectal administration reduces the effect by 50%. Intravenous drug delivery offers 100% bioavailability and generally results in a more rapid therapeutic effect.

Distribution

Serum pH, blood flow, protein binding, fat solubility, and the degree of ionization influence the distribution of a medication. With the exception of lithium, methylphenidate, and venlafaxine, most psychoactive drugs are bound to proteins 80%–95%, either albumin or α_1 glycoprotein. In general, only the unbound or free drug is pharmacologically active. Drugs such as divalproex sodium and barbiturates tend to bind to albumin, whereas more basic drugs, such as the tricyclic antidepressants (TCAs), amphetamines, and benzodiazepines, bind to globulins. Decreases in protein binding increase the availability of the drugs for therapeutic action and may increase the incidence of medication side effects. Drugs with a narrow therapeutic range, such as divalproex sodium, may be more susceptible to alterations in protein binding.

Albumin binding is decreased in many illnesses, including cirrhosis, pneumonia, malnutrition, acute pancreatitis, renal failure, and nephrotic syndrome. In patients with these conditions, albumin-bound drugs with a low therapeutic index may increase in concentration, causing toxicity. In other diseases, such as hypothyroidism, albumin binding may be increased. α_1 Glycoprotein plasma concentrations may increase in patients with Crohn's disease, renal failure, rheumatoid arthritis, surgery, and trauma. In general, if protein binding is affected by disease, it may be necessary to make adjustments to medication dosages.

Metabolism

Drugs are primarily metabolized in the liver and gastrointestinal tract and then excreted through the kidney. Water-soluble drugs are readily excreted by the kidneys, but fat-soluble drugs tend to accumulate until they are converted into water-soluble compounds or metabolized by the liver into inactive compounds. Drugs are absorbed from the gastrointestinal system, pass through the liver prior to entering the systemic circulation, and undergo first-pass metabolism in the liver and intestinal wall. Hepatic metabolism may be either phase I or phase II metabolism.

Phase I metabolism, which involves oxidation via the cytochrome P450 (CYP450) mono-oxygenase system, reduction, or hydrolysis, prepares the drug for excretion or further metabolism by the phase II pathways. Phase II metabolism consists of conjugation of the drug or its metabolites with hydrophilic compounds in pathways such as glucuronidation, acetylation, and sulfation. This produces a form of the drug that is more readily excreted. First-pass metabolism can result in significant changes in the activity of a medication and may explain why there is often a big difference in potency when medications are given parenterally rather than orally.

Hepatic metabolism may be limited by both the hepatic blood flow that delivers the drug to the hepatic metabolizing enzymes and the intrinsic capacity of the enzymes involved in metabolism. Hepatic blood flow may be altered in patients with liver disease due to portosystemic shunting and may be increased in those with chronic respiratory illness, acute viral hepatitis, or diarrhea, and in patients taking certain medications (e.g., clonidine). In practice, however, only severe cirrhosis has clinically significant effects on hepatic blood flow. Hepatic metabolism is also affected by enzyme inhibition or induction caused by specific medications, whereas hepatic diseases, such as acute viral hepatitis, may limit phase I metabolism. Liver disease does not generally have clinically significant effects on glucuronide conjugation reactions due to its large reserve of enzymes.

Elimination

Drugs and metabolites may be excreted through the kidneys as well as into the bile, feces, sweat, saliva, or tears. Lithium, gabapentin, amantadine, and topiramate are primarily excreted through the kidneys without hepatic metabolism. The half-life is a measure of the amount of time needed to excrete half of the drug from the plasma and determines the frequency of administration that is required to achieve a steady-state drug concentration. The half-life of highly protein-bound psychoactive drugs is greatly increased. Although the kidney is primarily involved in drug elimination, renal disease may also affect absorption, distribution, and metabolism of drugs.

Drug–Drug Interactions

Drug–drug interactions are a common cause of patient morbidity (Robinson and Owen 2005). They may be pharmacokinetic or pharmacodynamic. Pharmacokinetic interactions involve changes in the absorption, distribution, metabolism, or excretion that influence drug concentration. Pharmacodynamic interactions involve alterations in the pharmacological response to a drug and can occur directly or by alterations in drug receptor site binding.

Cytochrome P450 System

The CYP450 system is a family of mostly hepatic enzymes that perform oxidative phase I metabolism. CYP450 enzymes exist in a number of body tissues, including the gastrointestinal tract, liver, and brain. The hepatic CYP450 system is responsible for most metabolic drug interactions. The major CYP450 enzyme families that are active in humans are CYP1, CYP2, and CYP3. These families are further divided into subfamilies that include CYP1A2, 2C9, 2C19, 2D6, 2E1, and 3A4. Substrates are those agents that are metabolized by the cytochrome enzyme.

An inhibitor may decrease or block enzyme activity required for drug metabolism and cause an elevated concentration of the circulating drug with potential to increase therapeutic or toxic effects. An inducer increases the activity of the metabolic enzyme and results in a decreased concentration in the amount of circulating drug and increased concentration of metabolites. This may lead to decreased therapeutic effect or to increased toxicity due to toxic metabolites. Knowledge of whether a drug has an inhibitory or inductive effect on a specific enzyme may help predict potential drug interactions.

Uridine Glucuronosyltransferases

Phase II metabolism usually follows phase I metabolism and generally plays a minor metabolic role. There are some medications, such as lamotrigine, morphine, and lorazepam, that are primarily metabolized by phase II metabolism. Phase II reactions are conjugation reactions in which water-soluble molecules bind with the drug to make it more easily excreted. The most common phase II enzymes are the uridine glucuronosyltransferases (UGTs). The UGTs are further classified into 1A and 2B. These enzyme systems also have substrates, inhibitors, and inducers (e.g., glucuronidation of lorazepam is competitively inhibited by the nonsteroidal anti-inflammatory drugs).

P-Glycoproteins

P-glycoproteins participate in the transport of substances out of the body into the gastrointestinal tract, bile, and urine. They are involved in blocking gastrointestinal absorption and are part of the first-pass effect, functioning as "gatekeepers" for CYP3A4 metabolism. The P-glycoprotein transporter does not affect drug metabolism but rather influences drug bioavailability by removing P-glycoprotein substrates and returning them into the gut lumen. P-glycoprotein inhibitors antagonize this process and precipitate retention of P-glycoprotein substrates. For example, omeprazole, which is an inhibitor of the P-glycoprotein transporter system, may lead to increased serum concentrations of carbamazepine, a substrate for this system.

Identifying Drug Interactions

Most pharmacokinetic drug–drug interactions involve the effect of a drug on the CYP450-mediated metabolism of another agent. For these interactions to have clinical importance, the drug needs to have a narrow therapeutic index and only one primary P450 enzyme involved in its metabolism. Agents that interact with different CYP450 enzyme subfamilies do not influence the primary drug's metabolism.

The addition of an interacting drug to a medication regimen in which one drug is at a steady-state concentration may have important effects. If the new drug is an inhibitor of a P450 enzyme, substrate drug concentrations and the potential for toxicity will rise. By contrast, the addition of a drug that is an enzyme inducer will increase elimination of the substrate drug and lower its therapeutic effect. Similarly, withdrawal of an interacting drug from the drug regimen may have important results. Withdrawal of a drug that inhibits metabolism will result in increased metabolism of the substrate drug and lowered therapeutic effect. These changes may require alterations in the dosages of the primary substrate drug to maintain clinical efficacy and minimize potential toxic side effects. If a new, important substrate drug is introduced to a drug regimen that already contains an interacting drug, alterations to the dosage may also need to be made to obtain the desired therapeutic action. Monitoring of drug levels wherever possible helps facilitate safe clinical practice.

Drug interactions that affect renal elimination are important only if the drug is excreted primarily through the kidney. Changes in urine pH may modify elimination of specific drugs. For example, drugs such as antacids that alkalinize the urine may reduce the excretion of drugs such as amphetamine and TCAs.

Antidepressants

Antidepressants are widely used to treat depressive, anxiety, and somatoform disorders as well as insomnia, enuresis, and chronic pain (Tables 15–2 and 15–3). When initiating pharmacological treatment for depression, it is important to emphasize the need for a 6-week trial at full antidepressant dosages in addition to recommending combined treatment with psychotherapy. However, a recent meta-analysis of adult studies suggests that effects of antidepressants may be seen within the first 2 weeks of initiating treatment (Posternak and Zimmerman 2005).

The U.S. Food and Drug Administration (FDA) has directed that all antidepressant medications distributed in the United States have a black box warning that the medications "increase the risk of suicidal thinking and behavior (suicidality) in children and adolescent with major depressive disorder

Table 15–2.   Preparations and dosages of antidepressants

Medication	Brand name and preparation	Dosage	Schedule
Selective serotonin reuptake inhibitors			
fluoxetine	Prozac 10, 20, 40 mg; 20 mg/5 mL oral suspension	2.5–60 mg/day (0.25–0.7 mg/kg/day)	qd
sertraline	Zoloft 25, 50, 100 mg; 20 mg/5 mL oral suspension	25–200 mg/day (1.3–3 mg/kg/day)	qd
paroxetine	Paxil 10, 20, 30, 40 mg; 10 mg/5 mL oral suspension	10–40 mg/day (0.25–0.7 mg/kg/day)	qd
fluvoxamine	Luvox 25, 50, 100 mg	12.5–200 mg/day (1.5–4.5 mg/kg/day)	qd
citalopram	Celexa 20, 40 mg; 10 mg/5 mL oral suspension	10–40 mg/day (0.25–0.7 mg/kg/day)	qd
escitalopram	Lexapro 5, 10, 20 mg; 5 mg/5 mL oral solution	5–20 mg/day (0.125–0.35 mg/kg/day)	qd
Tricyclic antidepressants			
imipramine	Tofranil 10, 25, 50 75, 100, 125, 150 mg	1–5 mg/kg/day	qd/bid
desipramine	Norpramin 10, 25, 50, 75, 100, 125, 150 mg	1–5 mg/kg/day	qd/bid
nortriptyline	Pamelor 10, 25, 50, 75 mg	0.5–2 mg/kg/day	qd/bid
clomipramine	Anafranil 25, 50, 75 mg	2–3 mg/kg/day	qd/bid
amitriptyline	Elavil 10, 25, 50, 75, 125, 150 mg	1–5 mg/kg/day	qd/bid

Table 15–2. Preparations and dosages of antidepressants *(continued)*

Medication	Brand name and preparation	Dosage	Schedule
Alternative antidepressants			
bupropion	Wellbutrin 75, 100 mg	150–400 mg/day	tid
	Wellbutrin SR 100, 150 mg	150–400 mg/day	qd/bid
venlafaxine	Effexor 25, 37.5, 50, 75, 100 mg; Effexor XR 37.5, 75, 150 mg	1–3 mg/kg/day (2–4 mg/kg/day)	bid/tid
duloxetine	Cymbalta 20, 30, 60 mg	20–60 mg/day	qd/bid
trazodone	Desyrel 50, 100, 150, 300 mg	25–200 mg/day	qhs
nefazodone	Serzone 50, 100, 150, 200, 250 mg	50–300 mg/day	bid
mirtazapine	Remeron 7.5, 15, 30 mg	7.5–30 mg/day (0.2–0.4 mg/kg/day)	qhs
selegiline	Eldepryl 5 mg	10–15 mg/day	bid (morning and noon)

Note. bid=twice a day; qd=every day; qhs=at bedtime; tid=three times a day.
Source. Adapted from Martin A, Scahill L, Charney DS, et al: "Appendix: Pediatric Psychopharmacology at a Glance," in *Pediatric Psychopharmacology: Principles and Practice.* Edited by Martin A, Scahill L, Charney DS, et al. Washington, DC, American Psychiatric Publishing, 2002, pp. 757–764. Copyright 2002, American Psychiatric Publishing, Inc. Used with permission.

Table 15–3. Common side effects of antidepressants

Antidepressant	Common side effects	Notes
Selective serotonin reuptake inhibitors (SSRIs)	*Central nervous system:* anxiety, mania, irritability, headache, sedation, insomnia, tremors, dizziness, extrapyramidal effects (akathisia, dystonia, and parkinsonism), dose-related frontal lobe–like syndrome (apathy, indifference, loss of initiative) *Gastrointestinal:* nausea, vomiting, anorexia, gastric irritation, constipation, dry mouth *Endocrine:* sexual dysfunction, potential weight gain, syndrome of inappropriate antidiuretic hormone (SIADH), sweating *Hematological:* platelet dysfunction, bruising, epistaxis	Effects generally mild, dosage related, and diminish over time Safe in overdose even at doses more than 50–75 times prescribed dose Potential for serotonin syndrome Abrupt discontinuation may be associated with a discontinuation syndrome (headache, sleep disturbance, flu-like symptoms, gastrointestinal and psychiatric symptoms) Citalopram has fewer drug interactions and fewer side effects Citalopram may prolong QT$_c$ in combination with pimozide
Bupropion	*Central nervous system:* agitation, insomnia, anxiety, lowered seizure threshold, tremor, headache, exacerbation of tics *Gastrointestinal:* dry mouth, constipation, nausea, anorexia *Dermatological:* rash *Cardiovascular:* palpitations	Contraindicated in patients with arrhythmias, atrioventricular block, bulimia, and seizure history Dosage-related lowering of seizure threshold that may precipitate seizures in susceptible individuals Potential for serum sickness–like reaction

Table 15–3. Common side effects of antidepressants (*continued*)

Antidepressant	Common side effects	Notes
Nefazodone	*Central nervous system:* fatigue, blurred vision, afterimage *Gastrointestinal:* dry mouth, nausea, constipation *Hepatic:* hepatic failure *Cardiovascular:* lightheadedness, orthostatic hypotension	Potential for severe hepatotoxicity and contraindication in patients with preexisting liver disease Concurrent use of cisapride contraindicated due to risk of lethal QT_c prolongation and torsades de pointes
Trazodone	*Central nervous system:* sedation *Gastrointestinal:* dry mouth, nausea *Genitourinary:* priapism *Cardiovascular:* orthostatic hypotension, syncope	Priapism an infrequent but potentially serious adverse event Sedative effect useful in treatment of insomnia
Tricyclic antidepressants	*Central nervous system:* sedation, ataxia, dizziness, slurred speech, muscle fatigue, diplopia, tremor, mania, psychosis, lowered seizure threshold *Anticholinergic effects:* dry mouth, constipation, urine retention, decreased sweating, confusion, delirium, tachycardia, blurred vision *Cardiovascular:* postural hypotension, increased heart rate, increased blood pressure, heart block, arrhythmias, palpitations, syncope, heart failure, prolonged QT_c interval *Endocrine:* weight gain *Dermatological:* rash	Potential for inducing serotonin syndrome in combination with SSRIs Monitor electrocardiograms and serum drug levels Potential for fatal cardiac conduction abnormalities in overdose Potential for withdrawal symptoms associated with anticholinergic rebound (nausea, vomiting, headache, lethargy, abdominal pain)

Table 15–3.   Common side effects of antidepressants *(continued)*

Antidepressant	Common side effects	Notes
Venlafaxine	*Central nervous system:* sedation, dry mouth, dizziness, headache, initial anxiety, activation *Gastrointestinal:* nausea *Endocrine:* hyponatremia, SIADH, increased serum cholesterol *Cardiovascular:* dosage-related increase in cardiac conduction and heart rate, sustained hypertension	Indication for treatment of chronic pain Severe hepatic impairment may increase the elimination half-life by almost 200%.
Duloxetine	*Central nervous system:* somnolence, fatigue, dizziness *Gastrointestinal:* dry mouth, nausea, constipation, decreased appetite *Endocrine:* increased sweating *Cardiovascular:* dose-related increase in blood pressure similar to venlafaxine	Indicated for treatment of chronic pain and urinary incontinence
Mirtazapine	*Central nervous system:* sedation, somnolence *Gastrointestinal:* dry mouth, increased appetite, pancreatitis *Endocrine:* weight gain, increased serum cholesterol and triglycerides *Hepatic:* transient increases in liver enzymes *Cardiovascular:* orthostatic hypotension	Potential for use in the treatment of insomnia due to strong sedative effect Rare instances of agranulocytosis and neutropenia

Table 15–3. Common side effects of antidepressants (continued)

Antidepressant	Common side effects	Notes
Monoamine oxidase inhibitors	*Central nervous system:* dizziness, headache, sedation, insomnia, hypersomnia, tremor, hyperreflexia, myoclonic twitches *Gastrointestinal:* dry mouth, constipation *Endocrine:* weight gain *Renal:* urinary hesitancy *Cardiovascular:* orthostatic hypotension, hypertensive crises	Interaction between sympathomimetic or dopaminergic agents may precipitate hypertensive crises Potential for serotonin syndrome Potentiation of antihypertensive agents including diuretics

(MDD) and other psychiatric disorders" (U.S. Food and Drug Administration 2004). The FDA recommends that "ideally" a child receiving antidepressants will be seen by the prescribing physician once a week for the first 4 weeks of treatment; biweekly for the second month; and at the end of the twelfth week on medication. The frequency and nature of monitoring will need to be individualized in the pediatric setting. Adverse reactions to antidepressants are most likely to occur early in treatment. Careful monitoring by the consultant for new or more frequent suicidal ideation, anxiety/panic, agitation, aggressiveness, or impulsivity is critical.

Selective Serotonin Reuptake Inhibitors

Selective serotonin reuptake inhibitors (SSRIs) have become the drug treatment of choice for depression primarily due to their low side-effect profile. All SSRIs have a similar efficacy and mechanism of action, and the choice of a specific agent is directed by the side-effect profile, half-life, and potential CYP450-mediated drug interactions (Table 15–4). Fluoxetine, for example, may prolong the half-life of diazepam as well as lead to elevated levels of TCAs and carbamazepine. Fluoxetine remains the most commonly prescribed SSRI in children and adolescents, although citalopram and escitalopram (S-enantiomer of citalopram) tend to have a more favorable side-effect profile and fewer drug–drug interactions. Because the SSRIs tend to be activating, they are generally prescribed in the morning, and it may be necessary to add either a sedative-hypnotic or trazodone for insomnia.

Serotonin Syndrome

Serotonin syndrome is often described as a clinical triad of mental status changes, autonomic hyperactivity, and neuromuscular abnormalities, although not all of these findings are present in all patients with this disorder (Boyer and Shannon 2005; Brown et al. 2000). An excess serotonergic agonism of the central and peripheral nervous system serotonergic receptors is caused by a range of drugs, including SSRIs, monoamine oxidase inhibitors (MAOIs), valproate, dextromethorphan, lithium, meperidine, and fentanyl. Drug–drug interactions that can cause serotonin syndrome include linezolid (an antibiotic that has MAOI properties) and SSRIs as well as combinations of SSRIs, trazodone, buspirone, venlafaxine, ondansetron, metoclopramide, and sumatriptan (Boyer and Shannon 2005). Serotonin syndrome is often

Table 15–4. Comparison of side effects of selective serotonin reuptake inhibitors

SSRIs	Sedation	Gastrointestinal upset	Activation/ Agitation/ Insomnia	Half-life (including active metabolites)	CYP450 metabolism	CYP450 inhibition
Fluoxetine	+	+	++	7–14 days	2C9, 2D6, 3A4	1A2, 2C9/19, 2D6, 3A4
Sertraline	+	+	+	2–3 days	2C9/19, 2D6	2C9, 2D6 (weak)
Paroxetine	++	+	+	24 hours	2D6	2D6
Fluvoxamine	+	++	++	17–22 hours	1A2, 2D6	1A2, 2C9/19, 3A4
Citalopram	±	+	±	36 hours	2D6, 3A4	1A2, 2C19, 2D6 (minimal)
Escitalopram	±	+	±	36 hours	2D6, 3A4	1A2, 2C19, 2D6 (minimal)

Note. SSRIs=selective serotonin reuptake inhibitors.
Source. Adapted from Schatzberg et al. 2003.

Table 15–5.   Manifestations of severe serotonin, neuroleptic malignant, and anticholinergic syndromes

	Serotonin syndrome	Neuroleptic malignant syndrome	Anticholinergic syndrome
Medication	Serotonin agents	Dopamine antagonist	Anticholinergic agent
Time for condition to develop	<12 hours	1–3 days	<12 hours
Mental status	Agitation, coma	Stupor, alert, mutism, coma	Agitated delirium
Vital signs	Hypertension	Hypertension	Hypertension
	Tachycardia	Tachycardia	Tachycardia
	Tachypnea	Tachypnea	Tachypnea
	> 41.1°C	> 41.1°C	< 38.8°C
Pupils	Mydriasis	Normal	Mydriasis
Mucosa	Sialorrhea	Sialorrhea	Dry
Skin	Diaphoresis	Diaphoresis, pallor	Erythema
Neuromuscular tone	Increased (lower extremities)	"Lead-pipe" rigidity (all muscle groups)	Normal
Reflexes	Hyperreflexia	Bradyreflexia	Normal

Source.   Adapted from Boyer EW, Shannon M: "The Serotonin Syndrome." *New England Journal of Medicine* 352:1112–1120, 2005. Copyright 2005, Massachusetts Medical Society. All rights reserved. Used with permission.

self-limited and may resolve spontaneously after discontinuation of the sero-tonergic agents. Severe cases require the control of agitation, autonomic instability, and hyperthermia as well as the administration of $5\text{-}HT_{2A}$ antagonists (cyproheptadine). The syndrome can be difficult to clinically separate from neuroleptic malignant syndrome (NMS) and anticholinergic "toxidrome" (Table 15–5).

Tricyclic Antidepressants

There are few double-blind, placebo-controlled trials with TCAs and even fewer with positive results. This, along with safety concerns, has limited their current use in the treatment of depression, and they are not used as first-line treatments for pediatric depression. Currently, TCAs are most often used with children for chronic pain and enuresis (see Tables 15–2 and 15–3 for dosages and side effects of TCAs).

The TCAs can affect the heart's electrical conduction system, resulting in prolonged QT intervals (Brown et al. 2000). TCAs may enhance the effects of antiarrhythmic drugs such as quinidine and procainamide. Consultants should consider obtaining electrocardiograms and serum blood levels before dosage changes or if there are concerns about toxicity. Side effects may be compounded when TCAs are used in conjunction with medications that have sedative, hypotensive, antiarrhythmic, or anticholinergic properties. Anticholinergic effects include urinary retention, delayed gastric motility, and the precipitation of narrow-angle glaucoma. Concurrent administration of sympathomimetic agents may precipitate a potentially fatal reaction, with symptoms of increased temperature, sweating, confusion, myoclonus, seizures, hypertension, tachycardia, and arrhythmias.

TCAs are rapidly and completely absorbed from the gastrointestinal tract. They undergo extensive first-pass metabolism. They are highly protein-bound and compete for binding on the α_1 glycoprotein binding sites with aspirin, phenytoin, and phenothiazines. TCAs generally have a narrow therapeutic index, and their metabolism by either CYP2D6 or CYP3A4 results in the potential for toxic side effects when given with medications that inhibit these enzymes (e.g., SSRIs). Children generally metabolize TCAs more efficiently, but there is a significant proportion of patients who are "slow metabolizers" and who have wide variations in blood plasma levels following the administration of a single dose. These drugs are excreted through the urine, with the half-life ranging from 10 to 30 hours. Children usually have shorter half-lives than adults due to their more efficient hepatic metabolism.

Overdosing on these medications carries the risk of fatality from the cardiac conduction abnormalities. Cardiotoxicity should be anticipated if the QRS interval is greater than 120 msec or if plasma concentrations are greater than 1,000 ng/mL. Abrupt TCA discontinuation can result in a discontinuation syndrome that includes dizziness, lethargy, headaches, nightmares, and anticholinergic rebound. When TCAs are used in patients with a history of epilepsy, anticonvulsant levels should be checked more frequently due to the potential drug interactions between TCAs and anticonvulsants. Patients with head trauma and brain damage are at an increased risk of seizures during TCA treatment.

Bupropion

Bupropion's exact therapeutic mechanism of action is unknown. It does inhibit neuronal reuptake of serotonin, norepinephrine, and dopamine, but it is a weak inhibitor compared with the SSRIs and TCAs (Brown et al. 2000; Katic et al. 1998). It has been used in smoking cessation treatment and has an activating effect that helps some patients. Immediate-release bupropion is absorbed rapidly from the gastrointestinal tract, and peak levels are obtained 2 hours after ingestion. It undergoes extensive first-pass metabolism, and the half-lives of its active metabolites are 20 hours or more.

Bupropion has been found to have little effect on blood pressure, heart rate, or electrocardiography, and its use is only very rarely associated with orthostatic hypotension. It carries an increased risk for seizures, particularly for patients with bulimia or anorexia nervosa. To minimize this risk, single doses of immediate-release bupropion should not exceed 150 mg and should be separated by a minimum of 8 hours. Bupropion also inhibits CYP2D6. The extended release preparation of bupropion results in lower peak concentrations but equivalent therapeutic efficacy. Overdose of bupropion has been associated with neurological toxicity. Concurrent use of lithium and bupropion has resulted in some isolated cases of seizures, and delirium has been associated with the combination of fluoxetine and bupropion.

Venlafaxine

Venlafaxine inhibits the reuptake of both serotonin and norepinephrine. It has been used in a number of clinical situations including the treatment of depression, generalized anxiety disorder, panic disorder, and chronic pain. It is rapidly absorbed from the gastrointestinal tract and is metabolized via the CYP450 system to its active metabolites. The extended-release preparation results in a slower rate of absorption but no change in total amount of absorption. It is excreted through the kidney. Cardiovascular side effects are generally rare, although there is a dose-dependent effect on blood pressure, with the potential for sustained diastolic blood pressure elevations.

Trazodone

Although trazodone is classified as an antidepressant, its current use has been primarily for the treatment of insomnia. Trazodone has also been used for the treatment of disruptive behavior in children and adolescents. It is well absorbed following oral administration and achieves peak plasma levels 1–2 hours after ingestion. It undergoes first-pass metabolism in the liver and is prone to CYP450 interactions. Its half life is 5–9 hours, and it is excreted primarily in the urine. Caution should be exercised when it is used in patients receiving antihypertensive agents because of the side effect of orthostatic hypotension.

Nefazodone

Nefazodone was originally developed with the intention of improving the side-effect profile of trazodone. It is generally well tolerated and has been shown to improve sleep architecture. However, it has an FDA black box warning because of concerns about hepatic toxicity and liver failure. Nefazodone should not be administered to patients with active liver disease or those with elevated serum transaminase levels. Routine liver function tests should be carried out during treatment with nefazodone. Nefazodone inhibits reuptake of both norepinephrine and serotonin receptors. It is rapidly absorbed and undergoes extensive first-pass metabolism. The elimination half-life is approximately 4 hours. There are potential drug interactions mediated through the CYP450 system. Coadministration with alprazolam and triazolam may result in elevated serum levels of these benzodiazepines. Nefazodone should not be used in combination with cisapride because elevated levels may result in cardiac conduction abnormalities and *torsades de pointes*. Nefazodone may also increase serum levels of digoxin.

Mirtazapine

Mirtazapine is rapidly absorbed from the gastrointestinal tract and is metabolized via the CYP450 system. It has active metabolites with a half-life of approximately 20 hours. It is generally considered to be safe in overdose due to its wide therapeutic index. Mirtazapine has the potential to induce somnolence, particularly at lower dosages, and is sometimes used to treat insomnia. Mirtazapine may also stimulate appetite. Both these side effects may be used to therapeutic benefit in specific clinical situations. Agranulocytosis and neutropenia are rare but potentially serious side effects.

Monoamine Oxidase Inhibitors

MAOIs represent a third line of antidepressants. Three agents are available in the United States for treating psychiatric disorders: phenelzine, tranylcypromine, and isocarboxazid. Selegiline is available for the treatment of Parkinson's disease. Use of the MAOIs is limited by the potential for drug interactions and the need for specific dietary restrictions. Hypertensive crises may occur when patients on MAOIs consume food items containing tyramine, caffeine, or chocolate as well as specific medications that include the sympathomimetic amines, bronchodilators, psychostimulants, L-dopa, and buspirone. Moclobemide, a short half-life reversible inhibitor of monoamine oxidase type A, is less susceptible to dietary interactions when it is taken with food. MAOIs may also interact with the SSRIs and other serotonergic medications (e.g., meperidine) to produce severe serotonin syndrome.

Mood Stabilizers

Mood stabilizers are used to treat primary mood disorders as well as mood disorders associated with medical conditions or secondary to substances or medications (Tables 15–6 and 15–7). Lithium has also been commonly used to augment the effect of antidepressants. Selected agents also are used in the treatment of chronic pain syndromes—for example, gabapentin for neuropathic pain and divalproex sodium for migraine prophylaxis.

Lithium

Lithium is readily absorbed in the gastrointestinal tract, although absorption of lithium carbonate is delayed in extended-release preparations, with a peak

Table 15–6. Preparations and dosages of mood stabilizers

Medication	Brand name and preparation	Dosage	Schedule
lithium	Lithium carbonate 150, 300, 600 mg Lithium citrate elixir 300 mg/5 mL Lithobid 300, 450 mg Eskalith, Eskalith CR 300, 450 mg	10–30 mg/kg/day 0.6–1.2 mEq/L therapeutic level	bid/tid
divalproex	Depakene (valproic acid) 250 mg tablets; 250 mg/ 5 mL elixir Depakote 125, 250, 500 mg tablets; 125 mg sprinkles Depakote ER 500 mg	15–60 mg/kg/day 50–120 μg/mL therapeutic level	bid/tid
carbamazepine	Tegretol 100, 200 mg tablet; 100 mg chewable; 100 mg/ 5 mL elixir	10–20 mg/kg/day	bid
	Carbatrol (extended release) 100, 200, 300, 400 mg	4–12 μg/mL therapeutic level	
gabapentin	Neurontin 100, 300, 400, 600, 800 mg	100–2,400 mg/day	tid
lamotrigine	Lamictal 25, 100, 150, 200 mg tablet; 5, 25 mg chewable	75–400 mg/day	qd
topiramate	Topamax 25, 100, 200 mg tablet; 125 mg sprinkles	50–400 mg/day	bid

Note. bid=twice a day; qd=every day; tid=three times a day.
Source. Adapted from Martin A, Scahill L, Charney DS, et al: "Appendix: Pediatric Psychopharmacology at a Glance," in *Pediatric Psychopharmacology: Principles and Practice.* Edited by Martin A, Scahill L, Charney DS, et al. Washington, DC, American Psychiatric Publishing, 2002, pp. 757–764. Copyright 2002, American Psychiatric Publishing, Inc. Used with permission.

Table 15–7. Common side effects of mood-stabilizing agents

Mood-stabilizing agent	Side effects	Notes
Lithium	*Central nervous system:* headache, fatigue, ataxia, tremor, cognitive impairment *Gastrointestinal:* nausea, gastric irritation, diarrhea, abdominal pain *Cardiovascular:* T-wave depression and inversion, decreased heart rate, cardiac conduction abnormalities, cardiac arrhythmias *Renal:* polyuria, edema, polydipsia, interstitial fibrosis, tubular atrophy, glomerular sclerosis *Endocrine:* weight gain, hypothyroidism *Dermatological:* dry skin, acne, psoriasis, alopecia	Importance of monitoring renal and thyroid function Importance of careful monitoring of serum levels due to narrow therapeutic index Potential for neurotoxicity, including neuroleptic malignant syndrome, with concurrent use of antipsychotic agents Renal excretion without hepatic metabolism
Divalproex sodium	*Central nervous system:* sedation, ataxia, dizziness, muscle fatigue, tremor *Gastrointestinal:* nausea, diarrhea, vomiting, increased appetite *Endocrine:* weight gain, possible polycystic ovarian syndrome *Hematological:* mild leukopenia, thrombocytopenia, agranulocytosis, increased prothrombin time *Hepatic:* elevated liver enzymes, infrequent fatal hepatotoxicity *Dermatological:* benign skin rashes, alopecia, Stevens-Johnson syndrome, toxic epidermal necrolysis	Potential occurrence of fatal hepatotoxicity Monitor for presence of thrombocytopenia
Gabapentin	*Central nervous system:* somnolence, dizziness, asthenia, ataxia, aggressive behavior *Endocrine:* weight gain	Broad therapeutic range No significant drug interactions Renal excretion without hepatic metabolism

Table 15–7. Common side effects of mood-stabilizing agents *(continued)*

Mood-stabilizing agent	Side effects	Notes
Topiramate	*Central nervous system:* sedation, ataxia, dizziness, muscle fatigue *Gastrointestinal:* nausea, anorexia, diarrhea, vomiting *Hepatic:* elevated liver enzymes *Endocrine:* weight loss *Dermatological:* rash	Renal excretion without hepatic metabolism
Lamotrigine	*Central nervous system:* dizziness, ataxia, diplopia, headache, blurred vision, somnolence, exacerbation of seizures *Gastrointestinal:* nausea, vomiting *Dermatological:* Stevens-Johnsons syndrome (0.5% incidence), rash, acne	Risk of Stevens-Johnson syndrome
Carbamazepine	*Central nervous system:* sedation, ataxia, dizziness, slurred speech, muscle fatigue, diplopia *Gastrointestinal:* nausea, diarrhea, vomiting *Endocrine:* weight gain *Hematological:* transient leukopenia, aplastic anemia, thrombocytopenia *Hepatic:* elevated liver enzymes, acute hepatic necrosis, liver failure *Renal:* syndrome of inappropriate antidiuretic hormone (SIADH) *Dermatological:* benign skin rash, Stevens-Johnson syndrome, toxic epidermal necrolysis *Cardiovascular:* heart block, cardiac rhythm disturbances following overdose	Importance of close monitoring of blood count due to concerns about aplastic anemia (bruising, bleeding, sore throat, fever, lethargy, mouth ulcers, death)

serum concentration occurring between 4 and 12 hours. Younger children may have a shorter elimination half-life and higher total clearance. Lithium is not bound to plasma proteins and is almost entirely excreted through the kidneys. Nonsteroidal anti-inflammatory drugs, thiazide diuretics, tetracycline, metronidazole, calcium channel blockers, sodium depletion, and dehydration may all increase serum levels.

Common side effects include gastrointestinal distress and tremor, which tend to be mild and dosage related. These side effects may be minimized by dosage reduction, use of divided doses given with food, or the use of slow-release preparations of lithium. Hand tremors may be managed by dosage reduction or administration of low-dosage beta-blockers. Chronic use of lithium may be associated with renal and thyroid gland dysfunction. Elevated thyroid stimulating hormone is present in as much as 30% of patients treated with lithium on a chronic basis, whereas up to 20% of patients may develop clinical hypothyroidism requiring treatment with L-thyroxine (Jefferson et al. 1987). Lithium may also potentiate the adverse effects of other medications, including those with extrapyramidal symptoms and tremor side effects of their own. Lithium has also been associated with a serotonin syndrome.

Lithium has a narrow therapeutic range with significant toxicity when serum levels exceed 1.5 mEq/L. Initial symptoms that suggest impending toxicity include marked tremor, nausea, diarrhea, blurred vision, vertigo, confusion, increased deep tendon reflexes, coma, and cardiac arrhythmia. Treatment for lithium toxicity includes gastric lavage, volume resuscitation, and, in severe cases, hemodialysis.

Anticonvulsants

Most of the anticonvulsant medications used for mood instability have a similar profile of side effects that includes sedation, ataxia, dizziness, muscle fatigue, nystagmus, and diplopia (see Table 15–7). Psychotic symptoms and cognitive impairment have also been reported. Similarly, gastrointestinal distress (e.g., nausea, vomiting, dyspepsia, diarrhea, and anorexia) is common. Giving the drugs in divided doses and with meals may minimize this distress. The potential for hematological abnormalities requires careful monitoring. Transient elevations in liver enzymes may occur, but these are usually reversible with dosage reduction or drug discontinuation.

Carbamazepine

Carbamazepine is used in the treatment of bipolar disorder, epilepsy, and neuropathic pain. Carbamazepine is slowly absorbed from the gastrointestinal tract, with a peak plasma concentration between 2 and 8 hours. Extended-release preparations are available to reduce the frequency of dosing. In children, there is a poor correlation between dosage and plasma concentrations of carbamazepine. Carbamazepine is highly protein bound. Significant CYP450 interactions occur between carbamazepine and divalproex sodium. Carbamazepine's induction of hepatic enzymes may decrease the effects of other medications including anticoagulants, antipsychotic agents, oral contraceptives, and theophylline. Carbamazepine levels may be increased during coadministration with phenobarbital, phenytoin, primidone, diltiazem, and verapamil. Carbamazepine also induces its own metabolism resulting in a predictable decrease in carbamazepine blood levels after 3–4 weeks of treatment and the need for frequent dosage adjustments during the first few weeks of treatment. Carbamazepine may also compete for hepatic glucuronidation with medications such as morphine. Overdose is associated with drowsiness, nausea, vomiting, gait disturbance, nystagmus, confusion, and seizures.

Divalproex

Divalproex is widely prescribed in the treatment of bipolar disorder, epilepsy, disruptive behavior disorders, and migraine prophylaxis. It is absorbed through the gastrointestinal tract, although absorption is delayed by food. A peak serum level occurs 3 hours after ingestion. Divalproex is protein bound but easily saturates the binding proteins, with the result that the relationship between dosage and total serum level may vary. Divalproex is metabolized principally in the liver and is excreted as a glucuronide conjugate. It has an elimination half-life of 5–20 hours. It may also displace other protein-bound drugs, including warfarin, phenytoin, and tolbutamide. Coadministration of divalproex with clonazepam and other long-acting benzodiazepines may result in prolonging benzodiazepine metabolism and may induce absence seizures. Coadministration with carbamazepine may result in carbamazepine toxicity at therapeutic levels of carbamazepine due to the presence of an active metabolite. Aspirin may also raise the levels of both total and free valproate due to enzyme inhibition and displacement from protein binding sites with potential toxicity.

Antipsychotic Agents

Antipsychotic agents are widely used in the treatment of agitation, delirium, and psychosis (Table 15–8). They have been used to augment the pharmacological treatment of pain. This group of medications may be broadly classified into the typical low-potency agents (e.g., chlorpromazine and thioridazine), typical high-potency agents (e.g., haloperidol and fluphenazine), and atypical agents (e.g., clozapine, risperidone, and olanzapine) (Brown et al. 2000). Antipsychotic agents are well absorbed from the gastrointestinal tract, although increased gastric acidity and delayed gastric emptying may decrease absorption. They are highly lipophilic and protein bound, with their metabolism occurring primarily via the hepatic oxidation pathways.

The typical low-potency agents can cause α-adrenergic and histaminic receptor blockades, which result in orthostatic hypotension and sedation, respectively. These medications have a high incidence of anticholinergic side effects. Compared with other antipsychotics, the low-potency agents are more likely to have dermatological side effects (e.g., photosensitivity), cholestatic jaundice, and QT_c prolongation. For these reasons, the use of low-potency agents is generally avoided in physically ill patients. Both the typical high-potency and atypical agents are more commonly used in this population (Table 15–9).

Central Nervous System Side Effects

Acute Dystonic Reactions

Acute dystonic reactions, which include torticollis, tongue protrusion, opisthotonos, facial grimacing, and oculogyric crises, commonly occur when patients are treated for the first time with antipsychotic agents. The risk seems to be greater with the high-potency antipsychotic agents. Acute dystonic reactions may also occur with the antiemetic medications, such as metoclopramide, particularly when used intravenously and at high dosages. Acute dystonic reactions may be treated with intravenous diphenhydramine (25–50 mg) or benztropine (1–2 mg), which generally needs to be continued orally even after the antipsychotic has been discontinued because of the long half-life of many antipsychotic agents.

Akathisia

Akathisia is a common reaction to the antipsychotic agents, including some of the newer atypical agents (e.g., risperidone). Symptoms include intense, un-

Table 15–8. Preparations and dosages and of antipsychotic agents

Medication	Brand name and preparation	Dosage (mg/day)	Schedule
Low-potency typical antipsychotics			
chlorpromazine	Thorazine 10, 25, 50, 100, 200 mg tablet; 30, 100 mg/ mL oral concentrate; 10 mg/5 mL syrup; 25, 100 mg suppository	25–400	qd/bid/ tid
thioridazine	Mellaril 10, 15, 25, 50, 100, 150, 200 mg tablet; 30, 100 mg/mL oral concentrate; 25, 100 mg/5 mL oral suspension	25–400	qd/bid/tid
High-potency typical antipsychotics			
haloperidol	Haldol 0.5, 1, 2, 5, 10, 20 mg; 2 mg/mL oral concentrate	0.25–10	qd/bid/tid
thiothixene	Navane 1, 2, 5, 10 mg tablet; 5 mg/mL oral concentrate	1–40	qd/bid/tid
fluphenazine	Prolixin 1, 2.5, 5, 10 mg tablet; 2.5 mg/5 mL elixir; 5 mg/mL oral concentrate	0.25–10	qd/bid/ tid
Atypical antipsychotics			
risperidone	Risperdal 0.25, 0.5, 1, 2, 3, 4 mg tablet; 1 mg/mL elixir	0.25–10	qd/bid
olanzapine	Zyprexa 2.5, 5, 7.5, 10, 15 mg	2.5–20	qd/bid
quetiapine	Seroquel 25, 100, 200, 300 mg	25–800	qd/bid
ziprasidone	Geodon 20, 40 mg	20–160	qd/bid
aripiprazole	Abilify 5, 10, 15, 20, 30 mg	5–30	qd
clozapine	Clozaril 25, 100 mg	25–800	bid/tid

Note. bid=twice a day; qd=every day; tid=three times a day.
Source. Adapted from Martin et al. 2002.

Table 15–9.   Comparison of side effects of atypical antipsychotics

Antipsychotic	Prolongation of QT_c	Orthostatic hypotension	Weight gain	Sedation	Anticholinergic	CYP450
Risperidone	±	+	+	±	±	2D6
Olanzapine	±	++	++	++	+	1A2 Minimal 2D6
Quetiapine	±	+	+	++	±	Minimal 3A4, 2D6
Ziprasidone	+	±	±	±	±	3A4
Aripiprazole	–	–	±	–	±	2D6, 3A4
Clozapine	±	++	++	++	++	2D6, 1A2

Note.   ++=very common; +=common; ±=sometimes; –=rarely or not at all.
Source.   Adapted from Birmaher 2003.

pleasant subjective feelings of inner restlessness and associated motor restlessness in the legs and body that in some cases can be so distressing that patients may be motivated to attempt suicide. Akathisia is best treated with either beta-blockers such as propranolol (30–120 mg/day in divided doses) or with benzodiazepines.

Extrapyramidal Symptoms

More chronic extrapyramidal symptoms include signs of parkinsonism, including masked facies, pill-rolling tremor, cogwheel rigidity, bradykinesia, and drooling. These symptoms are much more common with the typical antipsychotic agents but also may occur with some of the newer agents when prescribed at higher dosages. The symptoms are best treated by dosage reduction whenever possible, switching to an atypical antipsychotic agent or concurrent administration of benztropine or trihexyphenidyl. However, it is important to be alert to the potential cumulative anticholinergic side effects of these medications when used in combination in patients with physical illness.

Tardive Dyskinesia

Tardive dyskinesia, characterized by the development of involuntary movements particularly affecting the lips and tongue, is rarely seen in children because it develops usually only after many years of treatment with antipsychotic agents. It is important to differentiate tardive dyskinesias from withdrawal dyskinesias that may emerge when the dosage of an antipsychotic agent is reduced or the medication discontinued.

Seizure Threshold

Antipsychotic agents, in particular clozapine, have the potential to lower the seizure threshold. Seizures, however, are generally uncommon, particularly in the absence of a seizure history.

Neuroleptic Malignant Syndrome

NMS is a rare and potentially fatal reaction that may occur during treatment with antipsychotic agents (see Table 15–5). NMS has been estimated to occur in 0.2%–1% of patients treated with dopamine-blocking agents. NMS has been reported in other neurological disorders (e.g., Wilson's disease and Parkinson's disease treated with dopamine-blocking agents). NMS may also occur in patients treated with dopamine antagonists given for nausea (i.e., metoclopramide and prochlorperazine). Malnutrition and dehydration in the context of an organic brain syndrome that are being treated with lithium and antipsychotic agents may also increase the risk. Mortality rates may be as high as 20%–30% due to dehydration, aspiration, renal failure, and respiratory collapse. Differential diagnosis of NMS includes malignant hyperthermia, lethal catatonia, serotonin syndrome, and anticholinergic toxicity (see Table 15–5).

Treatment of NMS involves early diagnosis, discontinuation of all antipsychotic agents, and supportive treatment in an intensive care unit. Treatment includes intravenous hydration, correction of electrolyte abnormalities, cooling of the body, protection of the airway, treatment of infections, and intubation. Medications such as dantrolene (8–10 mg/kg body weight, intravenous), bromocriptine (2.5–10 mg three times a day) or amantadine (100 mg orally two to four times a day) have been used. The use of intravenous lorazepam (up to 2 mg every 2–4 hours) as well as levodopa, carbidopa, and diphenhydramine has also been reported. There may be a 30% risk of recurrent NMS if antipsychotic agents are restarted.

Cardiovascular Side Effects

Antipsychotic agents have been associated with prolongation of the QT_c interval and increased risk of *torsades de pointes*. The antipsychotic agent should be discontinued if the QT_c is prolonged greater than 25% above baseline. Thioridazine, mesoridazine, and droperidol currently carry FDA black box warnings regarding the risk of sudden death related to these phenomena. Other cardiac side effects include potentially fatal myocarditis, cardiomyopathy, and heart failure, in particular during treatment with clozapine. The low-potency antipsychotic agents are also associated with hypotension because of their autonomic side effects.

Endocrinological and Metabolic Side Effects

Glucose Tolerance

Antipsychotic agents have been found to increase the risk of diabetes mellitus. They are associated with a metabolic syndrome, which includes weight gain and hypertriglyceridemia as well as increased serum levels of insulin, glucose, and low-density lipoprotein cholesterol (Lieberman 2004). This syndrome may place patients at increased risk of cardiovascular disease. There is an association between the atypical antipsychotic agents and the development of hyperglycemia, insulin resistance, new-onset type 2 diabetes, and ketoacidosis. These effects are not solely explained by weight gain. Risk factors include obesity, hypertension, inactivity, prior abnormalities in lipid levels, and a family history of diabetes mellitus.

Lipids

Low-potency and some of the atypical antipsychotic agents have been noted to be associated with elevated serum levels of triglycerides and cholesterol.

Hyperprolactinemia

The high-potency antipsychotic agents and risperidone commonly result in hyperprolactinemia, which may present with amenorrhea, irregular menses, galactorrhea, gynecomastia, and osteoporosis.

Weight Gain

All of the antipsychotic agents, with the possible exception of molindone, ziprasidone, and aripiprazole, have been associated with weight gain and its concomitant health risks, including hypertension.

Hematological Side Effects

Potential hematological side effects include agranulocytosis, aplastic anemia, neutropenia, eosinophilia, and thrombocytopenia, all of which are particularly associated with the low-potency antipsychotic agents. Agranulocytosis is the most significant hematological side effect seen with the typical antipsychotic agents and occurs more commonly with the low-potency agents. Clozapine-associated agranulocytosis may occur in 1%–2% of patients, with particularly high risk during the first 6 months of treatment necessitating weekly monitoring of the absolute neutrophil count.

Hepatic Side Effects

Liver function abnormalities are common with antipsychotic agents but are generally of little clinical significance and do not require discontinuation of treatment. Mild to moderate elevations in liver aminotransferases and alkaline phosphatase are particularly common. The use of low-potency antipsychotic agents has been associated with cholestatic jaundice.

Anxiolytic Agents

Benzodiazepines are the medications most commonly used for the treatment of anxiety, although buspirone has also been marketed for this purpose (Table 15–10). Antidepressant agents, in particular the SSRIs and venlafaxine, are often used as a first-line treatment of anxiety disorders. Less commonly, beta-blockers (e.g., propranolol), antihistamines, barbiturates, and antipsychotic agents are used for the treatment of anxiety.

Benzodiazepines

Benzodiazepines are commonly used for the treatment of anxiety, alcohol or benzodiazepine withdrawal, and as antiemetic agents for patients receiving chemotherapy. Benzodiazepines are generally very well tolerated, with sedation being the main side effect (Table 15–11). When using benzodiazepines with other medications in the pediatric setting, it is important to be aware of potential additive central nervous system effects, including sedation and respiratory depression. It is also critical to monitor for withdrawal signs when benzodiazepines are abruptly discontinued, as may occur when patients are transitioned from ventilators or from the intensive care unit. Withdrawal signs include symptoms of dizziness, sweating, shakiness, headache, blurred vision, tinnitus, hypertension, nausea, vomiting, muscle cramps, hallucinations, and seizures.

Benzodiazepines are rapidly absorbed from the gastrointestinal tract with a rapid onset of action (Table 15–12). Agents that delay gastric emptying can delay absorption. With the exception of lorazepam and midazolam, benzodiazepines are not well absorbed from intramuscular injections. Lorazepam is available in a sublingual form. Benzodiazepines are highly lipid soluble and protein bound. They quickly cross the blood-brain barrier. They are degraded by hepatic oxidation, although many of the benzodiazepines have active metabolites that have long half-lives. For example, desmethyldiazepam, an active metabolite of diazepam, has a half-life in excess of 50 hours.

Many of the benzodiazepines are metabolized via the CYP3A4 pathway and so are prone to fluctuations in serum levels when coadministered with other medications (e.g., fluoxetine and fluvoxamine). Substances that inhibit hepatic microsomal enzymes (e.g., alcohol, isoniazid, and cimetidine) result in increased benzodiazepine plasma concentrations. Conversely, those that in-

Table 15–10. Preparations and dosages of anxiolytics

Medication	Brand name and preparation	Dosage	Schedule
Benzodiazepines			
alprazolam	Xanax 0.25, 0.5, 1, 2 mg; 1 mg/mL oral concentrate Xanax XR 0.5, 1, 2, 3 mg	0.25–4 mg/day	tid
clonazepam	Klonopin 0.5, 1, 2 mg	0.25–3 mg/day (0.01 mg/kg)	qd/bid
diazepam	Valium 2, 5, 10 tablet; 5 mg/5 mL oral solution; 5 mg/mL oral concentrate	2–10 mg/day (0.04–0.25 mg/kg)	tid/qid
lorazepam	Ativan 0.5, 1, 2 mg; 2 mg/mL oral concentrate	0.5–6 mg/day (0.05 mg/kg)	tid/qid
midazolam	Versed 2 mg/mL oral liquid	0.025–0.05 mg/kg iv (max 0.4 mg/kg) 0.25–1 mg/kg po (max 20 mg)	—
oxazepam	Serax 10, 15, 30 mg	10–30 mg/day	bid/tid
Alternative anxiolytic			
buspirone	Buspar 5, 10, 15, 30 mg	15–60 mg/day	tid

Note. bid=twice a day; iv=intravenously; po=orally; qd=every day; qid=four times a day; tid=three times a day.
Source. Adapted from Martin A, Scahill L, Charney DS, et al: "Appendix: Pediatric Psychopharmacology at a Glance," in *Pediatric Psychopharmacology: Principles and Practice.* Edited by Martin A, Scahill L, Charney DS, et al. Washington, DC, American Psychiatric Publishing, 2002, pp. 757–764. Copyright 2002, American Psychiatric Publishing, Inc. Used with permission.

Table 15–11. Common side effects of the anxiolytics

Anxiolytic	Side effects	Notes
Benzodiazepines Alprazolam Clonazepam Diazepam Lorazepam Midazolam Oxazepam	*Central nervous system:* sedation, fatigue, weakness, ataxia, slurred speech, confusion, reduced motor coordination, memory impairment, behavioral disinhibition, anterograde amnesia, vertigo, blurred vision *Respiratory:* respiratory depression, apnea *Gastrointestinal:* nausea, vomiting, gastric distress	Physical tolerance and dependence occur with chronic use of benzodiazepines Risk of benzodiazepine withdrawal syndrome (insomnia, trembling, sweating, palpitations, dry mouth, hot flushes, anxiety, depression, withdrawal seizures) Contraindicated in obstructive sleep apnea
Buspirone	*Central nervous system:* dizziness, drowsiness, nervousness, nausea, headache, lightheadedness, agitation, paresthesias *Gastrointestinal:* nausea, diarrhea, dyspepsia	No potential for abuse or tolerance No respiratory depression Risk of serotonin syndrome in combination with monoamine oxidase inhibitors and selective serotonin reuptake inhibitors Delayed onset of action relative to benzodiazepines

duce hepatic enzymes (i.e., tobacco and rifampin) may decrease the duration of the benzodiazepines. Benzodiazepines have also been shown to increase the half-life of digoxin. In contrast to others, oxazepam, lorazepam, and temazepam are primarily eliminated by renal excretion, making them useful alternatives where hepatic impairment is present.

The choice of specific benzodiazepines is governed by the desired onset and duration of action (see Table 15–12). Lorazepam is widely used in the pediatric setting because it can be given orally and intravenously with a rapid onset of action. Clonazepam is a useful alternative for patients who experience excessive sedation with lorazepam because it is one of the least sedating benzodiazepines. The intermediate acting agents have fewer respiratory depressant effects and are preferred for patients with respiratory illness. Midazolam is a

Table 15–12. Onset and duration of action of benzodiazepines

Benzodiazepine	Onset of action	Duration of action	Half-life (hours)
Diazepam	Rapid	Long	20–80
Lorazepam	Rapid	Intermediate	10–20
Midazolam	Rapid	Very short	2–4
Flurazepam	Rapid-intermediate	Long	70–90
Alprazolam	Intermediate	Short	12–15
Chlordiazepoxide	Intermediate	Long	5–30
Clonazepam	Intermediate	Short	30–50
Triazolam	Intermediate	Short	2–3
Oxazepam	Intermediate-slow	Intermediate	8–12
Temazepam	Intermediate-slow	Short	8–25

Source. Adapted from Jachna JS, Lane RD, Gelenberg AJ: "Psychopharmacology," in *The American Psychiatric Press Textbook of Consultation-Liaison Psychiatry.* Edited by Rundell JR, Wise MG. Washington, DC, American Psychiatric Press, Inc., 1996, pp. 991. Copyright 1996, American Psychiatric Press. Used with permission.

common preanesthetic agent as well as an effective agent for procedures done under conscious sedation. It has an extremely rapid onset of action (3–5 minutes) when given intravenously and has a short duration of action (approximately 2 hours). Midazolam is also associated with anterograde amnesia, which may be a helpful side effect in patients undergoing stressful or painful procedures.

Buspirone

Buspirone is a nonbenzodiazepine anxiolytic that has the advantage of not causing sedation or physical dependency (see Tables 15–10 and 15–11). It has little potential for abuse. In addition, buspirone does not affect the seizure threshold, does not cause respiratory depression, and has no interaction with alcohol. Its primary indication is for patients with chronic anxiety, although the SSRIs are the first-line treatment for anxiety disorders. Its major disadvantage is that it takes 1–2 weeks for its anxiolytic properties to be felt, and it is consequently often perceived to be less effective than the benzodiazepines.

Buspirone is a lipophilic drug that is well absorbed but extensively metabolized by first-pass metabolism. It is highly protein bound, with a half-life of 1–11 hours. Metabolism and clearance are decreased in hepatic and renal dis-

Table 15–13. Preparations and dosages of hypnotics

Medication	Brand name and preparation	Dosage	Schedule
Hypnotics			
zolpidem	Ambien, 5, 10 mg	5–10 mg/day	qhs
zaleplon	Sonata, 5, 10 mg	5–10 mg/day	qhs
eszoplicone	Lunesta, 1, 2, 3 mg	1–2 mg/day	qhs
Alternative hypnotic			
chloral hydrate	Somnote, 500 mg tablet; 500 mg/5 mL syrup	25–50 mg/kg/day	qhs

Note. qhs = at bedtime.
Source. Adapted from Martin A, Scahill L, Charney DS, et al: "Appendix: Pediatric Psychopharmacology at a Glance," in *Pediatric Psychopharmacology: Principles and Practice.* Edited by Martin A, Scahill L, Charney DS, et al. Washington, DC, American Psychiatric Publishing, 2002, pp 757–764. Copyright 2002, American Psychiatric Publishing, Inc. Used with permission.

ease. It may displace less firmly protein-bound drugs, such as digoxin, and has the potential for a hyperpyrexia reaction when combined with MAOIs. The plasma concentration of buspirone is increased by verapamil, diltiazem, and erythromycin but reduced by rifampin.

Hypnotic Agents

First-line agents used in the treatment of insomnia include the hypnotics and chloral hydrate as well as trazodone and antihistamines. The nonbenzodiazepine sedatives zolpidem, eszoplicone, and zaleplon that are used in the treatment of insomnia are well-tolerated medications with short half-lives and very few adverse side effects (Tables 15–13 and 15–14). Tolerance to the hypnotic effects occurs less frequently than with the benzodiazepines. Chloral hydrate is an older medication that has been commonly used to treat insomnia. However, chronic use has resulted in gastritis and gastric ulceration as well as hepatic and renal toxicity. It can also cause gastrointestinal upset when taken on an empty stomach. Its use should be avoided in patients with gastritis or peptic ulcer disease. Overdose of chloral hydrate may result in hypertension, hyperthermia, respiratory depression, coma, hepatic failure, renal insufficiency, and death.

Table 15–14. Common side effects of the hypnotics agents

Sedative-hypnotic	Side effects	Notes
Zolpidem	*Central nervous system:* dizziness, lightheadedness, drowsiness, headache *Gastrointestinal:* nausea, dyspepsia *Respiratory:* respiratory depression at high dosages	Possible mild withdrawal symptoms
Zaleplon	*Central nervous system:* headache, dizziness, somnolence	Dose reduction is required during concomitant treatment with cimetidine Possible mild withdrawal symptoms
Eszoplicone	*Central nervous system:* headache, somnolence, dizziness *Gastrointestinal:* bitter taste, dry mouth	Possible mild withdrawal symptoms
Chloral hydrate	*Central nervous system:* drowsiness, dizziness, malaise, fatigue, confusion *Gastrointestinal:* epigastric distress, nausea, vomiting, gastric ulceration *Cardiovascular:* hypotension, arrhythmias	Avoid in patients with severe renal, cardiac, and hepatic disease; peptic ulcer disease and gastritis Highly protein bound with potential to displace other medications such as warfarin

Psychostimulants

The psychostimulants are used in a number of conditions, including attention-deficit/hyperactivity disorder and narcolepsy. They have also been used to augment the treatment of pain, fatigue, and depression in physically ill patients. Stimulants have been used anecdotally in patients following central nervous system stroke when inattention and focus are problematic. Clonidine has been added to a stimulant to reduce aggression, insomnia, and stimulant rebound as the medication wears off. There are several different formulations with differing half-lives and long-acting preparations that allow greater duration of effect with single daily doses (Table 15–15).

Table 15–15.   Preparations and dosages of psychostimulants

Medication	Brand name and preparation	Dosage	Schedule
Stimulants			
methylphenidate	Ritalin 5, 10, 20 mg	15–60 mg/day	bid/tid
	Ritalin SR 20 mg	(0.3–2 mg/kg/day)	qd
	Ritalin LA 20, 30, 40 mg		qd
	Focalin 2.5, 5, 10 mg		qd
	Focalin XR 5, 10, 20 mg		qd
	Methylin 5, 10, 20 mg		qd
	Methylin ER 10, 20 mg		qd
	Metadate ER 10, 20 mg		qd
	Metadate CD 10, 20, 30 mg		qd
	Concerta 18, 27, 36, 54 mg	18–54 mg/day	
dextroamphetamine	Dexedrine 5, 10 mg capsule	10–40 mg/day	bid/tid
	Dexedrine 5, 10, 15 mg Spansule (sustained release)	(0.3–1.5 mg/kg/day)	qd qd
	Dextrostat 5, 10, 15 mg (extended release)		
mixed amphetamine salts	Adderall 5, 7.5, 10, 12.5, 15, 20, 30 mg	10–40 mg/day (0.3–1.5 mg/kg/day)	qd/bid qd
	Adderall XR 5, 10 15, 20, 25, 30 mg		
pemoline	Cylert 18.75, 37.5, 75 mg	37.5–112.5 mg/day	qd
Alternative			
atomoxetine	Strattera 10, 18, 25, 40, 60, 80 mg	40–80 mg/day (0.5–1.2 mg/kg/day)	qd/bid
modafinil	Provigil 100, 200 mg	100–200 mg/day	qd

Note.   bid = twice a day; qd = every day; tid = three times a day.
Source.   Adapted from Martin A, Scahill L, Charney DS, et al: "Appendix: Pediatric Psychopharmacology at a Glance," in *Pediatric Psychopharmacology: Principles and Practice.* Edited by Martin A, Scahill L, Charney DS, et al. Washington, DC, American Psychiatric Publishing, 2002, pp. 757–764. Copyright 2002, American Psychiatric Publishing, Inc. Used with permission.

The most commonly reported side effects reported with the use of the psychostimulant medications are appetite suppression and sleep disturbance (Table 15–16). Psychostimulants have additive effects with other medications that produce central nervous system stimulation and tend to increase blood levels of TCAs due to hepatic enzyme inhibition. Concerns about the occurrence of a small number of fatalities related to the combination of clonidine with the psychostimulants have been raised, although careful review has not supported a causal relationship (Connor et al. 2000; Wilens et al. 1999). Symptoms of overdose of psychostimulant medications include flushing, palpitations, hypertension, arrhythmias, tachycardia, delirium, hyperreflexia, hyperpyrexia, and psychotic symptoms.

In 2005, Health Canada suspended sales of Adderall based on U.S. reports of 20 deaths, including 14 deaths in children and adolescents. The FDA has noted that there is insufficient data to reach a causative conclusion and has not removed the medication, although recommendations have been made for a black box warning. Although cardiovascular effects of increased heart rate and blood pressure are common with all stimulants, they are generally thought to be safe and effective (Alexander et al. 2005). Patients should be screened with a physical examination and a careful history for cardiac risk factors (i.e., syncope, fainting, palpitations, current/past heart disease, and a family history of cardiomyopathy or sudden death before age 40) (Alexander et al. 2005). Positive answers to this screening or known heart disease should prompt cardiology consultation. Routine electrocardiographic screening is not recommended (Alexander et al. 2005).

Psychostimulants are readily absorbed, and the immediate-release agents have therapeutic effects about 30 minutes after ingestion. The psychostimulants are not tightly protein bound. They have rapid extracellular metabolism. Excretion occurs by the kidneys and may be increased by acidification of the urine. Psychostimulants have a short duration of action that has resulted in the development of a number of longer-acting agents to reduce the frequency of dosing (see Table 15–15). There are also some more specific formulations of methylphenidate (e.g., Focalin [*d-threo*-methylphenidate], which is the d-isomer of methylphenidate and is effective at approximately half the milligram dosage of Ritalin).

Table 15–16.   Common side effects of the psychostimulants

Psychostimulant	Side effects	Notes
Methylphenidate Amphetamines	*Central nervous system:* insomnia, fatigue, headache, nervousness, social withdrawal, confusion, tremor, blurred vision, unmasking or induction of tics, possible growth velocity reduction *Gastrointestinal:* nausea, stomachache, anorexia, constipation *Cardiovascular:* elevated heart rate, elevated blood pressure, hypotension, palpitations, cardiac arrhythmias (at higher dosages)	Interaction with sympathomimetics and MAOIs to cause headache, arrhythmias, hypertensive crisis, and hyperpyrexia Concurrent use with beta-blockers may cause hypertension, reflex bradycardia, and heart block Adderall has been associated with cases of unexplained deaths in children with and without structural cardiac abnormalities Rebound or abstinence symptoms when the medications wear off May worsen psychosis and mania
Pemoline	Similar side-effect profile to other psychostimulants *Hepatic:* delayed hepatic hypersensitivity reaction	Rarely used due to black box warning regarding potential fatal hepatotoxicity
Atomoxetine	*Central nervous system:* insomnia, headache, rhinitis, dry mouth, dizziness *Gastrointestinal:* nausea, dry mouth, constipation, decreased appetite *Cardiovascular:* palpitations	50%–75% Dosage reduction in hepatic insufficiency Black box warning regarding potential increase in suicidality
Modafinil	*Central nervous system:* headache, syncope, visual changes, hypertonia, nervousness, dyskinesia, depression *Gastrointestinal:* nausea, vomiting *Cardiovascular:* arrhythmias, hypertension	50%–75% Dosage reduction in hepatic insufficiency Elevated liver transaminases May cause cataplexy May cause respiratory problems

Atomoxetine

Atomoxetine is a new alternative medication for the treatment of attention-deficit/hyperactivity disorder. It is technically an antidepressant and not a psychostimulant. It is well absorbed orally, metabolized through the CYP450 system, and excreted in the urine. It is generally very well tolerated, with only small elevations in blood pressure and pulse. Atomoxetine has no reported effect on the electrocardiogram (see Tables 15–15 and 15–16).

Modafinil

Modafinil is a recently released medication that is used to improve wakefulness in patients with excessive sleepiness associated with narcolepsy, obstructive sleep apnea/hypopnea syndrome, and shift work sleep disorder. It may be useful for patient experiencing malaise and fatigue due to physical illness, although it has not been used for this purpose with children or adolescents. Modafinil may interact with drugs that inhibit, induce, or are metabolized by CYP450 isoenzymes. It appears to induce CYP3A4, CYP1A2, and CYP2B6, and inhibits CYP2C19 and CYP2C9. Thus it may reduce cyclosporine and theophylline levels while increasing those of propranolol, phenytoin, and warfarin.

Psychotropic Medication Use in Specific Physical Illnesses

Hepatic Disease

Hepatic disease may affect drug distribution due to changes in hepatic blood flow, effects on protein binding, and changes in volume of distribution due to peritoneal ascites (Beliles 2000b). The primary effects are reduced availability of medications for drug metabolism and the potential for increased serum drug levels. In acute hepatitis, there is generally no need to modify drug dosage because drug metabolism is only minimally altered and the change is transient. In chronic hepatitis and cirrhosis, however, there is destruction of hepatocytes, and drug dosages may need to be modified. Mild elevations in liver transaminases (i.e., alanine transaminase and aspartate aminotransferase) are common and usually benign and require investigation only if elevated two

Table 15–17.   Medication use in hepatic disease

Medication class	Impact of hepatic disease on drug dosing	Potential drug effect on liver function
Antidepressants	Antidepressants that are metabolized by phase I hepatic oxidative metabolism require an approximately 50% dosage reduction. Dosages of bupropion should not exceed 75 mg/day in patients with cirrhosis. Trazodone requires dosage reduction due to prolonged clearance of trazodone in patients with hepatic disease.	Tricyclic antidepressants may exacerbate hepatic encephalopathy by anticholinergic action. Nefazodone use is contraindicated in hepatic disease. Minor elevations in transaminases are common and usually benign. Sertraline's short half-life and less potent inhibition of CYP2D6 make it the preferred selective serotonin reuptake inhibitor in hepatic disease.
Antipsychotics	Atypical antipsychotics that are metabolized by phase I hepatic oxidative metabolism require dosage reduction.	Chlorpromazine is associated with intrahepatic cholestasis and obstructive hepatic disease. Low-potency drugs may precipitate hepatic encephalopathy in patients with cirrhosis. Discontinue clozapine in patients with marked transaminase elevations or jaundice.
Anxiolytics/Hypnotics	Benzodiazepine half-lives are increased in hepatic disease. Lorazepam, oxazepam, and temazepam require no dosage adjustment in hepatic disease because they are metabolized by phase II hepatic oxidative metabolism. Zaleplon and zolpidem require dosage reduction.	Avoid use of benzodiazepines in patients at risk of hepatic encephalopathy.

Table 15–17. Medication use in hepatic disease (*continued*)

Medication class	Impact of hepatic disease on drug dosing	Potential drug effect on liver function
Mood stabilizers	Carbamazepine, divalproex, lamotrigine, and topiramate require dosage reduction and close monitoring. No dosage adjustment is required for gabapentin or lithium.	Depakote is associated with hepatic failure in 1 in 40,000 cases. Carbamazepine is associated with hepatitis. Carbamazepine and valproic acid are contraindicated in patients with preexisting hepatic disease.
Psychostimulants	Atomoxetine requires a 25%–50% reduction in dosage.	

Source. Adapted from Beliles 2000b; Jacobson 2002; Robinson and Owen 2005.

to three times above baseline. By contrast, elevations in bilirubin or alkaline phosphatase suggest involvement of the biliary tract and may require further evaluation.

Liver cirrhosis may distort liver architecture and alter hepatic blood flow. In severe disease, portosystemic shunting may affect 60% or more of portal vein flow that diverts circulating drugs away from the liver, resulting in decreased drug extraction and first-pass metabolism. By contrast, hepatic blood flow may be increased in viral hepatitis and in patients with chronic respiratory problems. Medications with high baseline rates of clearance by the liver (e.g., haloperidol, paroxetine, sertraline, nefazodone, venlafaxine, TCAs, and midazolam) are significantly affected by alterations in hepatic blood flow.

Albumin and α_1 glycoproteins that are produced in the liver may be reduced in patients with infectious and inflammatory hepatic disease, whereas surgery, trauma, and cirrhosis may result in elevated protein levels. Elevated serum bilirubin levels are found in acute viral hepatitis and primary biliary cirrhosis. Bilirubin has a strong affinity for albumin binding sites and may displace medications (e.g., divalproex sodium and phenytoin). In steady-state situations, changes in protein binding may result in elevated, unbound, active forms of a drug in the presence of normal serum total drug concentrations. Because it is often difficult to predict changes in drug protein binding, it is important to pay close attention to the clinical and toxic effects of psychotropic medications and not rely exclusively on serum drug concentrations.

In general, for patients with hepatic disease it is necessary to use lower dosages of medications (Table 15–17). Initial dosing of medications should be reduced in patients with hepatic disease, and titration should proceed more slowly. For drugs that have significant hepatic metabolism, intravenous administration may be preferred. In general, parenteral administration of drugs avoids first-pass metabolic effects, and the dosing and action of drugs are similar to those in patients with normal hepatic function.

Gastrointestinal Disease

Gastrointestinal disease primarily affects drug absorption (Beliles 2000b). Examples of conditions that affect absorption include diseases affecting gastrointestinal motility, surgical alteration of the gastrointestinal tract (e.g., bypass surgery, G-tube and J-tube placement), short bowel syndrome, and celiac disease. Any conditions that divert blood away from the gastrointestinal tract (e.g., congestive heart failure or shock) may also affect absorption. Administration of antacid medications may similarly reduce gastric absorption.

Gastric motility may be affected by a number of medical conditions and by specific medications. For example, gastric motility is delayed in patients with diabetes mellitus, gastritis, and pyloric stenosis. Anticholinergic medications delay gastric motility. A number of medications are given to increase gastrointestinal motility, including metoclopramide, cisapride, and propantheline. In general, slowed gastrointestinal motility results in better absorption of poorly soluble drugs and vice versa. Enteric-coated preparations of medications are likely to have increased rates of drug absorption in patients with reduced gastric acidity. Orally administered drugs may be poorly absorbed in patients with malabsorption syndromes. If absorption is an issue, liquid formulations of drugs and alternative routes of administration such as sublingual, intramuscular, and intravenous may be preferred. Gastrointestinal disease affecting the large intestines generally has little effect because most medications are absorbed more proximally.

Many psychotropic medications have the potential to cause gastrointestinal side effects. Medications with anticholinergic side effects can slow gastrointestinal motility, affect absorption, and cause constipation. By contrast, SSRIs increase gastric motility and may cause diarrhea. SSRIs also have a potential to increase the risk of gastrointestinal bleeding, especially when coadministered with nonsteroidal anti-inflammatory drugs. Using extended- or controlled-release preparations of medications may reduce gastrointestinal side effects, particularly in cases in which gastric distress is related to rapid increases in plasma drug concentrations.

Renal Disease

Renal insufficiency results in a functional loss of nephrons. This is generally a transient and reversible phenomenon in acute renal failure, but in chronic renal failure it may be permanent and lead to the need for dialysis. Pharmacodynamic effects of renal failure include increased receptor sensitivity, and pharmacokinetic effects include delayed drug clearance (Beliles 2000b). Renal insufficiency may result in decreased absorption of drugs from the small intestine due to the gastric-alkalinizing effects of increased ammonia levels that develop in the presence of excess urea. Renal insufficiency may increase the volume of distribution of water-soluble or protein-bound drugs, with a consequent reduction in plasma levels at normal drug dosages. Plasma protein binding of drugs may be reduced in nephrotic syndrome as a result of decreases in albumin concentration. Displacement of highly protein-bound drugs may result in increased availability of these drugs for renal filtration and excretion. Renal insufficiency may also be associated with decreased first-pass metabolism and influence hepatic clearance due to CYP2D6 inhibition. Renal excretion or clearance is reduced in renal failure and is significant for drugs that are cleared primarily by renal excretion. Renal blood flow may be altered by changes in glomerular vasculature, severe dehydration, and conditions affecting other organ syndromes (e.g., cirrhosis).

In general, initial dosages of medications should be reduced or dosing intervals lengthened in patients with renal failure (Table 15–18). The *rule of two-thirds* is that dosages of medications should be reduced by one-third of the normal dosage in patients with renal insufficiency. However, most psychotropic medications, with the exception of lithium and gabapentin, do not require significant adjustments to dosing in patients with renal failure. It is important to carefully monitor serum concentrations in patients with renal insufficiency, particularly for medications with a narrow therapeutic index. Lithium may be given to renal transplant recipients; however, cyclosporine may elevate serum lithium levels by decreasing lithium excretion, necessitating a dosage adjustment. Patients with renal failure and those on dialysis appear to be more sensitive to the side effects of the TCAs, possibly due to the accumulation of hydroxylated tricyclic metabolites. However, SSRIs have generally supplanted the use of TCAs in the treatment of depression in patients with renal insufficiency.

Hemodialysis

Special consideration should be given to patients on hemodialysis. During hemodialysis, there may be an initial lowering of the plasma drug concentration followed by a rebound after dialysis as the drug redistributes from the periphery to the circulation. Drugs that are highly protein bound (this includes most of the psychotropic agents with the exception of lithium, divalproex sodium, venlafaxine, gabapentin, and topiramate) are generally not significantly cleared by dialysis. Drugs such as lithium and gabapentin are completely removed by dialysis, and the common practice is to administer these medications after dialysis. Drugs with a narrow therapeutic index should be avoided wherever pos-

Table 15–18. Medication use in renal disease

Medication class	Impact of renal disease on drug dosing	Potential drug effect on renal function
Antidepressants	Tricyclic antidepressants, nefazodone, and selective serotonin reuptake inhibitors require no dosage adjustment except in severe renal insufficiency. Venlafaxine requires a 25%–75% reduction in dosage due to reduced renal clearance.	Patients with renal insufficiency are more susceptible to side effects of tricyclics, especially sedation and anticholinergic effects.
Antipsychotics	Risperidone requires dosage reduction.	Antipsychotic agents are generally safe.
Anxiolytics/Hypnotics	Benzodiazepines, especially chlordiazepoxide, require dosage reduction due to increased half-life in renal insufficiency. Lorazepam and oxazepam are preferred due to the absence of active metabolites. Buspirone is not recommended.	Barbiturates use should be avoided due to the risk of excessive sedation.
Mood stabilizers	Lithium, carbamazepine, topiramate, and gabapentin require 50%–75% reduction in dosage. Divalproex sodium requires no dosage adjustment.	Lithium is contraindicated in acute renal failure but is considered safe in chronic renal failure with a dosage adjustment. Lithium requires dosage reduction in patients on hemodialysis. Lithium should be given after dialysis.

Source. Adapted from Beliles 2000b; Jacobson 2002; Robinson and Owen 2005.

sible in patients who are on dialysis. In addition, patients on dialysis often have significant fluid shifts and are at risk of dehydration. NMS may be more likely in these situations. Another common issue is that of orthostatic hypertension, which occurs particularly following dialysis.

Cardiac Disease

Cardiac disease may influence the pharmacokinetics of medications. For example, congestive heart failure may result in decreased perfusion of drug absorption sites both in the gastrointestinal tract and in skeletal muscle, affecting drugs given both orally and by intramuscular injection (Beliles 2000b). Sympathetic activity may redistribute blood flow to the brain and heart, reducing perfusion of the liver, kidney, and other organs, with the potential to affect drug distribution. Local edema may also reduce epithelial permeability and increase drug absorption. Cardiac patients are commonly treated with anticoagulant medications (e.g., warfarin) that are highly protein bound. In these situations, it may be necessary to reduce the dosage of highly protein-bound psychotropic agents to reduce the potential risk of elevated levels of anticoagulants.

Potential cardiovascular side effects of psychotropic medications include orthostatic hypotension, conduction disturbances, and arrhythmias (Table 15–19). Orthostatic hypotension is one of the most common cardiovascular side effects that complicate the use of TCAs. The risk is increased in patients who have impaired left ventricular function. If TCAs are used in patients with cardiac disease, nortriptyline is thought to be less likely to result in orthostatic hypotension. Trazodone may result in orthostatic hypotension and exacerbate myocardial instability. As a result, SSRIs and bupropion are preferred as antidepressant agents in patients with cardiac disease.

There is the potential for increased cardiac morbidity and mortality particularly in patients with preexisting cardiac conduction problems such as atrioventricular block. Thioridazine and pimozide in particular should be avoided in patients with severe cardiac disease. Similarly, intravenous haloperidol has been associated with the development of the arrhythmias, including QT_c prolongation and *torsades de pointes,* and may depress cardiovascular function (Beliles 2000a). Both the TCAs and lithium may exacerbate congestive cardiac failure. Some of the calcium channel–blocking agents, such as diltiazem and verapamil, may slow atrioventricular conduction and may theoretically inter-

Table 15–19. Medication use in cardiac disease

Medication class	Impact of cardiac disease on drug dosing	Potential drug effect on cardiac function
Tricyclic antidepressants		Increased cardiac morbidity and mortality due to arrhythmias
		Side effects in healthy individuals limited to orthostatic hypotension
		Nortriptyline preferred due to lower likelihood of hypotension
		Potential for delayed cardiac conduction, increased heart rate, and heart block
		Prolonged PR interval, QRS duration, and QT_c interval
		Potential torsades de pointes in preexisting conduction disturbances
		Potential for ventricular tachycardia or fibrillation in Wolff-Parkinson-White syndrome
Selective serotonin reuptake inhibitors		Isolated reports of bradycardia and atrial fibrillation with fluoxetine
		Citalopram not recommended in cardiac disease with prolonged conduction times
Antipsychotics		Orthostatic hypotension associated with use of clozapine, quetiapine, and low-potency antipsychotics
		Pimozide, thioridazine, mesoridazine, droperidol, sertindole, ziprasidone, and high-dose intravenous haloperidol carry risk of prolonged QT_c interval
Anxiolytics/Hypnotics		Benzodiazepines and buspirone believed to be free from cardiovascular effects
Mood stabilizers	Lithium requires dosage reduction in patients with congestive heart failure.	Lithium may cause sinus node dysfunction or first-degree atrioventricular block.
		Carbamazepine is associated with atrioventricular conduction disturbances.
		Lamotrigine is associated with QT_c interval prolongation.
		Divalproex sodium is believed to be safe.
Psychostimulants		Methylphenidate and amphetamines are believed to be safe at low dosages.

Source. Beliles 2000b; Robinson and Owen 2005.

act with the TCAs. Patients with Wolff-Parkinson-White syndrome who have a short PR interval (less than 0.27 seconds) and widened QRS interval associated with paroxysmal tachycardia are at high risk of life-threatening ventricular tachycardia that may be exacerbated by the use of TCAs.

Quinidine-like effects of the TCAs and the antipsychotic agents may lead to prolongation of the QT_c interval with increased risk of ventricular tachycardia and ventricular fibrillation, particularly in patients with congenital heart disease. Patients with a baseline QT_c interval of greater than 440 msec should be considered at particular risk. The range of normal QT_c values in children is 400 msec ± 25–30 msec. A QT_c value that exceeds two standard deviations (>450–460 msec) is considered too long and may be associated with increased mortality (Labellarte et al. 2003). An increase in the QT_c of greater than 60 msec from baseline is also associated with increased mortality. It is important to keep in mind that computer readouts of the electrocardiogram are not reliable, particularly in situations of tachycardia or bradycardia. Situations that should prompt cardiology consultation include QT_c duration longer than 480 msec, QT_c prolongation longer than 60 msec over baseline, prolonged QT_c duration that continues after the medication has been discontinued, or the presence of cardiovascular symptoms.

Respiratory Disease

The benzodiazepines are the psychiatric medications of most concern in patients with pulmonary disease due to the risk of respiratory depression (see Table 15–20). There is particular concern in patients who retain carbon dioxide. Both buspirone and trazodone are good alternative medications for the treatment of anxiety and insomnia.

Conclusion

Overall, there remains a paucity of information in the literature pertaining to the pharmacological treatment of children and adolescents with physically illness. Studies to date have essentially excluded youngsters with comorbid general medical conditions. Clinical experience suggests that the target symptoms outlined in this chapter will respond to psychotherapy and medications. Psychiatric consultants working in the pediatric setting require a solid understanding of pediatric psychopharmacology. Nonprescribing consultants should

Table 15–20. Medication use in respiratory disease

Medication class	Potential drug effect on respiratory function
Antidepressants	Monoamine oxidase inhibitors may interact with sympathomimetic medications used in asthma treatment Need to monitor anticholinergic side effects Tricyclic antidepressants and selective serotonin reuptake inhibitors generally do not cause problems
Antipsychotics	Laryngeal dystonia that may affect respiratory status Clozapine has been associated with respiratory arrest and depression as well as allergic asthma Need to monitor anticholinergic side effects
Anxiolytics/ Hypnotics	Respiratory depression and failure possible with benzodiazepines Consider baseline blood gases prior to benzodiazepines Oxazepam, lorazepam, and temazepam have fewer respiratory depressant effects Buspirone, zolpidem, and zaleplon believed to be safe

Source. Adapted from Beliles 2000b; Jacobson 2002; Robinson and Owen 2005.

establish a consulting relationship with a child and adolescent psychiatrist familiar with the pediatric setting. As in all psychiatric practice, both patients and family members should be given full explanations of the indications for medication treatment as well as the potential risks and benefits. Informed consent should also always be obtained prior to starting a new medication.

References

Alexander M, Vaughan B, Urion D, et al: Adderall use in children and adolescents. Pediatric Views, 2005. Available at http://www.childrenshospital.org/views/june05/adderall.html. Accessed April 23, 2006.

Beliles KE: Alternative routes of administration of psychotropic medications, in Psychiatric Care of the Medical Patient, 2nd Edition. Edited by Stoudemire A, Fogel BS, Greenberg DB. Oxford, England, Oxford University Press, 2000a, pp 395–405

Beliles KE: Psychopharmacokinetics in the medically ill, in Psychiatric Care of the Medical Patient, 2nd Edition. Edited by Stoudemire A, Fogel BS, Greenberg DB. Oxford, England, Oxford University Press, 2000b, pp 272–394

Birmaher B: Treatment of psychosis in children and adolescents. Psychiatr Ann 33:257–264, 2003

Boyer EW, Shannon M: The serotonin syndrome. N Engl J Med 352:1112–1120, 2005

Brown TM, Stoudemire A, Fogel BS, et al: Psychopharmacology in the medical patient, in Psychiatric Care of the Medical Patient, 2nd Edition. Edited by Stoudemire A, Fogel BS, Greenberg DB. Oxford, England, Oxford University Press, 2000, pp 329–372

Connor DF, Barkley RA, Davis HT: A pilot study of methylphenidate, clonidine, or the combination in ADHD comorbid with aggressive oppositional defiant or conduct disorder. Clin Pediatr 39:15–25, 2000

Jacobson S: Psychopharmacology: prescribing for patients with hepatic or renal dysfunction. Psychiatric Times Nov:65–69, 2002

Jefferson JW, Greist JH, Ackerman DL, et al: Lithium Encyclopedia for Clinical Practice, 2nd Edition. Washington, DC, American Psychiatric Press, 1987

Katic A, Steingard RJ, Schmidt C: An update on adolescent psychopharmacology. Adolesc Med 9:217–228, 1998

Labellarte MJ, Crosson JE, Riddle MA: The relevance of prolonged QT_c measurement to pediatric psychopharmacology. J Am Acad Child Adolesc Psychiatry 42:642–650, 2003

Lieberman JA: Metabolic changes associated with antipsychotic use. Prim Care Companion J Clin Psychiatry 6(suppl 2):8–13, 2004

Martin A, Scahill L, Charney DS, et al: Appendix: pediatric psychopharmacology at a glance, in Pediatric Psychopharmacology: Principles and Practice. Edited by Martin A, Scahill L, Charney DS, et al. Washington, DC, American Psychiatric Publishing, 2002, pp 757–764

Posternak MA, Zimmerman M: Is there a delay in the antidepressant effect? A meta-analysis. J Clin Psychiatry 66:148–158, 2005

Robinson MJ, Owen JA: Psychopharmacology, in The American Psychiatric Press Textbook of Psychosomatic Medicine. Edited by Levenson JL. Washington, DC, American Psychiatric Publishing, 2005, pp 871–922

Schatzberg AF, Cole JO, DeBattista C: Manual of Clinical Psychopharmacology, 4th Edition. Washington, DC, American Psychiatric Publishing, 2003

U.S. Food and Drug Administration: FDA public health advisory: suicidality in child and adolescents being treated with antidepressant medications, October 15, 2004. Available at http://www.fda.gov/cder/drug/antidepressants/SSRIPHA200410 .htm. Accessed April 24, 2006.

Wilens TE, Spencer TJ, Swanson JM, et al: Combining methylphenidate and clonidine: a clinically sound medication option. J Am Acad Adolesc Psychiatry 38:614–622, 1999

16

Preparation for Procedures

Children are exposed to multiple invasive medical procedures, often starting on their first day of life. Healthy children receive two to four injections for immunization on five separate occasions between ages 2 and 15 months and again when entering school (Blount et al. 2003; Cohen 2002). Children with serious medical conditions such as cancer are at even greater risk for increased numbers of medical procedures. Some studies have estimated that the average cancer treatment requires more than 300 blood tests. Similarly, premature infants may have to endure invasive procedures including blood tests, spinal taps, and intubation as well as the placement of catheters and chest tubes. Studies of newborns born at less than 32 weeks of gestation have shown that they may receive an average of between 2 and 10 invasive procedures each day (Johnston et al. 1997).

Many invasive procedures that occur in pediatric intensive care units are conducted without anesthesia (Southall et al. 1993). These aversive medical procedures result in a cycle of pain and distress often accompanied by secondary anticipatory anxiety. More than 50% of children receiving blood tests report moderate to severe distress or pain. Pediatric cancer patients report that pain due to procedures may be of greater intensity than their illness-related pain (Ljungman et al. 1999). Poor management of pain in early childhood may alter the neuronal circuits that process pain and result in accentuated behavioral response to pain in later childhood (Ruda et al. 2000). Emotional factors, such as elevated levels of anxiety or fear, may increase pain perception and make subsequent medical procedures more stressful (Blount et al. 2003; McGrath 1994). Medical posttraumatic stress disorder has been diagnosed in one-fifth of young adult survivors of childhood cancer and may be associated with the avoidance of medical care in adulthood (Hobbie et al. 2000; Pate et al. 1996). This chapter provides guidelines on approaches to help reduce distress related to stressful and invasive medical procedures

Assessment

Prior to any intervention to reduce procedural anxiety it is important to assess the child's prior medical experiences and the techniques that may have been used to facilitate or improve their level of coping. Other issues that should be assessed include the child's understanding of the illness, the rationale for the procedure, the child's level of cognitive and emotional development, and the family's receptiveness to psychological intervention (see Table 16–1).

Preparation

Preparation for procedures should occur in a developmentally appropriate manner with interventions that are individualized to each child and that utilize the active participation of parents for support in the role of coaches. Good preparation has been shown to provide comfort to the child, reduce the child's level of distress both before and after hospitalization, and shorten the length of the procedure (Butler et al. 2005). Effective preparation for procedures includes providing information, modeling, and teaching of coping strategies. Involving children and their families in preparation programs has consistently been found to reduce levels of distress related to procedures, particularly those programs that allow the children to play an active role (Harbeck-Weber and McKee 1995). General principles for the preparation of children are outlined in Table 16–2.

Table 16–1. Assessment of children prior to painful procedures

1. Has your child had prior painful or stressful procedures?
2. How well does your child understand the procedure protocol?
3. Did your child experience anxiety or distress during these procedures? Rate on a scale from 1 to 5.
4. What aspect of the procedure was most distressing to your child?
5. Did your child report any distressing images, nightmares, or memories after the procedure?
6. What techniques has your child used to reduce his/her level of anxiety?
   Breathing
   Deep muscle relaxation
   Being held
   Massage
   Distraction
   Guided imagery
   Hypnosis
   Behavior modification
7. Rate the effectiveness of each technique in reducing your child's level of anxiety.
8. What is the optimal timing for your child to be prepared for a procedure?
9. Do you prefer to be present or absent during your child's procedure?
10. What behaviors indicate that your child is experiencing distress or pain?
11. Have you received any instruction on coping strategies to assist your child during the procedure?
12. What incentives would be helpful to reward your child after the procedure?

Education

Preparatory information is most effective if it includes a problem description of the types of sensations the child is likely to experience and a procedural description with the expected sequence of events. This can be accomplished with the use of dolls or puppets that are put through a simulated procedure similar to the one that the child has to go through. Parents are also given information and a chance to ask questions. Parents involved in such programs have been shown to be less anxious and more satisfied with the child's nursing care, and children similarly have been rated as showing fewer distress behaviors (Wolfer and Visintainer 1975).

Table 16–2. Preparation of children for painful procedures

Provide information and prepare the parent and child

Give step-by-step information of what will occur during the procedure.

Give sensory information about what the child will see, hear, and feel.

Use age-appropriate language and terminology and avoid medical jargon.

Avoid high-anxiety words such as *pain, hurt, cut, shot.* Use words such as *poking, freezing, squeezing* instead.

Do not insinuate that the procedure will definitely hurt.

Be aware of possible misinterpretations of words and phrases such as *dye* or *put to sleep.*

Address children's concerns (e.g., "taking all my blood").

Consider using books describing the procedure the child can read with the parent.

Give information before and during the procedure.

Be honest.

Parental involvement

Ask the parents how much distress they expect from the child.

Allow parents to remain present.

Do not ask the parent to help restrain the child.

Instruct the parent not to threaten the child (e.g., with additional shots).

Instruct the parent to use coping-promoting behaviors (e.g., distraction) and to avoid distress-promoting behaviors (e.g., reassurance).

Health care worker behavior

Be calm, confident, and in control.

Avoid reassurance, apology, criticism.

Avoid conversation with other health care workers and parents that may be distressing (e.g., describing possible adverse events) in front of the child.

Teach students how to perform the procedure outside the room to minimize discussion in front of the child.

Health care setting

Maintain a quiet, calm environment.

Avoid stressors such as beeping monitors.

Avoid long delays between informing the child of the procedure and performing it.

Avoid situations in which children can see or hear procedures performed on other children.

Table 16–2. Preparation of children for painful procedures *(continued)*

Procedural details

Allow comfort items such as favorite stuffed animals or blankets.

For venipunctures and intravenous cannulation in thumb-sucking children, avoid the arm of the preferred thumb.

Do not force the child to lie down if he or she does not want to and is not required to.

Consider giving the child a "job" (e.g., holding a gauze).

Give the child choices to increase the perception of control (e.g., right arm or left).

For long procedures (e.g., burn dressing changes), allow the child "time-outs" of a predetermined number and duration (e.g., three 20-second time-outs).

Allow the child to count down from 10 to 1 before a brief procedure.

Use automatic lancets for finger sticks.

Venipuncture, when feasible, may be less painful than heel lance.

Hospitalized children

Use a treatment room; keep the patient's room/bed as a "safe place."

Give hospitalized children a predictable "safe" time when procedures will not occur and a predictable time for procedures.

Plan ahead and draw all blood samples at once if possible.

Do not give pain medications by a painful route (i.e., intramuscular).

Source. Reprinted from Young KD: "Pediatric Procedural Pain." *Annals of Emergency Medicine* 4:160–171, 2005. Copyright 2005, Elsevier Inc. Used with permission.

Modeling

Modeling involves the use of videos showing a peer successfully completing the invasive procedure with the help of appropriate coping strategies. These techniques are particularly helpful for children who have negatively distorted expectations (Cohen et al. 2001). The effectiveness of modeling appears to be enhanced when the model is of a similar age and ethnicity to the patient (Melamed et al. 1976). Beneficial effects of preparation programs appear to last for at least a month, and children older than age 7 years appear to benefit more than younger children.

Coping Strategies

Coping strategies that may be used during the procedure itself include breathing, deep muscle relaxation, distraction, behavioral rehearsal, positive reinforcement, modeling, visual imagery, and hypnosis. These interventions have consistently been shown to reduce levels of distress and improve levels of cooperation in children and adolescents undergoing stressful procedures. The addition of training in the use of coping skills appears to have added benefits when compared with interventions that use only education or modeling.

General Principles

Whenever possible it is preferable to perform procedures in a treatment room rather than at the bedside in order to preserve the room or bed as a safety zone for the hospitalized child. Local anesthesia, including EMLA cream (lidocaine, 2.5%, and prilocaine, 2.5%), should be used for needle procedures. General anesthesia should be considered for particularly distressing procedures or for children who appear to have overwhelming anxiety. For procedural pain that is known to be severe and stressful, the use of pharmacological agents is important to reduce pain to levels that are acceptable levels for the child. This may include the use of analgesic agents, including local anesthetics and nerve blocks as well as anxiolytics or sedative medications to reduce anxiety. Although anxiolytics alone do not provide analgesia, their adjunctive use has been shown to reduce the child's level of distress not only during the procedure but also for subsequent procedures.

Parental presence is generally helpful. Parents should assist with nonprocedural talk, humor, distraction, and encouragement of coping strategies. Efforts to give the child a feeling of being in control may be used, such as the choice of which arm will be used for the blood test, what type of bandage they will get, or which coping strategies the child will use. Parents should be encouraged to repeat positive statements during the procedure to reinforce their child's coping. It is important to emphasize the importance of practice to help establish proficiency in the use of these techniques.

It is important to debrief the child after the procedure and to give praise for any successful efforts at coping, even if the overall experience was not positive. Giving the child a sense of success and accomplishment during the procedure may facilitate improved performance during subsequent procedures. It is important to discuss which parts of the intervention were successful and which were not so that the child can build on the experience to improve his or her coping skills. *Transformation* refers to the attempt to change the child's evaluation of the event from horrible or awful to simply irritating or unfortunate (Chen et al. 1999). The goal is to modify or change the frequency of unwanted thoughts and behaviors that result from pain, and it can be effective for children older than 8 years who can self-initiate and maintain its use. Medical play may have a role for children who have a history of previous trauma related to procedures or in cases where further trauma is unavoidable and the goal is to provide the child with a way to express his or her feelings and develop a sense of mastery or control.

Distraction

Distraction involves refocusing attention away from threatening or anxiety-provoking aspects of the medical treatment to nonthreatening and engaging or pleasant thoughts or situations (Blount et al. 2003). Techniques are adapted according to the age and developmental level of the child. Rocking, patting, and sucking on a pacifier can help distract infants. Toddlers respond well to blowing bubbles or party blowers or the imaginary blowing out of birthday candles. The use of pop-up books or singing can also be helpful. Young children like to hold stuffed animals or toys or be comforted by having their arm touched or stroked during the procedure.

With older children and adolescents, distraction techniques include listening to music through headphones, counting backward, playing video games, or watching videotapes during the procedure. Sometimes attention can be focused on parts of the body that are not in pain. Older children may respond well to the explanation of how difficult it is to pay attention to more than one thing at a time (e.g., doing homework when the television is on in the same room). Similarly, children may relate to the experience of not noticing an injury sustained during a sports game until after the game is over. It is helpful to teach several distraction strategies so that the child has the option of trying out different techniques as needed.

There are some children who are extremely vigilant and prefer not to be distracted from the procedure (Schultheis et al. 1987). In these cases, it may be more helpful to develop a plan in which the child's attention is very specifically focused on what is happening and the child verbalizes changes in sensations as the procedure progresses.

Breathing

Some of the distraction techniques, such as blowing bubbles, party blowers, or pinwheels, utilize the benefits of breathing that help promote muscle relaxation. Even children as young as 4 years of age can be taught to take slow, deep breaths with the emphasis on breathing out slowly and fully.

Diaphragmatic Breathing

Older children and adolescents can be taught the technique of diaphragmatic breathing by watching their hands move up and down on their stomachs during breathing. One technique that can be used to help teach children and adolescents the principle of diaphragmatic breathing is as follows. The child is asked to lie down on the floor or on the bed. A small book is placed on the child's stomach near the belly button. The child is asked to imagine that the book is a boat sitting on the child's stomach. The child is told that breathing in fills the stomach with air and makes a wave that causes the boat to rise up. As the child breathes out, the air leaves the stomach and the wave falls.

Alternate Nostril Breathing

To teach alternate nostril breathing, the child is asked to sit in a comfortable position with the left hand on the left knee and the right index and middle fingers in the center of the eyebrows. The child closes the right nostril with the right thumb and breathes in and out through the left nostril five times. The child then removes the hand from his or her face, places it on the right knee, and breathes in and out through both nostrils five times. This process is repeated three times. This is an easy and effective technique that children can quickly learn.

Progressive Muscle Relaxation

Progressive muscle relaxation is used to distract patients from their pain and to reduce the intensity of their pain experience (Abel and Rouleau 2000). Muscle relaxation results in a reduction of muscle tension. It may also reduce autonomic nervous system reactivity. In the tension-relaxation method, the child is taught to constrict the muscles for 5–10 seconds and then relax specific muscle groups (see Table 16–3). It can be combined with suggestions of relaxation, heaviness, and warmth and images of relaxing situations. With serial sessions, the number of muscle groups is reduced until the child can attain a state of relaxation using a relaxation cue word. In the suggestion method,

Table 16–3.   Progressive muscle relaxation exercise: sample script

Instructions

Have the patient sit (or lie) quietly in a comfortable position. With a calm and nonrushed approach, use the following script as a guideline for progressive muscle relaxation. This process of tensing and relaxing the muscles is repeated on the left side of the body and can also incorporate the muscles in the legs and in the face. The exercise should last 10–20 minutes. You may choose to record the session so that the patient can practice using the recording.

Suggested script

Close your eyes as you take in a deep breath through your nose, filling your lungs completely, and then slowly breathe out. Take another deep breath in and feel the air filling up your chest, like a big balloon.

Continue taking slow, deep breaths in three or four times through your mouth, noticing the feeling of the air as it flows gently and easily in and out of your body. Feel your body relaxing, with all the tension draining from your muscles, as you become softer and floppy like a big rag doll.

Now focus your attention on your right hand. Squeeze your hand tightly together, as tightly as you can, noticing the feeling of your fingernails pushing into the palm of your hand. Hold your hand tightly clenched as we count slowly …1…2…3…4…5… . Notice how your hand feels slightly warm and tense as you squeeze tightly. Notice how different it feels from your other hand.

Quickly relax your hand and notice the feeling of the blood rushing back into your hand, with a slight warm feeling, as your hand relaxes and sinks down on to the bed. Now bend your right arm at the elbow, tightening the muscles in your arm. Squeeze tightly as we count slowly…1…2…3…4…5…. Now release your arm and allowe it to become relaxed and floppy. Notice the difference in sensations between your right arm and left arm.

Now push your arm down into the bed and against the side of your body, squeezing very tightly as we count again slowly…1…2…3…4…5…. Release the muscles and allow the arm to sink back down into the bed, and notice the feeling of complete relaxation in that arm.

the patient is given repeated suggestions of calmness, relaxation, heaviness, and warmth combined with pleasant imagery, but without initially tensing the muscles. In the technique of differential relaxation, the child learns to relax one part of the body while maintaining tension in other part. For example, in the treatment of migraine headaches, the patient learns to relax the jaw and shoulders but keeps tension in arms and trunks. Patients may be given tapes to facilitate the use of the relaxation techniques at home.

Positive Statements

Children and parents should be encouraged to repeat positive thoughts or statements during the procedure. Positive statements assist the child in feeling more relaxed and calm, whereas negative messages may increase symptoms of anxiety and distress. Examples of positive statements to be repeated during a procedure include 1) this will be over soon, 2) I am going to get through this, 3) I am relaxed and calm, 4) I am a very strong boy/girl, 5) this is not going to hurt that much, 6) this gets easier each time I do it, and 7) the pain is not as bad as I thought.

Guided Imagery

Children are generally easily able to focus their attention and become absorbed in their own world of fantasy or imaginary play. Younger children in particular are able to shift backward and forward between fantasy and reality while listening to an absorbing story that is being told to distract them from the procedure. Guided imagery with younger children generally involves the use of storytelling. Older children and adolescents may respond to more conventional scripts that contain pleasant or relaxing images. Some children prefer calm soothing images such as lying in bed or rocking in a chair or hammock. Others prefer more active images in which they participate as a character in a story. The ability to engage in this technique is facilitated if the child has a feeling of trust in the consultant.

Behavior Modification

Children of all ages will respond to incentives given to reward completion of a stressful procedure. The should include verbal encouragement and praise and age-appropriate rewards such as the use of sticker charts for young children and more concrete items for older children.

Medical Hypnosis

Medical hypnosis has been used in a number of settings to treat children and adolescent patients, including children as young as age 3 years. Children are generally found to be highly hypnotizable. The types of problems successfully treated include pain, procedural anxiety, enuresis, asthma, and habit disorders (Olness and Kohen 1996). Hypnosis has been used to reduce anticipatory nau-

sea related to chemotherapy in oncology patients and to treat procedural anxiety in children undergoing invasive and stressful procedures, including bone
marrow aspirations and lumbar punctures. Hypnosis has been shown to result
in a decreased need for hypnotic and anxiolytic agents and decreased incidence
of anxiety in subsequent procedures (Maldonado and Spiegel 2000). Hypnosis
has been associated with lower ratings of postoperative pain and shorter hospital stays (Kuttner and Solomon 2003). Hypnosis can also be used for patients who have phobias about specific medical procedures.

Components of Hypnosis

Hypnosis is a psychophysiological state of attentive, receptive concentration in
which there is a relative suspension of peripheral awareness (Spiegel et al.
2000). Hypnotic phenomena occur spontaneously, and the alteration of consciousness that hypnotized individuals may experience has a variety of therapeutic applications (Spiegel and Spiegel 1978). Hypnosis can be used to help
alter thoughts, feelings, expectations, attitudes, and perceptions. Although
hypnosis is not a treatment in itself, it is often used to complement other types
of medical therapy and to facilitate the use of distraction and relaxation to reduce procedural anxiety. Three processes describe the hypnotic experience: absorption, suggestion, and dissociation (Maldonado and Spiegel 2000).

Absorption

Absorption is the tendency to engage in a state of focused attention. It describes a state in which the individual is immersed in a central experience with
decreased peripheral awareness. During a state of absorption, peripheral perceptions, thoughts, and memories become less important.

Suggestion

Individuals in a state of hypnosis develop a heightened responsiveness to suggestions provided by the consultant. Individuals will accept instructions in a less
critical manner while in a state of hypnosis; they may question the reasons for actions less and respond more automatically. This process may be used by the consultant to bypass the patient's defenses in an effort to bring about symptom relief.

Dissociation

During a state of hypnosis, individuals are able to keep many routine experiences out of consciousness. Emotional states and sensory experiences may be

dissociated from the individual's conscious experience during a state of hypnosis. The dissociation can also prevent access to memories, resulting in states of dissociative amnesia.

Hypnotic Responsiveness in Children

Children are often adept at learning techniques of hypnosis, partly due to their natural ability to enter into states of imagery and imagination (Kuttner and Solomon 2003; Morgan and Hilgard 1979). Children often enter into spontaneous states of self-hypnosis or imaginary play, for example, when they are bored or distracted. Children may spontaneously use fantasy to modify unpleasant situations or to prepare for creative activities and new achievements. In addition, children are often motivated to try out new experiences and are responsive to suggestions during a state of hypnosis.

Early studies of hypnosis suggested that there is a curvilinear relationship between age and hypnotic susceptibility, with a peak in the 8- to 12-year age range (Olness and Kohen 1996). More recent work, however, has suggested that children of all ages are quite hypnotizable and the failure to recognize this may be more of an artifact of the scales used to assess hypnosis. Responsivity to hypnosis in children is more accurately assessed by looking at the child's ability for active imagination in addition to more formal induction techniques such as eye closure and relaxation, which are the basis of assessment in adults. In particular, eye closure is one of the more difficult items for children because it may trigger negative attitudes and concerns related to sleep as well as limiting opportunities for the child's natural curiosity in motor phenomena that may occur during hypnosis. Similarly, items described as "challenge items" that are used with adult patients, such as arm immobilization, may remove control from the child and provoke oppositional behavior or resistance to hypnosis. Behaviors that suggest susceptibility to hypnosis include quiet wakeful behavior, involvement in vivid imagery, heightened attention to a narrow focus, and the capacity to follow posthypnotic suggestions.

Factors Compromising Hypnotic Responsiveness

Several factors may compromise hypnotic responsiveness in children (Olness and Kohen 1996), including misconceptions about hyponosis, parental attitudes, and situational variables.

Misconceptions About Hypnosis

Negative portrayals of hypnosis in the media or misconceptions based on knowledge of hypnosis used for entertainment may interfere with a child's willingness to enter hypnosis. Some families may also have objections based on religious beliefs. Children may equate hypnosis with loss of autonomy or experience anxiety with certain induction techniques that involve experiences of loss of control. Children may resist hypnosis because of previous negative experiences with the technique, an unwillingness to give up a specific symptom because of secondary gain or defensiveness (Olness and Kohen 1996), or negative feelings directed toward the therapist.

Parental Attitudes

Negative attitudes or misinformation on the part of parents and other adult figures may influence the child's responsiveness to hypnosis. Both parents and medical colleagues require education about the use of hypnosis, including education about the need for adequate preparation time for procedures. Last-minute requests for intervention are often associated with failure of the technique in the child for whom the technique might otherwise be helpful. By contrast, positive attitudes on the part of parents may promote the use of hypnosis in children.

Situational Variables

Certain situational variables, such as extreme anxiety or pain or lack of adequate time for training, may interfere with the use of hypnosis in specific clinical situations.

Hypnotic Induction

It is helpful to present hypnosis to children and families as a skill that they may already have but that they are not aware of using. In pediatric hypnosis, one goal is to help children develop their own abilities and control over the use of the hypnotic techniques. Parents are usually involved to help support the child's efforts, to act as coaches, and to help decrease feelings of anxiety. Children's ability to enter a state of hypnosis results in increased suggestibility to techniques of imagery rather than those of relaxation. Images such as taking part in a sports activity, being in a favorite room of the house, or imagining themselves as a cartoon character are examples of techniques used to help children dissociate themselves psychologically from experiences of pain and anxiety (Maldonado and Spiegel 2000).

Prehypnotic Interview

It is important to introduce the concept of medical hypnosis to children and their parents with a full explanation of the applications and techniques. During this didactic discussion, the therapist should elicit and respond to specific concerns of the child and the parents. Any concerns or misconceptions regarding hypnosis should be clarified during this initial interview. It is important to demystify hypnosis and to explore and clarify some of the differences between the use of hypnosis for medical versus entertainment purposes. It may be helpful to define *hypnosis* as a state of mind that combines relaxation and concentration on a specific focus such that undesired thoughts or anxieties fade into the background. The ability to shift attention can be demonstrated by asking the child or parents to focus on sounds in the medical unit that were not previously noticed. The heightened attention that occurs during hypnosis can also be highlighted by describing everyday events that parents may be more attentive to—for example, the cry of an infant in distress. Further discussion includes emphasizing the specific goals of hypnosis for the child, such as helping the child focus on comfort to reduce the experience of pain. Education about the principles of relaxation training and guided imagery is included.

Inclusion of Parents

Most therapists suggest involving the child's parents in the hypnosis sessions, either from the beginning or after the child has received some training in self-hypnosis. Younger children generally prefer to have their parents present during the initial sessions, because their presence can reduce feelings of anxiety. Older children, by contrast, may find the presence of parents more likely to increase anxiety, and it may be better to conduct initial sessions alone. Parental presence, however, clearly helps diminish parental anxiety and builds rapport between the family and the consultant. Parents who have observed the sessions are able to act as coaches for their children when they practice the techniques. Many parents will also spontaneously allow themselves to enter into a state of hypnosis during the training or request self-instruction and experience their own benefits from the technique.

Assessment of Hypnosis

There is a considerable variation in the hypnotizability of individual patients. Patients who are easily hypnotizable can be expected to benefit from techniques of hypnosis, whereas those who are less receptive to this technique should be directed toward other approaches such as biofeedback or relaxation. There are some objective tests that can be used to determine the patient's level of hypnotic responsivity. There are a number of clinical scales that have been used to assess the patient's ability to enter a state of hypnosis, including the Hypnotic Induction Profile (Spiegel and Spiegel 1978). This scale involves a structured hypnotic induction followed by an assessment of the patient's response to suggestions. The Children's Hypnotic Susceptibility Scale (London 1963) has been developed based on the items in the Stanford Hypnotic Susceptibility Scale, Form A (Weitzenhoffer and Hilgard 1959). Morgan and Hilgard (1979) also developed the Stanford Hypnotic Clinical Scale for Children, which has a version for both younger and older children. It is helpful to use a structured script to induce hypnosis that incorporates suggestions for relaxation, imagery, and posthypnotic suggestion prior to efforts to address the child's particular symptom. This exercise may be somewhat less threatening and may help establish a sense of confidence in the technique by both the patient and the parents. After the assessment session, the consultant will debrief with the patient by discussing which components of the induction were most successful or appealing to the child.

Hypnotic Induction Techniques

There are a number of different methods used to induce a state of hypnosis that rely on techniques of relaxation and imagery (Ollness and Kohen 1996). Children respond to a large variety of hypnotic induction techniques, and the choice depends on the age and personality characteristics of the individual child as well as the experience of the therapist. Techniques need to be adapted based on the age of the child, and success in the induction of hypnosis is enhanced by knowledge of the child's preferences, which should be assessed prior to starting the child's training in hypnosis. Compared with adults, children are more likely to open their eyes, make spontaneous comments, and move around, giving the impression that they are resistant to the procedure. The consultant is likely to be more successful if these behaviors are permitted or reinforced during the induction rather than resisted. It may also be important to deemphasize the use of words such as *sleepy* because younger children may be resistant to falling asleep. It is also important to avoid the use of authoritarian methods and phrases because children generally have a greater need to remain in control. Use of the phrases such as "you may…" rather than "you will…" are likely to be better received.

Visual Imagery Techniques

There are a number of visual imagery techniques used to induce hypnosis in children. The child may be asked to imagine a favorite place, either real or imaginary. The therapist may enhance the imagery by adding specific details, including suggestions about sounds, physical sensations, temperature, and color. The child may choose to have friends or family members present in the imaginary place. The child may talk with the therapist about the place they are in during hypnosis to help reinforce the cooperative nature of the relationship. In the cloud-gazing technique the child is asked to imagine clouds floating in the sky that change in shape and color. Suggestions are made that the child may become part of one of the clouds with feelings of comfort, lightness, and calmness. With the television fantasy the child is asked to imagine him- or herself watching a favorite video or television program. The suggestion is made that the child has the remote control for the television and may turn the movie on or off and play out certain scenes, including those of the child involved in pleasurable activities. It is also possible to ask the child to imagine playing different videos, starting with one of them lying on their hospital bed followed by a video of a more pleasurable scene. The child may be asked to notice differences in sensations of pain or anxiety between each videotape to help the child establish a sense of control over his or her symptoms.

Movement Imagery

In the *magic carpet* technique the child is asked to imagine him- or herself sitting on a magic carpet. Suggestions are made that the child will be able to control the movement of the carpet and to take the carpet up into the air with images of grass, trees, or clouds. The child is able to take the carpet to favorite places or to visit friends. Friends or family members may accompany the child on the magic carpet ride. In the *sports activity* technique, the child is asked to imagine him- or herself playing a favorite sport. The child may be prompted to imagine him- or herself at a later age, perhaps playing for a favorite professional team and wearing the team colors. Suggestions are made about the physical sensations experienced by the child as he or she plays the sport. Suggestions may also be made about the response of the crowd and teammates as the child helps the team win the game. In the *bouncing ball* technique, the child is asked to imagine him- or herself as a bouncing ball that bounces in any direction the child chooses. The ball may bounce out of the hospital and go on a journey to the child's favorite places.

Ideomotor Techniques

Ideomotor techniques involve suggestions in which the child is asked to imagine particular movements, generally of parts of their body, after which the movements generally start to occur. These techniques are particularly effective because they give the child a physical demonstration of their own ability to utilize hypnosis to control a physical movement in their body. In the *arm levitation* technique, a suggestion is made that a balloon is tied around one of the child's wrists. Suggestions about lightness or floating sensations are used to help the child allow his or her arm to float into a vertical position. In the *fingers moving together* technique, the child is asked to clasp his or her hands together with the two index fingers pointing forward, separated by about 1 inch. The suggestion is made that the fingers get drawn together, either with the image of a rubber band tied around both fingers or of magnets pulling the fingers together. As the fingers slowly move together and touch, suggestions are made for the child to drift off into a state of heightened relaxation.

Application to Pain and Procedural Anxiety

Several techniques and images can be used to help decrease symptoms of pain and anxiety related to invasive procedures. It is important to adapt the technique based on the age and developmental level of the child. It is also helpful for the child to have training in several different techniques of induction and pain relief so that he or she has a choice of techniques at the time of the procedure.

Hypnoanesthesia

In hypnoanesthesia, suggestions are made about feelings of numbness that begin in a part of the child's body and then spread to incorporate the area being affected during the procedure. Suggestions may include numbness that can be induced by the image of a cold block of ice, of painting on a local anesthetic, or of pulling a "magic glove" or "magic stocking" over one of the hands or feet of the child. The child may also learn the technique of transferring feelings of numbness from one part of the body to another by touching him- or herself with the "anesthetized" hand. The child may also be asked to imagine nerves that pass from the brain to different areas of the body and are controlled by pain switches in the brain. After the child has identified a specific nerve pathway, which may be designated by a color, the child is asked to imagine a dimmer switch or control that can be used to reduce sensations to and from that particular part of the body.

Distancing Suggestions

The child may be asked to imagine the painful arm or body parts floating away and becoming detached from his or her body. As the body part is dissociated, sensations of pain are diminished. Pain may also be transferred from a part of the body, such as the back during a lumbar puncture procedure, to another part, such as a finger, that is then also detached and dissociated. The technique of watching a videotape can be incorporated, with the child asked to visualize a tape of him- or herself undergoing the procedure and then turn off the tape and play a tape of a favorite place or activity instead. Suggestions are made for decreased experiences of pain while the child is watching the pleasant videotape.

References

Abel CG, Rouleau JL: Behavioral therapy strategies for the medical patients, in Psychiatric Care of the Medical Patient, 2nd Edition. Edited by Stoudemire A, Fogel BS, Greenberg DB. Oxford, England, Oxford University Press, 2000, pp 61–71

Blount RL, Piira T, Cohen LL: Management of pediatric pain and distress due to medical procedures, in Handbook of Pediatric Psychology, 3rd Edition. Edited by Roberts MC. New York, Guilford, 2003, pp 216–233

Butler LD, Symons BK, Henderson SL, et al: Hypnosis reduces distress and duration of an invasive medical procedure for children. Pediatrics 115:e77–85, 2005

Chen E, Zeltzer LK, Craske MG, et al: Alteration of memory in the reduction of children's distress during repeated medical procedures. J Consult Clin Psychol 67:481–490, 1999

Cohen LL: Reducing infant immunization distress through distraction. Health Psychol 21:207–211, 2002

Cohen LL, Blount RL, Cohen RJ, et al: Children's expectations and memories of acute distress: the short and long-term efficacy of pain management interventions. J Pediatr Psychol 26:367–375, 2001

Harbeck-Weber C, McKee DH: Prevention of emotional and behavioral distress in children experiencing hospitalization and chronic illness, in Handbook of Pediatric Psychology, 2nd Edition. Edited by Roberts MC. New York, Guilford, 1995, pp 167–184

Hobbie WL, Stubler M, Meeske K, et al: Symptoms of posttraumatic stress in survivors of childhood cancer. J Clin Oncol 18:4060–4066, 2000

Johnston CC, Collinge JM, Henderson SJ, et al: A cross-sectional survey of pain and pharmacological analgesia in Canadian neonatal intensive care units. Clin J Pain 13:308–312, 1997

Kuttner L, Solomon R: Hypnotherapy and imagery for managing children's pain, in Pain in Infants, Children and Adolescents, 2nd Edition. Edited by Schechter NL, Berde CB, Yaster M. Philadelphia, PA, Lippincott Williams & Wilkins, 2003, pp 317–328

Ljungman G, Gordh T, Sorensen S, et al: Pain in paediatric oncology: interviews with children, adolescents in their parents. Acta Paediatr 88:623–630, 1999

London P: Children's Hypnotic Susceptibility Scale. Palo Alto, CA, Consulting Psychologists Press, 1963

Maldonaldo JR, Spiegel D: Medical hypnosis, in Psychiatric Care of the Medical Patient, 2nd Edition. Edited by Stoudemire A, Fogel BS, Greenberg DB. Oxford, England, Oxford University Press, 2000, pp 73–87

McGrath PA: Psychological aspects of pain perception. Arch Oral Biol 39:55–62, 1994

Melamed BG, Meyer R, Gee C, et al: The influence of time and time of preparation on children's adjustment to hospitalization. J Pediatr Psychol 1:31–37, 1976

Morgan A, Hilgard ER: The Stanford Hypnotic Clinical Scale for children. Am J Clin Hypn 21:148–169, 1979

Olness K, Kohen DP: Hypnosis and Hypnotherapy with Children, 3rd Edition. New York, Guilford, 1996

Pate JT, Blount RL, Cohen LL, et al: Childhood medical experience and temperament as predictors of adult functioning in medical situations. Children's Health Care 25:281–296, 1996

Ruda MA, Ling Q, Hohmann A, et al: Altered nociceptive neuronal circuits after neonatal peripheral inflammation. Science 289:628–631, 2000

Schultheis K, Peterson L, Selby V: Preparation for stressful medical procedures and person × treatment interactions. Clin Psychol Rev 7:329–352, 1987

Southall DP, Cronin B, Hartmann H, et al: Invasive procedures in children receiving intensive care. BMJ 303:1512–1513, 1993

Spiegel H, Spiegel D: Trance and Treatment: Clinical Use of Hypnosis. New York, Basic Books, 1978

Spiegel H, Greenleaf M, Spiegel D: Hypnosis, in Kaplan and Sadock's Comprehensive Textbook of Psychiatry, Vol 2, 7th Edition. Edited by Sadock BJ, Sadock VA. Philadelphia, PA, Lippincott Williams & Wilkins, 2000, pp 893–904

Wolfer JA, Visintainer MA: Pediatric surgery patients' and parents' stress responses and adjustment as a function of psychologic preparation and stress-point nursing care. Nurs Res 24:244–255, 1975

Delirium Rating Scale–Revised–98

This is a revision of the Delirium Rating Scale (Trzepacz et al. 1988). It is used for initial assessment and repeated measurements of delirium symptom severity. The sum of the 13 item scores provides a severity score. All available sources of information are used to rate the items (nurses, family, chart) in addition to examination of the patient. For serial repeated ratings of delirium severity, reasonable time frames should be chosen between ratings to document meaningful changes because delirium symptom severity can fluctuate without interventions.

DRS-R-98 Severity Scale

1. Sleep-wake cycle disturbance
Rate sleep-wake pattern using all sources of information, including from family, caregivers, nurses' reports, and patient. Try to distinguish sleep from resting with eyes closed.

0. Not present
1. Mild sleep continuity disturbance at night or occasional drowsiness during the day
2. Moderate disorganization of sleep-wake cycle (e.g., falling asleep during conversations, napping during the day or several brief awakenings during the night with confusion/behavioral changes or very little nighttime sleep)

3. Severe disruption of sleep-wake cycle (e.g., day-night reversal of sleep-wake cycle or severe circadian fragmentation with multiple periods of sleep and wakefulness or severe sleeplessness.)

2. Perceptual disturbances and hallucinations
Illusions and hallucinations can be of any sensory modality. Misperceptions are "simple" if they are uncomplicated, such as a sound, noise, color, spot, or flashes; and "complex" if they are multidimensional, such as voices, music, people, animals, or scenes. Rate if reported by patient or caregiver, or inferred by observation.

0. Not present
1. Mild perceptual disturbances (e.g., feelings of derealization or depersonalization; or patient may not be able to discriminate dreams from reality)
2. Illusions present
3. Hallucinations present

3. Delusions
Delusions can be of any type, but are most often persecutory. Rate if reported by patient, family, or caregiver. Rate as delusional if ideas are unlikely to be true yet are believed by the patient who cannot be dissuaded by logic. Delusional ideas cannot be explained otherwise by the patient's usual cultural or religious background.

0. Not present
1. Mildly suspicious, hypervigilant, or preoccupied
2. Unusual or overvalued ideation that does not reach delusional proportions or could be plausible
3. Delusional

4. Lability of affect
Rate the patient's affect as the outward presentation of emotions and not as a description of what the patient feels.

0. Not present
1. Affect somewhat altered or incongruent to situation; changes over the course of hours; emotions are mostly under self-control

2. Affect is often inappropriate to the situation and intermittently changes over the course of minutes; emotions are not consistently under self-control, though they respond to redirection by others
3. Severe and consistent disinhibition of emotions; affect changes rapidly, is inappropriate to context, and does not respond to redirection by others

5. Language
Rate abnormalities of spoken, written, or sign language that cannot be otherwise attributed to dialect or stuttering. Assess fluency, grammar, comprehension, semantic content, and naming. Test comprehension and naming nonverbally if necessary by having patient follow commands or point.

0. Normal language
1. Mild impairment including word-finding difficulty or problems with naming or fluency
2. Moderate impairment including comprehension difficulties or deficits in meaningful communication (semantic content)
3. Severe impairment including nonsensical semantic content, word salad, muteness, or severely reduced comprehension

6. Thought process abnormalities
Rate abnormalities of thinking processes based on verbal or written output. If a patient does not speak or write, do not rate this item.

0. Normal thought processes
1. Tangential or circumstantial
2. Associations loosely connected occasionally, but largely comprehensible
3. Associations loosely connected most of the time

7. Motor agitation
Rate by observation, including from other sources of observation such as visitors, family, and clinical staff. Do not include dyskinesia, tics, or chorea.

0. No restlessness or agitation
1. Mild restlessness of gross motor movements or mild fidgetiness
2. Moderate motor agitation including dramatic movements of the extremities, pacing, fidgeting, removing intravenous lines, etc.

3. Severe motor agitation, such as combativeness or a need for restraints or seclusion

8. Motor retardation
Rate movements by direct observation or from other sources of observation such as family, visitors, or clinical staff. Do not rate components of retardation that are caused by parkinsonian symptoms. Do not rate drowsiness or sleep.

0. No slowness of voluntary movements
1. Mildly reduced frequency, spontaneity, or speed of motor movements, to the degree that may interfere somewhat with the assessment.
2. Moderately reduced frequency, spontaneity, or speed of motor movements to the degree that it interferes with participation in activities or self-care
3. Severe motor retardation with few spontaneous movements

9. Orientation
Patients who cannot speak can be given a visual or auditory presentation of multiple-choice answers. Allow patient to be wrong by up to 7 days instead of 2 days for patients hospitalized more than 3 weeks. Disorientation to person means not recognizing familiar persons and may be intact even if the person has naming difficulty but recognizes the person. Disorientation to person is rare and is most severe when one doesn't know one's own identity. Disorientation to person usually occurs after disorientation to time and/or place.

0. Oriented to person, place and time
1. Disoriented to time (e.g., by more than 2 days or wrong month or wrong year) or to place (e.g., name of building, city. state), but not both
2. Disoriented to time and place
3. Disoriented to person

10. Attention
Patients with sensory deficits or who are intubated or whose hand movements are constrained should be tested using an alternate modality besides writing. Attention can be assessed during the interview (e.g., verbal perseverations, distractibility, and difficulty with set shifting) and/or through use of specific tests (e.g., digit span).

0. Alert and attentive
1. Mildly distractible or mild difficulty sustaining attention, but able to refocus with cueing; on formal testing, makes only minor errors and is not significantly slow in responses
2. Moderate inattention with difficulty focusing and sustaining attention; on formal testing, makes numerous errors and either requires prodding to focus or finish the task
3. Severe difficulty focusing and/or sustaining attention, with many incorrect or incomplete responses or inability to follow instructions. Distractible by other noises or events in the environment

11. Short-term memory
Defined as recall of information (e.g., three items presented either verbally or visually) after a delay of about 2–3 minutes. When formally tested, information must be registered adequately before recall is tested. The number of trials to register as well as effect of cueing can be noted on scoresheet. Patient should not be allowed to rehearse during the delay period and should be distracted during that time. Patient may speak or nonverbally communicate to the examiner the identity of the correct items. Short-term deficits noticed during the course of the interview can be used also.

0. Short-term memory intact
1. Recalls 2/3 items; may be able to recall third item after category cueing
2. Recalls 1/3 items; may be able to recall other items after category cueing
3. Recalls 0/3 items

12. Long-term memory
Can be assessed formally or through interviewing for recall of past personal (e.g., past medical history or information or experiences that can be corroborated from another source) or general information that is culturally relevant. When formally tested, use a verbal and/or visual modality for three items that are adequately registered and recalled after at least 5 minutes. The patient should not be allowed to rehearse during the delay period during formal testing. Make allowances for patients with less than 8 years of education or who are mentally retarded regarding general information questions. Rating of the severity of deficits may involve a judgment about all the ways long-term

memory is assessed, including recent and/or remote long-term memory ability informally tested during the interview as well as any formal testing of recent long-term memory using three items.

0. No significant long-term memory deficits
1. Recalls 2/3 items and/or has minor difficulty recalling details of other long-term information
2. Recalls 1/3 items and/or has moderate difficulty recalling other long-term information
3. Recalls 0/3 items and/or has severe difficulty recalling other long-term information

13. Visuospatial ability
Assess informally and formally. Consider patient's difficulty navigating one's way around living areas or environment (e.g., getting lost). Test formally by drawing or copying a design, by arranging puzzle pieces, or by drawing a map and identifying major cities, etc. Take into account any visual impairments that may affect performance.

0. No impairment
1. Mild impairment such that overall design and most details or pieces are correct; and/or little difficulty navigating in his/her surroundings
2. Moderate impairment with distorted appreciation of overall design and/or several errors of details or pieces; and/or needing repeated redirection to keep from getting lost in a newer environment despite trouble locating familiar objects in immediate environment
3. Severe impairment on formal testing; and/or repeated wandering or getting lost in environment

DRS-R-98 Optional Diagnostic Items

These three items can be used to assist in the differentiation of delirium from other disorders for diagnostic and research purposes. They are added to the severity score for the total scale score but are not included in the severity score.

14. Temporal onset of symptoms

Rate the acuteness of onset of the initial symptoms of the disorder or episode being currently assessed, not their total duration. Distinguish the onset of symptoms attributable to delirium when it occurs concurrently with a different preexisting psychiatric disorder. For example, if a patient with major depression is rated during a delirium episode due to an overdose, then rate the onset of the delirium symptoms.

0. No significant change from usual or longstanding baseline behavior
1. Gradual onset of symptoms, occurring over a period of several weeks to a month
2. Acute change in behavior or personality occurring over days to a week
3. Abrupt change in behavior occurring over a period of several hours to a day

15. Fluctuation of symptom severity

Rate the waxing and waning of an individual or cluster of symptom(s) over the time frame being rated. Usually applies to cognition, affect, intensity of hallucinations, thought disorder, or language disturbance. Take into consideration that perceptual disturbances usually occur intermittently but might cluster in period of greater intensity when other symptoms fluctuate in severity.

0. No symptom fluctuation
1. Symptom intensity fluctuates in severity over hours
2. Symptom intensity fluctuates in severity over minutes

16. Physical disorder

Rate the degree to which a physiological, medical, or pharmacological problem can be specifically attributed to have caused the symptoms being assessed. Many patients have such problems but they may or may not have causal relationship to the symptoms being rated.

0. None present or active
1. Presence of any physical disorder that might affect mental state
2. Drug, infection, metabolic disorder, central nervous system lesion or other medical problem that specifically can be implicated in causing the altered behavior or mental state

DRS-R-98 SCORESHEET

Name of patient: _____   Date: ___ / ___ / ___   Time: _____

Name of Rater: _____

SEVERITY SCORE: [   ]   TOTAL SCORE: [   ]

Severity Item	Item Score				Optional Information
Sleep-wake cycle	0	1	2	3	Naps Nocturnal disturbance only Day-night reversal

Perceptual disturbances	0	1	2	3	Sensory type of illusion or hallucination:
					    auditory visual olfactory tactile
					Format of illusion or hallucination:
					    simple complex

Delusions	0	1	2	3	Type of delusion: persecutory Nature: poorly formed systematized
Lability of affect	0	1	2	3	Type: angry anxious dysphoric elated irritable
Language	0	1	2	3	Check here if intubated, mute, etc.
Thought process	0	1	2	3	Check here if intubated, mute, etc.
Motor agitation	0	1	2	3	Check here if restrained *Type of restraints:*
Motor retardation	0	1	2	3	Check here if restrained *Type of restraints:*
Orientation	0	1	2	3	Date: Place: Person:
Attention	0	1	2	3	
Short-term memory	0	1	2	3	Record # of trials for registration of items: Check here if category cueing helped
Long-term memory	0	1	2	3	Check here if category cueing helped
Visuospatial ability	0	1	2	3	Check here if unable to use hands
Diagnostic Item	**Item Score**				**Optional Information**
Temporal onset of symptoms	0	1	2	3	Check here if symptoms appeared on a background of other psychopathology
Fluctuation of symptom severity	0	1	2		Check here if symptoms only appear during the night

Source.   Reprinted from Trzepacz PT, Mittal D, Torres R, et al: "Validation of the Delirium Rating Scale-Revised-98: Comparison With the Delirium Rating Scale and the Cognitive Test for Delirium." *Journal of Neuropsychiatry and Clinical Neurosciences* 13:229–242, 2001. Used with permission.

Index

Page numbers printed in **boldface** type refer to tables or figures.

Medical team *(continued)*
    pretransplant assessment and
        relationship with, **210**, 213
    role of consultation psychiatrist in
        supporting, 3, 6
    sources of information for
        assessment and, 33
Medications. *See also*
    Psychopharmacology
    anxiety and, **133**
    delirium and, 81, **84–85**, 87
    polypharmacy during bone marrow
        transplantation and, 253–254
Membrane stabilizers, and pain, **190**,
    196
Memory
    delirium and, 77–78
    treatment adherence and, 238
Mental status examination, 41–42, 56
Mesoridazine, 334
Metabolism, and psychopharmacology,
    308–309, 334–335
Methylphenidate, **342**, 343, **344**
Mexiletine, 196
Midazolam, 336, **337**, 338–339
Migraines, 171, 196.
    See also Headaches
Mini-Mental State Examination
    (MMSE), 83
Mirtazapine, **313**, **316**, 324
Mixed amphetamine salts, 342
Mixed type delirium, 79
Moclobemide, 324
Modafinil, **342**, **344**, 345
Modeling, and preparation for medical
    procedures, 361

Monitoring, family adjustment to
    illness and degree of, 286
Monoamine oxidase inhibitors, 324,
    317, **355**
Mood disorder(s). *See also* Depression;
    Mania
    assessment of, 113–114
    clinical considerations in, 98–103
    definition of, 96, **97**, **99**
    differential diagnosis of depression,
        organic mood disorder, and,
        114
    due to a general medical condition,
        105–111, **107**
    laboratory tests and, 114, **115**
    prevalence of, 95
    primary mood disorder, 103
    as reaction to medical illness,
        103–105
    substance-induced, **110–111**,
        111–113
    treatment of, 115, 117
    treatment adherence and, 233
Mood scales, 37, **39**
Mood stabilizers
    cardiac disease and, **353**
    hepatic disease and, **347**
    preparations and dosages of, **325**
    principles of use, 324, 328
    renal disease and, **351**
    side effects of, **326–327**, 328
Morbidity. *See also* Survival rates
    cardiac disease and side effects of
        psychoactive drugs, 352
    depression and, 102–103
    treatment adherence and, 228